The AIDS Epidemic

THE AIDS EPIDEMIC

Social Dimensions of an Infectious Disease

William A. Rushing
Vanderbilt University

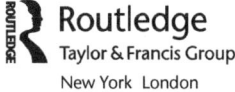
Routledge
Taylor & Francis Group
New York London

First published 1995 by Westview Press

Published 2018 by Routledge
605 Third Avenue, New York, NY 10017
2 Park Square, Milton Park, Abingdon, Oxon OX14 4RN

Routledge is an imprint of the Taylor & Francis Group, an informa business

Copyright © 1995 Taylor & Francis

Library of Congress Cataloging-in-Publication Data
Rushing, William A.
   The AIDS epidemic : social dimensions of an infectious disease /
William A. Rushing.
      p.   cm.
   Includes bibliographical references and index.
   ISBN 0-8133-2044-5—ISBN 0-8133-2045-3 (pbk.)
      1. AIDS (Disease)—Social aspects.   2. AIDS (Disease)—
Epidemiology.   I. Title.
RA644.A25R86   1995
614.5'993—dc20   95-828
                                                                   CIP

ISBN 13: 978-0-8133-2045-8 (pbk)

Contents

Tables and Figures

Preface

Infectious diseases had been declining for many years in the United States when an apparently new infectious disease, acquired immune deficiency syndrome, or AIDS, suddenly appeared in the early 1980s. This is the most serious disease to appear in modern times, and as of this writing, neither vaccine nor cure is in sight. From a sociological point of view, AIDS is perhaps the most important disease in American history, and it is certainly one of the most important in all history.

Although most scientific experts on AIDS agree that a virus called human immunodeficiency virus (HIV) is the basic cause of AIDS, social factors are significant in the extent to which and the way in which the virus is transmitted. Some populations with certain social and cultural characteristics have much higher rates of HIV-AIDS. To date in the United States, HIV-AIDS has been predominantly a male disease and is disproportionately concentrated among male homosexuals (gays), injecting drug users (IDUs), and some racial-ethnic groups. A virus obviously does not discriminate against people because of their sexual orientation, drug use, or skin pigmentation. Rather, social and cultural factors explain why HIV-AIDS has become so prevalent in these populations. They also explain why HIV-AIDS in sub-Saharan Africa is far more prevalent than in the United States and why it is about evenly distributed between males and females in Africa. Furthermore, that the epidemic has slowed in the United States in recent years but not in sub-Saharan Africa (and other developing regions) also points to the role of social and cultural factors in the transmission of HIV.

Sociologically, one of the most significant aspects of any disease is its social meaning as distinct from its medical meaning and how the former affects the way some people react to those who have the disease. The social meaning of and societal reactions to HIV-AIDS have been unusually negative and extreme. Ostracism—the sociologist's favorite topic—has been common; persons who have HIV-AIDS have not always been treated as persons with a medical pathology but rather as moral deviants and outcasts. Although experts agree that education and prevention programs would slow the spread of HIV in the United States, the social meaning of the disease leads some people to oppose those very programs. At the same time, others have charged the government with refusing to support research and prevention programs because government officials do not care about the plight of the populations in which HIV-AIDS is most prevalent. Some gays and African Americans have even claimed that HIV-AIDS is a genocidal plot against them. Such extreme reactions are simply not in keeping with the way a civil society based on humane and rational values typically reacts to disease.

These and other social aspects of AIDS have been topics of myriad news columns, television programs, technical reports, books, and journal articles since the mid-1980s; the social aspects of HIV-AIDS have been analyzed more in this short time period than have the social aspects of any other disease in history. Recently, however, concern about AIDS has begun to decline. The viral cause of AIDS is now known, the major types of high-risk behaviors have been identified, the rate of increase of new AIDS cases is slowing (at least in the United States), the ostracism of people with AIDS has become milder in tone, and the demonstrations and accusations by AIDS activists have been muted. Hence, *New York Times* reporter Jeffrey Schmalz, who died from AIDS, wrote in a posthumously published *New York Times Magazine* article ("Whatever Happened to AIDS?", November 28, 1993) that AIDS was old news and that interest had waned. The social crisis of AIDS had been analyzed and reanalyzed; there seemed to be little new to say.

Why, then, in the mid-1990s, publish a book on social aspects of AIDS? Such a book is needed because this disease is still not very well understood sociologically. Despite all the attention that social factors in the etiology of AIDS and the societal reactions to the AIDS epidemic have received, their study in terms of the concepts and principles of sociology has been extremely limited. True, scientific experts agree that to attribute the cause of AIDS to a particular virus, while medically valid, oversimplifies and ignores the fact that certain behaviors associated with particular groups and populations are major factors in the etiology of AIDS. But such behaviors are anchored in the cultural norms and social institutions of those groups and populations. High-risk behaviors for transmitting HIV have not been examined extensively from this perspective.

Societal reactions to the AIDS epidemic are also anchored in cultural beliefs and social institutions. Modern society is indeed more civil than its predecessors, but the social forces typical of past societies are latent in the structure of today's society. When an epidemic like AIDS appears, such forces emerge and lead people to act as their ancestors did to previous epidemics. No less than the etiology of HIV-AIDS, the societal reactions to the AIDS epidemic pose important social problems that are as vexing as are the medical aspects of the disease.

By examining the two major social dimensions of HIV-AIDS—its social etiology and societal reactions to the disease—with concepts and principles of sociology, I show how HIV-AIDS is more complex and socially embedded than many have assumed. Although I bring little original evidence to bear on the epidemic (experts on HIV-AIDS and much of the public are aware of most of the basic facts about the disease), I hope that by interpreting these facts in terms of sociological concepts and principles, I can shed a different light on HIV-AIDS. The insights that such an interpretation brings can provide a broader understanding of HIV-AIDS and the course the epidemic has taken. Perhaps these insights will also help clinicians, public health officials, policymakers, and AIDS activists in dealing with the problems of this terrible disease.

—William A. Rushing

Acknowledgments

Several people deserve mention for their help. My longtime friend and colleague, Jack Gibbs, read the entire manuscript, and his suggestions—substantive and editorial—were very helpful, as was his encouragement. My wife Betty also read the entire manuscript, and her questions and comments helped me clarify my thoughts in a number of places, as did those of two anonymous reviewers for Westview Press. George Becker's comments on Chapters 1 and 3 and portions of Chapter 7 were helpful. I thank Dean Eaton for assisting with the graphics and Elizabeth Ziolko and Charles Parish for helping locate and retrieve library material. I thank Linda Norfleet, Linda Willingham, and, especially, Joyce Ogburn for their clerical assistance with early drafts.

Finally, a word of thanks to the editors of Westview Press. This book took longer to bring to a close than the editors and I had originally planned; I thank them for their patience.

W.A.R.

Sociology and AIDS

In the early 1980s an apparently new disease, acquired immune deficiency syndrome, appeared in the United States and spread rapidly. Almost all biomedical scientists believe AIDS is caused by a virus; for most patients the infection is lethal. Because most scientists also agree that an effective vaccine or cure for the disease is not imminent, many future AIDS deaths are inevitable. The disease has already taken a heavy toll in the United States. According to the Centers for Disease Control (CDC), reported cases of AIDS rose from 295 in 1981 to almost 42,000 in 1991, an increase of more than 14,000 percent, and reported AIDS deaths increased from 126 to more than 30,000, an increase of more than 23,000 percent (CDC, 1993a:17).[1] In the United States AIDS is now the leading cause of death for men aged twenty-five to forty-four years of age and the fourth leading cause for women twenty-five to forty-four (CDC, 1993d). The AIDS epidemic is the most serious epidemic to appear in the United States since the Spanish flu of 1918, which took many lives but lasted only a few months. The AIDS epidemic continues.

The disease first became evident among male homosexuals and intravenous drug users, and in the United States it remains disproportionately concentrated in these two populations. However, in most developing countries AIDS is found spread throughout the entire population; death tolls of holocaustal proportions seem likely. According to a 1992 projection of the International AIDS Center of the Harvard School of Public Health, up to 110 million people may be infected worldwide by the year 2000 (up from about 13 million in 1992), 90 percent of whom will be in Third World countries (Mann et al., 1992:3, 103, 107–108).

AIDS, The Disease

Almost all experts believe that AIDS is caused by the human immuno-deficiency virus, or HIV. Usually when a person is attacked by an infectious microbe (bacterial, viral, fungal, protozoan), his or her immune system will release immunocytes to fight the infection. HIV, however, is a special kind of microbe. It is a retrovirus, which inactivates the immune system and destroys its ability to produce certain immunocytes, namely, CD4 T cells. This makes the body helpless against a variety of infections, known as opportunistic infections, that healthy persons can usually throw off. A syndrome of such infections constitutes AIDS. The syndrome includes a rare form of pneumonia (*Pneumocystis carinii,* or PCP), skin cancer (Kaposi's sarcoma, or KS), herpes simplex or cold sores (with esophagitis, pneumonitis, or mucocutaneous ulcers), candidiasis of the esophagus and trachea, blood poisoning, and infections of the brain and nervous system (CDC, 1993a:16). All persons who have AIDS do not suffer from all of the diseases, however; and resistance may be strengthened with proper exercise, rest, and good nutrition (Root-Bernstein, 1993:49–56, 359–360). In time, however, most infected persons typically suffer from several infections, the cumulative effects of which cause death.

There are two known variants of HIV: HIV-1 and HIV-2. Both variants cause AIDS, but HIV-1 appears to be more virulent and may lead to AIDS faster (Ewald, 1994:130–132). Globally, HIV-1 is also more prevalent. HIV-2 is most often found in West Africa, though sporadic cases have been observed in the Americas, India, and a few European countries (Mann et al., 1992:79, 89, 275–276).[2] Nonetheless, for our purpose the general term HIV suffices.

HIV may vary widely from individual to individual and over time within the same individual (Ewald, 1994:125–130); it mutates very rapidly, even faster than influenza viruses. Consequently, even if an effective drug were developed for one HIV strain, it might not be effective for another. Certain drugs may suppress HIV or fortify the immune system, and hence slow the progress of opportunistic infections, but at present medicines cannot make people who have HIV noninfectious or prevent their deaths. Some biologists believe the mutating character of HIV is such that any vaccine or cure would soon be ineffective (Ewald, 1994:179–180).

HIV, ARC, and AIDS

HIV infections do not immediately result in AIDS. After infection occurs, a period variably estimated at two to fifteen years (McLaughlin, 1989:18; Anderson and May, 1992:62; Root-Bernstein, 1993:55; and Ewald, 1994:128) elapses before AIDS appears. The period from infection to onset of disease is longer than for most infectious microbes. Eventually, however, most infected persons develop AIDS-related complex (ARC), in which some opportunistic infections appear. In time, the ability of the immune system to produce CD4 T cells is destroyed, and infected persons contract various diseases; these people have "full-blown" AIDS.[3] Since all persons infected with HIV do not have AIDS, in many instances the generic term HIV-AIDS is the appropriate term to use (though some writers prefer "HIV disease").[4]

Sometimes, however, it is appropriate to refer just to HIV, as in "HIV-infected person." In other instances, the term AIDS is more appropriate, as in "AIDS epidemic" rather than "HIV-AIDS epidemic" or "HIV disease epidemic." This usage is consistent with medical convention, in which an epidemic is named by the disease rather than by the microorganism that causes the disease, as in "cholera epidemic" rather than "*Vibrio cholerae* epidemic" or "*Vibrio cholerae* disease epidemic."

Almost all AIDS statistics for the United States come from CDC publications. The number of AIDS cases has increased over time, partly because the definition of AIDS has been expanded. In particular, the number of conditions that meet the CDC's criteria for AIDS changed in 1993, resulting in a substantial increase in the number of cases. However, most statistics in this book are for the years prior to 1993.

As of December 31, 1992, the CDC (1993a:17) had reported 253,448 cases since 1980, of which 171,890 resulted in death. As for the number of persons in the United States who are infected with HIV, a seroprevalence survey, in which a test is done on blood drawn from participants, conducted by the National Center for Health Statistics (NCHS) for 1988–1991 (reported in December 1993) indicated that the number could be less than 1 million (Altman, 1993), which is much less than the public and many experts had believed. Previous overestimations affected societal reactions to HIV-AIDS significantly.

A Blood-borne Disease

HIV infection occurs when an infected person's blood or other body fluid (e.g., semen, plasma) enters another person's bloodstream (Friedland and Klein, 1987; Rothenberg, 1988:286). The most efficient mode of transmission is the entry of a large amount of infected blood into the bloodstream, as in a blood transfusion. However, the most common transmission mode is through sexual intercourse, from male to female, female to male, or male to male. Sex between males is the most frequent mode of transmission in industrialized countries; sharing of contaminated syringes by drug users is the second most common mode. In developing countries sex between males and females is the dominant mode of transmission.

Infection may also occur through placental transfer to a fetus and through receipt of blood products (as in treatment of hemophilia) and when infected blood enters a person's bloodstream via skin cuts and abrasions. The latter mode is much rarer, but health care workers have greater risk because of their contact with AIDS patients.[5] Although the virus has been isolated in saliva and tears (Fujikawa et al., 1985), the amount is miniscule, and there is no evidence that anyone has been infected from this source.

HIV-AIDS is thus not a common "everyday" infectious disease. HIV is not transmitted through the air, like the microbes in tuberculosis and influenza. It cannot be transmitted through physical touch, like many fungal infections are. It is not transmitted in contaminated water and food, like cholera, dysentery, and typhoid fever. The virus is not transmitted by an insect, as are plague (flea) and malaria (mosquito). Even the risk from mucous membrane contact, as with syphilis and other sexually transmitted diseases (STDs), is very low. In sum, HIV cannot be transmitted through casual contact (Lifson, 1988) and is not easy to "catch" or "pick up." It almost always requires the active participation of an individual in activity in which body fluid is exchanged with one or more persons.

Scientific Disagreements

Although most HIV-AIDS experts agree that HIV is necessary and sufficient to cause AIDS, some scientists dissent.[6] They note that cases of AIDS may exist in which HIV has not been detected and that some people infected with HIV may actually fight it off (Root-Bernstein, 1993:21–30, 49–56). Also, immunosuppression and AIDS may be due to factors other than HIV (Root-Bernstein, 1993:110–147). For example, when semen gets into the bloodstream of a sex partner, it may suppress the immune system by itself (Root-Bernstein, 1993:115–116). Nevertheless, even most critics agree that HIV is a dominant factor in AIDS even if it is not necessary and sufficient to cause AIDS. There are very few cases of AIDS in which HIV is not present (and most experts believe there are not any).

Most of the scientific disagreements concern how physiological processes are involved in the progression of HIV to AIDS rather than whether certain types of behavior are related to the transmission of HIV.[7] Even if some of the critics are correct, their criticisms are of little consequence for understanding the social aspects of HIV-AIDS. For example, the most thorough critic of the orthodox formulation does not deny the importance of behavior, such as certain types of sex acts, that the orthodox view emphasizes (Root-Bernstein, 1993:110–147). Whether semen causes immunosuppression by itself or via HIV is immaterial to the social dynamics of risky sexual behavior and its roots in social institutions.

The Sociological Significance of HIV-AIDS

The major premise of the sociological study of disease is that, even though all diseases are medical phenomena, they cannot be adequately understood in medical (or biological) terms alone. Diseases also have social features that can be understood only in terms of sociological concepts and principles. HIV-AIDS is no exception.

The immediate cause of any infectious disease is a microorganism. However, social factors influence person-to-person transmission and may explain why the prevalence of a disease varies between populations. Thus, although HIV is the (apparent) biological cause of AIDS, social factors determine the behavior that is crucial in most transmissions of HIV and explain why some groups and populations have higher rates than other groups and populations. The major groups with high rates of HIV-AIDS are well known—gays[8] and drug injectors in the United States and men and women in sub-Saharan Africa (referred to in this book as Africa). Certain types of person-to-person contacts are common among gays and drug injectors in the United States, whereas other types of contacts are common between men and women in Africa. For this reason, most experts on HIV-AIDS agree that differences in prevalence between populations are due to differences in certain behaviors. This is a valid idea. But unless the social conditions, such as cultural norms and social institutions, that regulate these behaviors are also specified, it is a limited idea. Sociological analysis of behavioral differences between populations is generally guided by the principle that these differences are related to variations in social conditions. Such analysis seeks to understand the dynamics of the relationship between social conditions and individual behavior. The principle that behavioral differences are related to social conditions is the central principle in the analysis of the social etiology of a disease. It applies to HIV-AIDS no less than to other diseases.

One aspect of the social etiology of HIV-AIDS concerns the *emergence* of HIV. No one knows how old HIV is, but experts in infectious diseases have long believed that changes in social conditions have played a role in the origin of infectious microbes. Significantly, dynamic social changes occurred in the American gay and drug subcultures and in Africa in the 1960s and 1970s, shortly before the AIDS epidemics in these regions began. This raises the question of whether changes in social conditions may have contributed to the emergence of HIV as well as to its epidemic spread in the different populations.

Understanding the social etiology of HIV-AIDS is important to understanding where HIV-AIDS is headed. It seems clear now that the rate of increase in HIV-AIDS is slowing in the United States but continues to accelerate rapidly in Africa. These trends are obviously not due to differences in access to vaccines or medical cures. Instead, they are due to differences in the effect of social factors on the behavior through which HIV is transmitted.

Sociologically, the societal reactions to HIV-AIDS, especially during the 1980s, are as significant as the social etiology of the disease. Persons with HIV-AIDS, particularly gays, have been deserted, denied proper medical care, and physically brutalized. Children with HIV-AIDS have been prohibited from attending school and church, and children with hemophilia who have contracted HIV have been stigmatized and treated as outcasts. To many people, persons with HIV-AIDS are morally impaired. At the same time, on the other side members of groups with high rates of HIV-AIDS have charged the government with genocide. And some scientists, members of the medical community, and persons in positions of political and moral authority have made alarming statements about HIV-AIDS—namely, that millions of Americans would die from AIDS by the 1990s. None of these responses has any basis in the biology of HIV-AIDS and its medical definition. They are based instead on the social conditions under which the AIDS epidemic has occurred.

History records similar reactions to epidemics in the past. But by the 1980s infectious diseases were no longer considered to be even mild health threats in the United States. Epidemics of influenza still occurred, of course, but flu symptoms were mild and did not last long. The death rate from infectious diseases in 1980 was a tiny fraction of what it had been in 1900 (McKinlay and McKinlay, 1977). Americans simply thought massive killer epidemics were past history and could not occur in their society. HIV-AIDS undermined people's security, and many responded in extreme ways, as society had in earlier times. As in the past, people responded to the *social meaning* of a disease, not to its biological features and medical definition. And since the social meaning of a disease is determined by the social conditions under which that disease occurs, it follows that certain social and cultural conditions of the United States in the 1980s were not unlike those that had existed in past epidemics. But at the same time, social conditions were also very different, and so specific reactions to HIV-AIDS were also different. In many ways, then, HIV-AIDS and the AIDS epidemic are manifestations of society, not simply the activity of a virus. If any disease or epidemic could be called a sociological disease or epidemic, it would certainly be HIV-AIDS.

Sociological Perspectives

As with any disease, a sociological analysis of HIV-AIDS may proceed in one of two ways. It may examine how sociological concepts and principles can be used to make programs of prevention and treatment more effective (Huber and Schneider, 1992). Or it may use sociological concepts and principles to achieve a deeper understanding of the social aspects of HIV-AIDS. That is the approach of this book.

Sociology consists of a number of specialties that focus on specific phenomena, such as deviant behavior and deviant subcultures, riots and other forms of collective disruption, interaction networks, or cross-cultural differences in social institutions. The different specialties draw on many of the same concepts and principles that are general to sociology, but each specialty has its own conceptual framework or perspective (and sometimes methodology) for analyzing social and cultural phenomena. And any one phenomenon may sometimes be analyzed from several perspectives. This is true for the AIDS epidemic. Consequently, each of the chapters in this book examines a different social aspect of HIV-AIDS from a specific sociological perspective.

The book is organized in two parts in accordance with a basic distinction medical sociologists make in the social dimensions of disease. Part One is concerned with social etiology and Part Two with societal reactions. Within each part are four chapters devoted to an analysis of a separate social aspect of HIV-AIDS.

NOTES

1. These are only the reported cases. However, since AIDS almost always requires intensive medical and hospital care, a high percentage of cases are probably reported to the CDC by local, state, and territorial health authorities. According to the CDC (1993a: 22, 1994a: 31), studies indicate that reported cases in most areas are more than 85 percent complete and that 70–90 percent of AIDS deaths in men twenty-five to forty-four years old (the highest age-sex risk group) are reported. Studies of homosexual men in New York and San Francisco indicate the percentage for deaths may be higher than this (Koblin et al., 1992).

2. Some have speculated about a third AIDS virus (sometimes referred to as the "isn't" virus), but the consensus of experts is that no such virus exists (Culliton, 1992).

3. Usually, the time between infection and onset of a disease is known as the incubation period, during which time the microbe is latent or dormant. However, two separate studies reported in January 1995 (Ho, et al., 1995; Wei, et al., 1995) reveal that HIV does not incubate and lie dormant. The relatively long period between infection and onset of AIDS is due, instead, to the particular dynamic between HIV and the immune system. After entering a person's bloodstream, HIV replicates rapidly, producing billions of progeny in short order. The person's immune system fights back by producing CD4 T cells, which kill billions of HIV. Unfortunately, however, a larger proportion of the CD4 T cells than the microbes are killed in the process. Although CD4 T cells are replenished, microbes are also replenished, and since a larger proportion of CD4 T cells get destroyed in the battle, in time the microbes get the upper hand. The immune system is overwhelmed by HIV and its ability to reproduce CD4 T cells and hence to fight off infections is impaired. Diseases associated with AIDS then begin to appear.

4. Others recommend the phrase, people living with AIDS (PLWA). The phrase is medically unorthodox since a person with a disease is usually referred to as a person

who has or is a victim of a disease. The phrase might also have a disastrous effect on some individuals: Some naive people may interpret PLWA to mean that AIDS is similar to certain other chronic diseases, such as diabetes, that one can live with if it is managed with medication, rather than a disease that is lethal. The results could be tragic if the interpretation caused those individuals to be less diligent in trying to avoid contracting HIV.

5. By the end of 1992, 33 health care workers with documented and possibly occupationally acquired HIV-AIDS infections had been reported (CDC, 1993a:19).

6. Critics claim that in scientific studies in which HIV is identified as the cause of AIDS, the investigators have not obeyed cardinal rules of procedure for biological research on infectious disease (namely, the postulates of Koch and Henle) (Duesberg, 1988; Root-Bernstein, 1993).

7. An exception is the argument by Peter Duesberg (1990, 1992), which maintains that drug use (which need not be from drug injection) is the cause of AIDS diseases. In a thorough test of the drug use hypothesis, M. S. Ascher et al. (1993) found no empirical evidence for it.

8. There is no convention in the use of the terms *homosexual* and *gay*. Some use the terms interchangeably so that gay refers to male and female alike (gay men and gay women), whereas others limit gay to males (female homosexuals are referred to as lesbians). I use the terms interchangeably. However, since female sexual orientation is not related to HIV-AIDS, in this book the term *gay* always refers to male homosexuals.

PART ONE

SOCIAL ETIOLOGY

For all but a tiny span of time in human history, infectious diseases have been the major diseases and causes of death, and they are still widespread in developing countries (World Health Organization, 1992:15). Sociologists have not studied these diseases very much.[1] One reason is that the etiology of these diseases is dominated by a single factor (a germ), whereas the etiology of the leading diseases in developed countries (e.g., heart disease, cancer) is more complex and involves a range of behavioral and social factors.[2] These factors, however, may also be important in infectious diseases, especially HIV-AIDS. Therefore, to comprehend the social etiology of this disease, we must understand some sociological principles regarding the etiology of infectious diseases in general.

The sociological approach to the etiology of disease is an extension of epidemiology, which studies the differences between populations in the prevalence of disease and the distribution of diseases between sectors (subpopulations) of one population. In this way hypotheses about the etiology of disease may be developed. The basic concepts of this approach are agent, host, and environment.

Agent, Host, and Environment

The immediate cause of an infectious disease is an invisible parasite or microbe called the agent (virus, bacteria). The agent attacks the host (e.g., people) and feeds on or in the tissues, organs, skin, and secretions of the host. In the absence of a medical cure, the host usually gets sick and sometimes dies. However, since the immune system of the host normally fights back, the host may survive and develop immunity to future attacks.

Germ theory led to the discovery that microorganisms cause infectious diseases. It also gave rise in medicine to the doctrine of specific etiology, which holds that for each disease there is one cause (Dubos, 1959:101–110). However, infectious diseases are more complicated than the doctrine suggests. The character of the population and the environment of the population are also important factors.

9

Some populations (and subpopulations) have stronger immune systems than other populations. For example, although the effect of inadequate nutrition on the immune system and hence on susceptibility to infectious diseases is complex, in general malnourished populations are more susceptible to many infectious diseases than are other populations (Ulijaszek, 1990; Chandra, 1983). Also, populations with a low prevalence of diseases have more resistance to new agents than do populations in which diseases are widespread because immune systems in the latter may already be compromised by so many diseases. Features of the environment may also be important. For example, person-to-person transmission of an agent is more likely to occur in environments in which individuals live in crowded conditions. The presence of an agent is thus not sufficient to cause a disease to be widespread in a population or subpopulation. How prevalent it is will depend on characteristics of the population and the environment. In comparison to the biomedical approach to infectious disease, the epidemiological approach places greater emphasis on these characteristics than on the characteristics of the agent.

The sociological approach to the etiology of disease builds on this idea. For this reason the approach is sometimes referred to as social epidemiology. Its focus is on the social characteristics of the population and the environment.[3]

Major Social Factors in Infectious Disease

Two demographic variables, population size/density and migration, are the most general social factors in the etiology of most infectious diseases. In addition, social norms and customs, social cohesion, social institutions, and social change may be significant.

Population Size/Density and Migration

Some infectious diseases exist only when populations reach a certain size and density. The larger the population is, the greater are the chances of host-to-host transmission of infectious agents. Consequently, many infectious diseases were probably very rare or nonexistent when hunting and gathering societies were universal (Black, 1975; Cockburn, 1977:89–90; Cassidy, 1980:120). As populations grew, especially with the development of cities, infectious diseases increased. Beginning with urbanization, societies were repeatedly wracked with devastating epidemics (McNeill, 1976).

As people move from place to place, they may carry infectious agents and introduce them to new populations. In this way the centuries-long rural-to-urban migration led to the spread of infectious diseases, as did the development of intercontinental travel, which continues to be a factor in the spread of many infectious diseases.[4]

Social Norms and Customs

Social norms and customs may be important in the spread of disease. Habits of poor personal hygiene and the custom of living near domesticated animals are obvious examples. The social dynamics behind poor health habits may be less obvious. For instance, a study in rural India showed that a major source of disease stemmed from the fecal contamination of food and water due to the custom of defecating in the open field. To rectify the problem, public health officials installed public latrines, which people—especially women—promptly ignored. Using the open field to defecate was an important social activity. "Every morning and afternoon women go to the field, not only to relieve themselves but also to take time off from busy domestic routines, to gossip and exchange advice about husbands and mothers-in-law. ... The linked habits of going to the field for social gathering and for toilet ... meet a strongly felt need for community living" (Paul, 1977:235).

Social Cohesion

Since the 1970s a wide range of studies have found that individuals with extensive and cohesive networks of social relations have lower mortality rates from a variety of diseases than do individuals who have smaller and less cohesive networks (for a general review, see House et al., 1988).[5] Significantly, noninfectious diseases have been the focus of these studies. A much different relationship probably exists for infectious diseases. Other things being equal, since wider and more cohesive networks of social relations bring people together, social cohesion probably increases opportunities for host-to-host transmission of infectious agents.

Social Institutions

Social institutions are the frameworks within which people conduct their day-to-day routines of living and working. Some institutions facilitate person-to-person contact and hence opportunities for infectious agents to move from host to host. For example, the extended family of early (and present-day) simple agricultural societies involved more extensive contact between people than does the nuclear family unit, which some anthropologists believe was typical in the hunting and gathering societies that preceded early agricultural societies (Dumond, 1977). This contact may have been a major factor in the emergence of so many infectious diseases in early agricultural societies as well as in many developing countries today.

Social institutions, such as religion, that lead to the gathering of people are also implicated in disease transmission. For example, ceremonial baths as part of religious pilgrimages have contributed to cholera epidemics in India (Briggs, 1961:81; McNeill, 1976:46). Likewise, most social institutions are associated with physical structures in which people gather (e.g., schools, business firms, hospitals, churches).

Social Change

Since the agent is produced in the environment, it follows that changes in the environment may lead to changes in infectious diseases. According to T. Aidan Cockburn (1977:95), a medical and anthropological expert on infectious diseases, "Every change in the environment or culture is reflected in the patterns of the infectious diseases of the population." Changes in population size/density or migration patterns may change the prevalence of infectious diseases, as may an increase in social cohesion and population responses to changes in customs and norms. All were involved in the historical transition from hunting and gathering to agriculture about ten thousand years ago. Population size and densities increased, people began to live near animals, extended and cohesive kinship systems emerged, and infectious diseases increased (Cockburn, 1977; McKeown, 1979:45; Murdock, 1980:7). The transition led to *new* infections as well as facilitated the transmission of old ones (Cockburn, 1977:95). Some scholars believe that early agriculture led to the emergence of many common infectious diseases (e.g., rubella, smallpox, mumps, poliomyelitis, and chickenpox). Since agents for these diseases can exist only by rapid transmission from one host to another, they probably did not exist prior to agriculture and the existence of populations large enough to permit rapid transmission (Cockburn, 1977:89). It was not until the emergence of cities that the population threshold was reached for some infectious agents to thrive (Black, 1975; McNeill, 1976:50–51; Cockburn, 1977). For example, since it may take a population of about 1 million people in contact with one another (a single city or several populations close together) before the threshold is reached, many present-day common infectious diseases (e.g., measles) may have come into existence only when populations of this size emerged (Cockburn, 1977:91).

In addition, rural immigrants brought their rural customs to the city. They brought domesticated animals (Rosenberg, 1962:103, 191; Furnas, 1969: 455–456; Braudel, 1981:487; Evans, 1987:111, 114) and made no effort to collect and dispose of garbage and excreta (human and animal), frequently allowing both to pile up on the street (Burnet and White, 1972:13; Cornell, 1982: 204; Lyons and Petrucelli, 1987:55). (Much of the garbage was eaten by domesticated animals, just as in the countryside [Rosenberg, 1962:103].) Sewers were nonexistent or inadequate, and water was often contaminated (Lyons and Petrucelli, 1987:90, 203, 315). These conditions facilitated the spread of old microbes and could have led to the emergence of new ones.

Social Change and the Prevention of Infectious Diseases

Social and cultural change may contribute to a decline in infectious diseases. In societies that value science and have faith in knowledge based on science, people may change their behavior to avoid getting an infectious disease when medical science identifies how the agent is transmitted. For example, the development of germ theory led to segregating infectious patients, cleaning food, boiling water, practicing better personal hygiene, and improving infant feeding (Preston, 1976:86). Norms of behavior changed, preventive behavior increased, and infectious diseases declined.

Individual Infection and Epidemics

The focus of physicians and biomedical scientists is the physiological processes by which the agent causes an individual to get a disease. These processes are universal regardless of the environment in which the individual exists or the character of the population of which the individual is a member.

However, sociological phenomena, not just the agent, determine how widespread the infection becomes. Given the presence of the agent, the prevalence of a disease will vary depending on social norms and other characteristics of the population. For example, the greater the cohesion is, the more widespread a contagious disease is apt to be. Therefore, even though a microbe may be a necessary and sufficient condition for an individual to get infected, and a necessary condition for an epidemic to occur, it is not sufficient to cause an epidemic. Social cofactors must also be present.

The issue here is fundamentally different from the argument that HIV is not a sufficient (or necessary) condition for AIDS, in which different conceptions of the physiological causes of AIDS are the central issue (Root-Bernstein, 1993). That argument concerns the physiology of the disease itself, not the social factors that contribute to its epidemic form. The physiological action of HIV is the same for all individuals who are infected (though the speed of the action may vary between individuals). But before HIV could have led to the AIDS epidemic, social cofactors had to have been in place.

Guenther Risse (1988:55) stated that "epidemics are the result of a complex interplay of biological and social factors which at certain points in our history create favorable ecological niches for given diseases to thrive and therefore decimate humankind." This proposition guides the analysis in the next four chapters, which explore the social epidemiology of HIV-AIDS, the possible origin of HIV, and the trends and containment of the disease.

NOTES

1. For example, the index of the highly acclaimed *Handbook of Medical Sociology* (Freeman and Levine, 1989) contains no reference to infectious disease or to specific infectious diseases (other than AIDS), though numerous references appear for chronic illness, specific chronic illnesses (e.g., heart disease, cancer, stroke), stress, and mental illness.

2. Another reason is that when medical sociology became a recognized specialty in sociology after World War II, infectious diseases constituted only a small proportion of all diseases. In 1950 only one of the ten major causes of death was an infectious disease. This remains the case today (the disease is pneumonia-influenza, of which 98 percent of the deaths are from pneumonia [U.S. Bureau of the Census, 1988:77]).

3. The framework of agent, host, and environment is not limited to infectious disease. It is also used to conceptualize noninfectious diseases, though agent is frequently replaced by the more general term *pathogen*.

4. The colonization of the Americas highlights the social and cultural significance of intercontinental travel for the spread of infectious diseases. Europeans brought many infectious diseases against which Native Americans had little immunological resistance. This led to depletions of populations and, indeed, to the disappearance of entire civilizations in the New World. William McNeill (1976:204) gave an example of just how devastating infectious disease can be. In 1903 a previously isolated tribe of Caypao Indians of Brazil accepted a European Christian missionary into the tribe, which numbered at least 6,000 members. The spread of infectious diseases reduced the tribe to 500 by 1918 and to 27 by 1927. In 1950 there were only 2 descendants left.

5. The reasons for the relationship are not exactly clear, though two general hypotheses—the main effects hypothesis and the buffering hypothesis—have been posited. The former stipulates that a weak or weakened network of social relations has a direct effect on the individual state of health (e.g., death of a spouse may create stress, which leads to premature death). The latter stipulates that a wider and more cohesive network serves to support the individual in time of crisis and provide a buffer against its consequences (Berkman, 1985).

1. High-risk Groups in the United States

The first question social epidemiologists ask about a disease or cause of death is whether it is unevenly distributed in a population, as between age-sex categories, ethnic groups, social classes, or other populations with distinctive social or cultural characteristics. If this is the case, social factors are probably part of the disease's causation. Early in the history of AIDS in the United States, the disease was found to be unusually prevalent in certain groups, which were subsequently designated "high-risk groups."

High-risk Groups

In June 1981 the CDC (1981a) reported that five homosexual young men had *Pneumocystis carinii* pneumonia, which usually occurs only in individuals whose immune systems have been seriously damaged. A month later the CDC (1981b) reported that during the previous two-and-a-half years twenty-six gays had been diagnosed with Kaposi's sarcoma, which is also associated with a weakened immune system. A few months later the afflictions were also found among persons who had injected drugs, Haitians and Africans living in the United States, and persons who had received blood transfusions and blood products. Further statistics soon revealed a very high concentration of PCP, KS, and other afflictions among gays, so the syndrome of diseases that later came to be called AIDS was believed to be associated with male homosexuality and was originally called gay-related immunodeficiency disease (GRID).

Although it is generally believed that the earliest known adult cases of AIDS were homosexuals who did not inject drugs, repeated serological analysis of stored blood samples taken from drug injectors from forty-two states and the District of Columbia in 1971–1972 revealed the presence of HIV in a number of them (the number varied depending on the test), whereas all tests for a control group of nondrug abusers were negative (Moore et al., 1985). Another study of the stored blood of persons in drug treatment programs in Manhattan found that HIV had been present in 1975–1976 (Des

Jarlais et al., 1989). Also, many of the early AIDS cases who identified themselves as gay were also injecting drugs, so infection may have been needle transmitted rather than sexually transmitted (Root-Bernstein, 1993:8). Even if HIV did appear first among gays, its appearance among drug injectors occurred not long after. Its presence among drug injectors may have gone undetected longer because drug addicts may not have sought medical care as frequently as gays.

Early findings led male homosexuals and drug injectors to be designated as high-risk groups for AIDS, a labeling that some have criticized. One criticism contends that the high-risk label for gays and drug injectors stigmatizes HIV-AIDS. It does stigmatize HIV-AIDS, but this is because the disease is disproportionately concentrated in certain groups. No such stigma would be attached to a disease disproportionately concentrated among groups with no preexisting stigma, such as members of the American Legion who contracted Legionnaires' disease (because they happened to attend a convention in a certain hotel in a particular city).

Another criticism is that such labeling deflects attention away from specific behaviors that put a person at risk and suggests that all persons in a high-risk group are at high risk of being infected. This, however, is not what the term *high-risk group* means in epidemiology. High-risk group simply refers to a group in which the rate of a disease is unusually high and that a member of this group has a greater likelihood of being exposed to the cause of the disease than members of most other groups. To identify gays (and drug injectors) as a high-risk group does not imply that all (or even most) gays (or drug injectors) are inherently at greater risk of contracting HIV than other groups or that all gays (or drug injectors) engage in high-risk behavior. (As will become clear, gays and drug injectors are at risk only if they engage in certain high-risk behaviors.)

In addition to male homosexuals and drug injectors, the CDC recognizes two other high-risk groups in the United States. One consists of persons who receive blood tranfusions and blood products. However, donor blood has been screened for HIV since 1985 and is largely free of HIV today. The percentage of all reported cases of AIDS in people who had received a blood transfusion or blood product (e.g., persons with hemophilia) had constituted only 3 percent of all reported cases of AIDS by December 31, 1992 (CDC, 1993a:9), and the number of cases reported each year has decreased slightly since 1988 (CDC, 1991b:361). With the continued screening of donor blood, the decline will continue. Since the only factor that distinguishes these persons from the rest of the population is a preexisting medical condition, I do not consider them further.

The other high-risk group consists of persons who were born in a country (Africa and certain Caribbean countries) that the CDC refers to as a "pattern II" country. In a pattern II country, the predominant mode of transmission is through heterosexual intercourse. Through 1992, less than 1 percent of the cases were in this category (in 1993, the CDC discontinued this classification). Such persons are assumed by the CDC to have gotten AIDS through heterosexual contact, and heterosexual transmission of HIV in the United States is examined in Chapter 4.

Gays and drug injectors are subpopulations with distinct subcultural and social characteristics. The role these characteristics play in the transmission of HIV is examined in this chapter, with most attention given to gays. In addition, ethnic, racial, and class differences in HIV-AIDS are examined.

Sex, Drugs, and the Behavioral Basis for the Transmission of HIV

Anal sex is a favored sexual practice for many gays. Since the anal tract is apt to tear during sexual intercourse and semen (which has a high concentration of blood cells) from the inserter seeps into the receiver's bloodstream, anal sex is especially high risk for the receiver to contract HIV (Coxon, 1988). Other common sexual practices among male homosexuals, such as fisting (inserting the hand and arm up the anus), may also result in tears to the anal tract, further increasing the risk of infection from anal intercourse. The urethral wall of the inserter may also tear, allowing blood from the receiver to enter the inserter's bloodstream, although the risk to the inserter is far less than to the receiver (Levy, 1993). Because anal intercourse is also high risk for all sexually transmitted diseases (in the rectal as well as genital regions), the incidence of STDs (besides HIV-AIDS) in the gay population is unusually high (Rompalo and Handsfield, 1989; Ostrow et al., 1983). STDs also create lesions in the genital and anal regions. Since the lesions give HIV a convenient portal entry into a person's bloodstream, STDs are themselves serious risk factors in the transmission of HIV.

Virtually all experts now agree that in comparison to anal intercourse, penile-vaginal intercourse is a very inefficient (even rare) mode of transmitting HIV (Padian et al., 1990; Root-Bernstein, 1993:32; see also Booth, 1988 and Hearst and Hulley, 1988). The walls of the vagina are thicker and tougher than those of the anal and urethral tracts and hence are less apt to tear during sexual intercourse. Nevertheless, the presence of STDs does increase the chances of contracting HIV from an infected partner in penile-vaginal intercourse. Males may be infected by the vaginal secretions (e.g., menstrual blood) of an infected partner, but this is rare in the United States. The female is probably at greater risk than the male (Padian et al., 1991) since infected semen may remain in her genital tract for a period of time, giving the agent an opportunity to penetrate tissue and enter the bloodstream. How-

TABLE 1.1   AIDS Cases by Sex and Exposure Category, Reported Through December 31, 1992 (thirteen years and older)[a]

Sex/Exposure Category	Number	Percent
Males	221,714	89.0
Females	27,485	11.0
Males		
Homosexual/bisexual	142,626	64.3
Injecting drug user	43,786	19.7
Homosexual and injecting drug user	15,899	7.2
Heterosexual[b]	4,343	2.0
Has had sex with injecting drug user	2,585	1.2
Born in pattern II country	2,076	0.9
Other/undetermined[c]	12,984	5.9
Females		
Injecting drug user	13,626	49.6
Heterosexual[b]	8,949	32.6
Has had sex with injecting drug user	5,896	21.5
Born in pattern II country	886	3.2
Other/undetermined[c]	4,024	14.6

[a]Figures reflect reporting delays.

[b]This category includes people who have had sex with members of certain high-risk categories, such as drug injectors and HIV-infected persons, risk not specified, and excludes persons born in a pattern II country.

[c]This category includes persons with hemophilia/coagulation disorder and recipients of blood transfusion.

SOURCE: CDC (1993a:117).

ever, in the United States the most frequent way females contract HIV is from injecting drugs (this is the second most frequent mode of transmission for males). The second leading risk category for females is having sex with a drug injector.

It is clear, therefore, that most HIV-AIDS infections have a behavioral basis, specifically male homosexual behavior and/or drug injection. This can be seen in the CDC statistics reported in Table 1.1, which gives the percentage of all AIDS cases of adults and adolescents (persons thirteen years of age and over) as of December 31, 1992. For males, 91.2 percent were classified as a homosexual/bisexual and/or drug injector. No female was classified as a homosexual/bisexual, but 49.6 percent were drug injectors. (All statistics reported by the CDC [and NCHS] reflect "reporting delays." There is a lag of several months between when many AIDS cases are diagnosed or deaths occur and when they are reported [in some instances, several years may lapse]. Therefore, Table 1.1 and all subsequent tables based on statistics reported by the CDC [and NCHS] reflect these delays.)

Thus, the mode of transmission is such that HIV-AIDS is largely a male disease in the United States. Although the percentage of female cases has increased in recent years, 86.5 percent of all cases thirteen years and older reported in 1992 were male (CDC, 1993a:9). Also, because of the significance of sexual activity and drug use to the transmission of HIV, HIV-AIDS is highly concentrated among the young and middle-aged adults, with almost 80 percent of those infected between twenty-five and forty-four years old (CDC, 1993a:13).

The basic premise of the social epidemiologic perspective is that social and cultural factors may be involved in the etiology of disease. At one level, the factors involved in HIV-AIDS are gay sexual behavior and drug use. However, since such behavior did not begin to contribute to HIV-AIDS until the 1980s, this means that changes in the behavior of gays and drug injectors had to have occurred. Such changes, in turn, stemmed from social changes in the gay and drug subcultures.

Gay Subcultures and the HIV-AIDS Epidemic

Distinctive gay subcultures with special institutions, meeting places, a special argot, and distinctive folklore exist in many urban areas today (Plummer, 1975:154–174; Goodwin, 1989).[1] These subcultures became widespread especially during and after the 1970s, the period when the gay liberation movement first emerged, but their development occurred over a very long time. Several works have described various aspects of this history (for the most comprehensive treatment, see Greenberg, 1988). The following is a very general outline.

Social Oppression and Gay Subcultures

Homoerotic tendencies and relationships have existed for thousands of years. Homosexuality exists in tribes, bands, and other simple, nonliterate societies today and was probably present when these were the only societies in the world. It was also present in ancient civilizations and the feudal period in Europe. However, as a group phenomenon in which homosexuals are tied through a network of relationships, homosexuality did not exist until much later (Greenberg, 1988:14, 25–298; Weeks, 1990:2). For example, in classical Greece homosexual relations were legally and socially accepted and appear to have been universal among males in Sparta. A man's desire for sex with men was not seen as incompatible with a desire for sex with women. As revealed in writings and especially vase paintings (Dover, 1978), homosexual relations were accepted alongside heterosexual relations and were integral aspects of Greek society (Greenberg, 1988:141–151). Consequently, there were no distinct groups or separate communities of homosexuals (Greenberg, 1988:143–144).

Networks of homosexuals first appeared in the late-fourteenth-century European city (Greenberg, 1988:305, 306). By the eighteenth century, networks with distinctive customs and special meeting places (e.g., taverns) existed in urban areas (Greenberg, 1988:313, 314; Dynes and Donaldson, 1992). By the middle of the twentieth century, homosexual subcultures were common to urban areas throughout the United States. In 1949 urban sociologist Ernest Burgess (1949:234) wrote, "Every city has its [separate] homosexual world with its rendezvous, parties, and celebrities. This world has its own language, incomprehensible to outsiders. It has its own literature, group ways, and code of conduct. It is a world where members find moral support, sympathy, and fellowship."

Many ethnographies in the 1950s and 1960s revealed that homosexuality was present in American cities "as a way of life with distinctive manners, customs, and institutions" (Greenberg, 1988:464). Sex institutions in particular were common. They included bars especially, but massage parlors, porno shops, movie theaters, and certain parks, beaches, and public restrooms ("tearooms") in or around the city were also places where homosexuals commonly met and had sex. The subcultures occupied their own physical and social space in the city. Most people were unaware of these subcultures and certainly unaware of much of the sexual activity within them. They were figuratively walled off from the rest of the city and hence out of sight to most people.

Gay subcultures were specific to urban environments. Only in cities was there a population base large enough for the number of males who desired same-sex erotic relations to reach the critical mass necessary to sustain a subculture. In addition, cities provided general anonymity, impersonality, and a loosening of social controls; the impersonality of cities allowed for networks of gays to emerge in which the anonymity of the individual was preserved. In rural areas and small towns male homosexuals were so secretive that separate gay communities rarely existed; most of the male homosexuals in these settings did not even know each other as late as the 1970s (Harry and DeVall, 1978:140–143). In a questionnaire survey in 1970, Martin Weinburg and Colin Williams (1974:131–146) found that in comparison to gays in San Francisco and New York City, gays in "outlying areas" (places with 25,000–250,000 people) were less involved with other gays—had less gay sex and fewer gay friends, had more heterosexual friends, were more fearful of being discovered, and hence were more circumspect in concealing their identity. As gays in rural areas and towns and small cities learned about the gay subcultures in urban areas, many migrated to large cities (Verghese et al., 1989; D'Emilio, 1992:93). However, since cities had existed for thousands of years, urban environments, while necessary, were not sufficient to account for the emergence of gay subcultures. Social repression was also central (Greenberg, 1988:301–346; see also Plummer, 1975:167–171).

For much of history, as in classical Greece, male homosexuals were not oppressed. However, they have been the object of hostility in the West since at least the fourteenth century, and the hostility deepened during the industrial age (Greenberg, 1988:301–396; on England in the eighteenth century, see Senelick, 1992; see also Weeks, 1988:2). It continued into the twentieth century. Almost everyone believed male homosexuals were immoral, even criminal, or sick, and for a man to be known as a homosexual almost always put his occupational future and social status in danger. Many professional accreditation associations barred gays from practicing on the ground of "moral turpitude." Consequently, in most places male homosexuals lived in the shadows of society and felt compelled to keep their sexual orientation secret; they lived in "the closet." Even though urban environments were less intolerant, most gays still did not feel safe in being open about their sexual orientation (Greenberg, 1988:457).

Gay subcultures solved this problem. Since they were largely invisible to the rest of the community, gays did not need to hide their sexual orientation within the subcultural settings (where a person could "come out" of the closet). Men who desired sex with other men could openly engage other like-minded men safe from community surveillance and controls (for a general discussion, see Plummer, 1975:167–171; for an early study, see Leznoff and Westley, 1956). In this setting homosexuality was normal and gays were socially accepted.

But the burdens of concealment and social isolation remained. Most people still considered male homosexuals as criminals and moral deviants, and gays were still treated with scorn (Weinberg and Williams, 1974:18–21; Greenberg, 1988:457). For example, a 1969 Harris poll reported that 63 percent of a national sample believed homosexuals were "harmful to American life" (*Time,* October 31, 1969:61). "Fear of ostracism, divorce, unemployment, hellfire, or a guilty conscience" was still pervasive (Greenberg, 1988:457). And gay subcultural institutions were frequently raided by police and the patrons harassed, arrested, and in danger of having their homosexual identities publicly revealed (Humphrey, 1970; D'Emilio, 1992:86–88). The problem declined with the gay liberation movement in the late 1960s and 1970s.

Gay Liberation

Gays began to resist oppressive social and police measures. The most well-known resistance was the Stonewall riot in New York City. On the evening of June 27, 1969, the police raided a popular gay bar, Stonewall Inn, in

Greenwich Village. The raid itself was not unusual, but this time the gays fought back, hurling slogans and objects at the police. This touched off numerous protest demonstrations by gays, including a huge parade down Fifth Avenue (Fettner and Check, 1984:226). In the months and years to follow, gay pride parades were held in cities to commemorate the event and indeed "became the order of the day" (Gregersen, 1983:175). Gays organized politically and gained political power, and with this more legal rights (gay rights) (Marotta, 1981; Gregersen, 1983:176). (On developments in San Francisco, see D'Emilio, 1992.)

Central to the gay rights movement was the demand that homosexuals be socially recognized and accepted as nondeviant and normal. The more radical gay rights groups "called for a rethinking of human sexuality and its place in society [and] insisted that everyone was capable of homosexual response and argued that homosexuality could achieve equal status with heterosexuality only when that capability was realized" (Greenberg, 1988: 458). In short, homosexuality was just another sexual orientation.

The movement enjoyed significant success. Although various forms of sex common to gays (e.g., sodomy) are still illegal in a number states, many communities began to relax antigay statutes in the 1960s and 1970s.[2] The American Psychiatric Association eliminated homosexuality from its list of mental disorders, thus declaring that homosexuality was not an abnormal condition and a form of sickness. Social attitudes toward homosexuals also began to change, and the social acceptance of homosexuals increased. By 1992–1993, according to two nationwide polls, by *Newsweek* and the *New York Times/* CBS, a substantial minority, 41 percent and 36 percent of respondents, respectively, considered homosexuality an "acceptable alternative life style"; 35 percent of the *Newsweek* respondents approved of legally sanctioned homosexual marriage; and 32 percent approved of homosexual couples adopting children (Turque et al., 1992; Schmalz, 1993a). Nevertheless, public opinion is still negative, a large proportion of Americans believe sex between same-sex individuals is immoral, and opposition by religious and political conservatives is especially intense, as is that of people from small towns and rural areas (for a review, see Greenberg, 1988:465–475). However, starting in the 1960–1970 period, homosexuals were less apt to be defined as deviant, criminal, or mentally ill. Oppressive practices by community officials and the police declined, and more people (but not a majority) considered homosexuality a form of sexual orientation or "lifestyle" rather than a form of sexual deviance.[3]

Consequently, gays had less need to conceal their identities. Same-sex couples appeared more frequently in public, as did gays who participated in public demonstrations. Gays began to appear on television, and homosexual organizations sprang up on college campuses. And gay subcultures flourished. In addition to bars (which were central), networks of friends, sex institutions, a special argot, and folklore, the subcultures included political organizations, community centers and social clubs (e.g., church and theater groups), and a range of products and services that catered to gays, such as newspapers, bookstores, restaurants, discos, T-shirts, sex aids, travel agencies, publications listing gay bars by city and types of sex one could find, and legal services (Harry and DeVall, 1978:146-149; Altman, 1982:8; Gregersen, 1983:174; Goodwin, 1989). The subcultures became more vibrant, elaborate, and open to community view. Anthropological sexologist Edgar Gregersen (1983:174) referred to this transition as a change from "a secret ... subculture, to a fairly public 'satellite culture,' with spin-offs into the heterosexual world."

Such a range of activities represented "a sense of shared values," but it also indicated "a willingness to assert one's homosexuality as an important part of one's whole life rather than something private and hidden as was traditionally the case" (Altman, 1982:8). Social cohesion among gays was thus strengthened (on social cohesion in the gay community, see Tessina, 1989:24), and this helped resolve the problem of social isolation along with pangs of guilt and self-identity (e.g., the "Who am I?" question) (Goodwin, 1989). The migration of homosexuals to urban subcultures accelerated (D'Emilio, 1992:101).[4] This enlarged and strengthened the subcultures, which, in turn, gave more gays a sense of acceptance and more opportunities to express their sexual orientation in the open.

Several factors contributed to the success of gay liberation (Harry and DeVall, 1978:165–182; Greenberg, 1988:459–475; D'Emilio, 1992). The cohesiveness of gays gave them political power. But the increase in sexually permissive attitudes in the overall population was perhaps the most significant factor. Casual or "recreational" sex and sex in which the sole purpose is pleasure were increasingly accepted by more people (Greenberg, 1988:461–462) (though not to the extent that many conservative moralists were claiming). The number of unmarried young adults openly living together increased. Coed dorms on college campuses were permitted. To some people, especially religious conservatives and persons from small towns and rural areas, these developments were decadent and immoral (Greenberg, 1988:465–475). But their increasing acceptance made it hard to deny gays the same right (Greenberg, 1988:462), just as gays were demanding.[5] Relative to the past, gays were liberated.

Paradoxically, then, while social oppression was central in the origin of gay subcultures, once the subcultures were developed, the easing of oppression allowed them to flourish. The range of activities and institutions expanded. In some cities gay communities were relatively self-contained. True "gay ghettos" existed in which most or all the residents, home owners, and owners or operators of commercial establishments were gay (Harry and DeVall, 1978:134–146). And as the notion of liberation indicates, harassment of the residents and patrons of these areas declined, and there was less need for gays to keep their sexual orientation a secret. But another social paradox of gay liberation was also unfolding: Changes in gay sexual activity were destined to be factors in the AIDS epidemic.

Gay Liberation and Sex-positive Subcultures

In an analysis of sexual orientation in society, George Becker (1984) distinguished between two polar types of society: "sex-negative" societies and "sex-positive" societies. In the former, sex is repressed and is restricted to single partners, and monogamous relations are the normative ideal. Victorian England is one example. In the latter, sex is viewed as pleasurable and recreational, and polygamous relations are the normative ideal. An example is the Mangaians of Polynesia, among whom sex is exalted and "the normative expectation is to be sexually active with numerous partners" (Becker, 1984:57). Americans took a step in a sex-positive direction in the 1960s and 1970s, though it overstates the matter to say that they developed an extremely sex-positive orientation in which numerous partners were exalted as a normative expectation (Fumento, 1990:227–234). It does not overstate the matter with respect to gay subcultures, however. This is especially clear from the development of gay commercial sex institutions.

Sexual Institutions. Establishments where sexual activity took place increased. Robert Padgug (1989:303) stated, "Not surprisingly, when gay people asserted their right to exist in the gay liberation period that began in the 1960s, sexual institutions expanded astronomically." The extent of the increase is suggested by the following statistic: *The Address Book,* a publication of gay institutions in the United States, grew in listings from 690 in 1964 to 5,800 in 1983 (Darrow et al., 1986:97–98). Although not all of these were sex institutions, many were.

The most well-known sex institutions were the bathhouses ("baths" or "tubs") and bars with dark back rooms or basements ("fuck" rooms). The variety of bathhouses increased, as did bars (e.g., dancing, private, or "leather" [where customers wore motorcycle costumes with studded belts and caps and exhibited macho demeanor]) and other sex institutions and settings where sexual activity took place: porno theaters, massage parlors, tearooms, discotheques, Sexual Freedom League (group sex) parties, public parks, beaches, and various combinations of these (for sociological studies of tearooms and baths in particular, see Humphreys, 1970; Weinberg and Williams, 1975; Kinsella 1989:175–176). These institutions provided instant, accessible, and impersonal sex with multiple partners (Plummer, 1975:168), giving "room for sexual experimentation and creativity, [which] expanded immensely" (Padgug, 1989:303).[6]

The sex-positive character of these sex institutions is depicted in the writings of a number of gay authors. Seymour Kleinberg (1980:172) wrote that gay bars and baths in particular were "created to expedite sexual liaison and devoted to libertinism." A handbook on gay sex and gay relationships, written in 1982 and updated in 1991, states that the bathhouse "and its spin-off institutions [are] wholeheartedly dedicated to the pleasures of masculine and sexual promiscuity" and "represent an Eden of sensuality" (Muchmore and Hanson, 1991:73). Dennis Altman (1982:17, 79) described the bathhouses of the early 1980s as "large-scale luxurious pleasure palaces where everyone is potentially an immediate sexual partner," where men "rarely talk much, [where] it is quite common for sex to take place without words, let alone names, being exchanged." Such statements are supported by sociologists' observations of activity in bathhouses and interviews with the patrons (see Weinberg and Williams, 1975, especially on the "orgy room" of bathhouses; Kinsella, 1989:175–176, on the "sling room"). Weinberg and Williams (1975:129) concluded that "everyone at a gay bath is a potential partner." In sum, as sexual freedom grew, sex institutions emerged to meet sexual desire.

But they also stimulated sex, as in the erotic rooms and orgy rooms where group sex could take place (Weinberg and Williams, 1975:127). As Altman (1982:80) stated, they "increased sexual expectations." The number of sexual partners an individual might have could be very high. One survey of male homosexuals in San Francisco in the 1970s found that over 80 percent of the respondents claimed they had had fifty or more partners over the course of their lifetime, about 70 percent had had one hundred or more, and about 25 percent reported one thousand or more. More than 50 percent had had sexual activity with a male, on average, at least two to three times a week (more than 5 percent had had sex an average of seven times or more), and 75 percent said more than 50 percent of their male partners had been strangers (only 2 percent reported not having sexual partners who had been strangers) (Bell and Weinberg, 1978:298, 308). This same study reported that 79 percent had five or more partners annually (Bell and Weinberg, 1978:312). Similar results were reported by a study of a cohort of 8,906 gays in New York City who were recruited from clinics, gay organizations, and bathhouses and via mobile vans sent to areas of the city populated largely by gays. At the time of the first interview in 1977–1978, the median number of partners in the prior six months was ten, with 28 percent having twenty or more (Koblin et al., 1992:649).

In comparison, the number of partners heterosexuals generally had was far less. A study of a cohort of about one thousand twenty-five- to fifty-four-year-old single men in San Francisco in 1984 found that whereas 27 percent of homosexuals and 21 percent of bisexual men reported more than ten male partners during a six-month period in 1984, only 3 percent of heterosexual men reported ten or more female partners (Winkelstein et al., 1987). And in a comparison of couples (married heterosexuals, unmarried heterosexuals, gays, and lesbians) who volunteered to participate in a survey in the early 1980s, Philip Blumstein and Pepper Schwartz (1983) reported that gays were far more apt to be nonmonogamous or polygamous than other couples. For example, whereas a small minority of heterosexuals had had sex with an outside partner the previous year, about 75 percent of homosexual men had done so (Blumstein and Schwartz, 1983:276). And when polygamous behavior among heterosexuals did occur, it usually did not happen repeatedly, whereas for gays it did ("The only couples who adopt [polygamy] as a way of life are gay men" [Blumstein and Schwartz, 1983:278]).[7] A national survey of sexual practices in 1990–1991 found that only 7 percent of the adult heterosexual respondents had had more than one sexual partner in the previous year (Catania, Coates, Stall, et al., 1992:1103).[8] Evidence for attendees at STD clinics in Great Britain was similar. More than 50 percent of homosexual men said they had had five or more partners in the previous five years in comparison to 14 percent of heterosexual men (percentages with three or more partners were 83 percent to 18 percent) (Johnson et al., 1992:411).

It is clear, then, that by the 1970s the gay subcultures were decidedly sex positive in orientation and that sex institutions played a central role in this. Jeffrey Weeks (1988:8), who studied changes in the gay subcultures that accompanied gay liberation, stated, "The 1970s [witnessed] an explosion of what has been described as 'public sex' amongst gay men," with the sex institutions and clubs becoming places "where casual, recreational sex with multiple partners became the norm. ... [This] clearly represented ... a normalization in a new way of sex as recreation and pleasure."

Gay subcultures have probably always had a strong focus on sex and sexual need (Weeks, 1990:232), but by the 1970s the focus on sex was extreme. According to Mary Bateson and Richard Goldsby (1988:44), "Some gay men became sexual athletes, and group sex with multiple contacts was common, so that we hear of hundreds of different sexual contacts within a year that heterosexual men shake their heads in astonishment."[9] In the urban gay enclaves many men were having sex with many men who were also having sex with many men. This is not to say that all or even most gays had polygamous partners or that none had monogamous relations (Sonenschein, 1968). However, there is little disagreement that casual sexual activity and sex institutions in urban gay subcultures soared in the 1960s and 1970s and that much of the gay subcultures was organized around sex institutions, especially bathhouses, which provided places where casual, polygamous sex could be located, sustained, organized, and financed.

In writing about these institutions, some gay writers expressed approval (Muchmore and Hanson, 1991), some were ambivalent (Altman, 1982), but others expressed outright concern about the dangers and also raised moral questions (Kramer, 1977; Holleran, 1978; Shilts, 1987; Kirk and Madsen, 1989).[10] Still others, while also critical, primarily searched for a psychocultural understanding of why casual sex exploded in the 1970s and took some of the forms it did (Kleinberg, 1980:145–212).

Especially troubling to some writers was the commercialization of sex by bathhouses and other sex institutions (Kramer, 1977; Holleran, 1978; Shilts, 1987). It was not that the institutions were places where a person usually paid directly to have sex, as in a brothel. Rather, sexual activity was supported indirectly by the commercialization of other products and services. Many establishments charged a fee to enter and provided other services for a charge, including entertainment, saunas, towels, recreational facilities, meals, drinks, private rooms, and other amenities. These institutions were generally very successful commercially; they have been described as an example of "the triumph of consumer capitalism" (Altman, 1982:79–107). Even national chains of bathhouses emerged (Weinberg and Williams, 1974: 26). Therefore, in meeting sexual desire, sex institutions were manifestations of the economics of supply and demand. But these institutions were also *social* in nature.

Sex Institutions as Social Institutions

The extensive casual networks of gays engaging in sex apparently for the sole purpose of sensuous pleasure, and in so many different ways, went far beyond anything that had occurred before in the United States or elsewhere or that anyone could have imagined just a few years previously. Without question, "the sexual style of gay communities in the 1970s and early 1980s was a specific historic phenomenon" (Bateson and Goldsby, 1988:44). But to view it as historically specific does not explain it.

This phenomenon was not due to an unusually strong sex drive among gays; homosexuals had been around for many centuries, and there was no record of such activity previously. Greater social acceptance of gays was certainly a factor, but only a small percentage of the public accepted such behavior (very few even knew about it). Furthermore, in previous periods in history when homosexuality had been widely accepted socially, as, for example, in classical Greece, there had been no sexual practices remotely resembling those associated with the gay subcultures of the 1970s and 1980s. The factors motivating the sex-positive orientation of these decades involved the *social meaning* of sex-positive behavior and sex institutions.

Sex Institutions as Symbols of Sociosexual Freedom. Gay sex institutions had symbolic significance beyond sexual economics. Since they were tolerated by the community (even if most people did not know what took place in them), to many gays they symbolized the social acceptance of homosexuals by society. For example, Ronald Bayer (1985:596) stated that the gay bathhouse became "a powerful symbol of the struggle for greater social toleration for homosexuality." More specifically, they symbolized sexual freedom and the removal of sociosexual oppression.

In sociology, the study of meaning relates behavior and the institutions that structure behavior to cultural beliefs and normative attitudes, which the behavior and institutions symbolize. Sometimes the meanings are self-evident and sometimes not. Regardless, meanings contribute to the motivation of behavior and thus sustains institutions that are frameworks for behavior. To date, sociologists have not studied the normative and cultural symbolism of gay sex institutions and activities as they have the way the activities in sex institutions were organized (Weinberg and Williams, 1975).[11]

The abrupt lifting of oppressive measures after so many years of persecution and denial probably contributed to the extreme form that sexual expression took. "Repressed socially, sexually, and psychically for so long, like the children of the Victorians, the gays let it all loose" (Fettner and Check, 1984:226). Similarly, Padgug (1989:303) viewed the heightened sexual expression "as a protest against the earlier suppression of homosexuality, and as a genuine, although sometimes utopian, attempt to fashion a society under new conditions of freedom." For gays who had been closeted, gay liberation was "the beginning of a mass coming-out" (Fettner and Check, 1984:226; Kinsella, 1989:179).[12]

Many gays began to view sex as an end in itself. For example, Andrew Holleran (1988:24) wrote that "the idea of restraints on sex [was] anathema" to the gay community during the gay liberation years, and he referred to "the exhilarating suspicion that we [gays] were pioneers in the pursuit of human happiness and no one had found [the limits to sex] yet." Emile Durkheim (1949) noted many years before, however, that the pursuit of ends with no limits—a condition of anomie—is an endless and meaningless endeavor in which satisfaction is never realized. Thus, Kleinberg (1980:149, 148) wrote of the sexual activity among gays during the 1970s in terms of "pseudo men [gays dressing in leather motorcycle costumes and acting macho] in search of nothing" (which he thought was no better or worse than the closeted, more oppressive period of "pseudo [effeminate] men in search of pseudo women"). And other writers "were warning of [the] emptiness at the heart of the new sexual culture" (Weeks, 1990:233).

When sex is unbounded by love, affection, tenderness, and some degree of permanence, or, as Weeks (1988:8) put it, when there is a "decoupling of sex and intimacy," sex appears empty indeed and devoid of meaning. Nevertheless, practices and customs associated with particular groups and societies have significant social meaning and cultural significance to the participants, even if these activities appear to be socially empty and to reflect a condition of anomie. Sex institutions were more than places for (unlimited or "empty") sexual gratification. They also symbolized a newfound sexual freedom and the removal of sociosexual reoppression.

Sex Institutions and Social Cohesion. Sex institutions were also socially significant because they enabled gays to discover other gays:

> Those gay institutions largely devoted to sexual activity—bars, baths, public spaces—were of great importance [to gay life]. ... The fundamental link among gay persons was, after all, sexual, but these institutions have represented far more than sites of sexual activity. Such places have developed a far greater symbolic and social significance to the gay community than is readily understood by non-gays. For decades they represented the only public spaces that could in any sense be termed homosexual and where homosexuals could discover each other as well as a wider homosexual world (Padgug, 1989:303).

Sex institutions were more than places where gays had sex. They also promoted social bonds and gay cohesion. Altman's (1982:79) description of bathhouses captures this nicely:

> Even the most transitory encounters [in bathhouses] are part of a heightened eroticism that pervades the building; there is a certain sexual democracy, even camaraderie, that makes the sauna attractive. The willingness to have sex immediately, promiscuously, with people about whom one demands only physical contact, can be seen as a sort of Whitmanesque democracy, a desire to know and trust other men in a type of *brotherhood*. (Emphasis added.)

Therefore, Bateson and Goldsby (1984:44–45) stated, "sex [in sex institutions] became an expression of unity and solidarity in the gay community, linking hundreds of men to each other, much as it links couples in happy marriages." Weeks (1990:232) described sex and sexual need as the "glue" that held gay subcultures together.

At the individual level, social cohesion gives the individual a sense of belonging. The significance of sex institutions in this regard is revealed in a frequently cited statement that a gay made to Barry Dank (1971:188) in his study of the coming out process around 1970: "I walked into this bar and saw a whole crowd of groovy, groovy guys. [I then realized] that not all gay men are dirty old men or idiots, silly queens, but there are some just normal looking and acting people. ... I saw gay society and I said, 'Wow, I'm home.'" Many gays, unless they have gay friends, live in social isolation and have no real "home."

Polygamous sexual relations in sex institutions helped fill the void. "Though 'everyone knew' that the baths were 'for' quick, unencumbered sex," they also opened "interactions with a range of people never met in the comparatively encapsulated everyday life of home and work. New buddies, friends, and lovers came out of the baths as they did in other sites of gay contact" (Adam, 1992:181). Cindy Patton (1990a:47) wrote that sex with many partners became "a symbolic badge of belonging." Altman (1982:21) stated, "For homosexuals, bars and discos play the role performed for other groups by family and church. ... [Here] homosexuals first meet others like themselves and are able to express themselves in ways denied them in other areas of their lives. [These settings provide] a sense of identity and even community that only a relatively small number of homosexuals find in alternative institutions."

In sum, gay sex institutions and the sexual activity in them became the functional social equivalent of family, friends, and community: They promoted social bonds that gave gays a sense of belonging and social support. The lack of such bonds may be particularly evident to gays who have lost many of their friends to AIDS. As one expressed it, "For a gay man friends are everything; it's not like we have kids and families" (Navarro, 1993b:A-1). Of course, some gays have stable relationships with lovers, not all gays are rejected by their kin, and a few gay couples have adopted children. But for many gays, especially in the 1970s and 1980s, sexual relations with multiple partners constituted social and not just sexual bonds and gave the individual a sense of cohesion with the gay community. And since sex institutions fostered sociosexual bonds, they were significant factors in filling the void of social isolation that many gays had historically experienced.[13] Altman (1982:21) observed that critics of commercialized sex missed this very point.

Gay Pride and Gay Liberation. Sex institutions also served to enhance gay pride and identification with the gay liberation movement. Ann Fettner and William Check (1984:226) wrote that gays "chose to express formally [openly] forbidden sexual interest in other men partly as an expression of what has come to be called 'gay pride.' " Such pride was related to sociosexual freedom. For example, a physician and reporter for the gay publication the *New York Native,* stated in 1981 that "sexual freedom was essential to being gay" (Kinsella, 1989:29). Since male sexual preference for another male was the focus of homosexual oppression, when oppressive measures were lifted, sexual freedom and gay pride were joined. Hence, sex institutions and clubs "symbolized a new hedonism, where sexual pleasure was placed at the heart of the new gay identity" (Weeks, 1990:232). "Gay liberation meant release from loneliness and exclusion, becoming members ... of a movement which rapidly became international" (Bateson and Goldsby,

1988:45). Sex institutions facilitated the sense of belonging to this social movement.

This symbolic meaning of sexual expression and sex institutions is exemplifed by the statement of a homosexual victim of AIDS in the early 1980s: "Whenever I threw my legs in the air, I thought I was doing my bit for gay liberation" (Altman, 1986:142–143). It thus "appears that for many gay men, establishing the gay liberation movement also meant developing uniquely homosexual types of sex (such as fisting) and specific places, such as bath houses and sex clubs, in which this liberation could be explored. Sex became, in a sense, a political statement" (Root-Bernstein, 1993:286).

But sex was also more than this. Polygamous gay sex symbolized the lifting of sociosexual restraints, and it was a way for gays to bond themselves to the gay community, to express their gay identity, and to manifest solidarity with the gay liberation movement.

Sex Institutions, Normative Boundaries, and Social Norms. Members of groups want their own identity, and to this end they strive to draw a distinction between themselves and the wider society in normative and cultural terms. Sex institutions and the activity within them did this for gays.

The normative ideal for heterosexual men is to marry; even with a high percentage of marriages ending in divorce, during the course of marriage exclusive bonds to mates are socially and legally sanctioned. In contrast, "there *are* no real sanctions to support" exclusive relationships for gay couples and "no clear role definitions as to who should do what." It is thus "easier for gay couples to experiment with unusual arrangements, and to maintain relationships that allow more flexibility and freedom than ... conventional [heterosexual] coupledom" (Altman, 1982:188). Since sex institutions provided settings where casual sexual encounters with multiple partners could take place, they supported sexual experimentation, flexibility, and freedom, and hence they served to symbolize the differentiation of gays from nongays. The bath "is a unique institution, with no real equivalent in the straight world," and as a normative boundary, it "stands as perhaps the best organized and most complete rejection of puritan values that exists in America today" (Muchmore and Hanson, 1991:74).[14] Altman (1982:211) certainly overstated when he wrote that "we [gays] organize our everyday lives in radical opposition to the sexual norms of the wider [heterosexual] society." Gays organize their everyday lives much as nongays do. But with respect to gay sex institutions and the sexual activity that took place in them, Altman's is not an overstatement. Despite the claim made by some that a distinct gay identity involves more than sex, it is in terms of sex institutions, sexual activity, and norms of sexual behavior that differences between gay subcultures and a predominantly heterosexual society are usually drawn—by gays as well as nongays.[15]

Some contend that polygamous sexual activity and institutions also involved deep psycho-cultural-sexual dynamics.[16] The point is, however, that impersonal and casual sexual networks were widespread among gays during gay liberation and that participation in such networks constituted a new social norm separating many gays from straight society. Indeed, Altman wrote in 1982 (pp. 17, 180) that "the assumption that it is desirable to have frequent and varied sex partners is increasingly seen as a positive part of the gay life style" and that "the image of 'groovy' sex [e.g., sadomasochism, bondage, or fist fucking and the use of amyl nitrite, or poppers, in connection with sex] has taken on a momentum and become a standard to which numbers of gay men feel pressure to conform."[17] Michael Fumento (1990:231) wrote that having many partners had become "a badge of honor." So even if the underlying motivation for the new norm involved deeper psycho-cultural-sexual dynamics, the fact is that the subcultures were sex positive in orientation; sex was exalted, and "the normative expectation [was] to be sexually active with numerous partners" (Becker, 1984:57). This norm helped establish a normative boundary between gays and the dominant nongay society.

The Sex-positive Gay Subcultures and HIV-AIDS

Once HIV existed, the sex-positive norms of polygamous sex guaranteed that HIV would spread rapidly through the gay population, which it did. Of course, monogamous sex with an infected partner increases an *individual's* chances of contracting HIV (or other STDs) more than many encounters with multiple partners, only some of whom are infected, do. But a monogamous relationship limits the infectious agent to no more than two people. Multiple partners give the agent opportunities to find a home in multiple hosts and thus increase the spread in the *population*. In addition, since the partners of a polygamous gay relationship were apt also to have multiple partners, the risk of contracting HIV in a particular sexual episode was unusually high. Just how fast the epidemic was growing among gays in some cities with strong gay subcultures is reflected in the percentage of gays attending an STD clinic in San Francisco who tested positive for HIV: 1 percent in 1978, 25 percent in 1980, and 65 percent in 1984. For a cohort of Pittsburgh gays, HIV infection went from 10 percent in 1983 to 28 percent in 1984 (Landesman et al., 1985:521). (HIV was not identified until 1984, of course, but blood samples stored prior to 1984 were tested.) And the importance of multiple partners in HIV infection is clear from a case-controlled study of fifty of the first seventy cases of male homosexuals with AIDS from San Francisco, Los Angeles, New York City, and Atlanta and two control groups of male homosexuals without AIDS (one control group was from an STD clinic, and one was from private physicians) (Jaffe et al., 1983). The median number of annual partners for the AIDS group was sixty-one in comparison to twenty-three and twenty-four for the control groups, respectively. And the fact that the median proportion of sex partners from bathhouses the previous year was fifty for the AIDS group in comparison to twenty-three and four for the controls, respectively, indicates how important sex institutions were in transmitting HIV.

Nevertheless, the gay subcultures arose out of social forces that were independent of sex institutions (Goodwin, 1989:xiii). In the absence of the symbolic and normative aspects of polygamous sex, sex institutions alone would not have caused polygamous behavior to be so widespread. James Kinsella (1989:179) stated, "Although anonymous sex at the baths undoubtedly contributed to the epidemic, the most important factor was an overriding sexual more of the gay culture ... that encouraged promiscuity and unsafe sex." Nevertheless, by providing a setting where casual polygamous sex could take place, sex institutions contributed to the development of the norm and helped sustain it. Further, psychologist Walt Odets (1994:13), in an editorial in *AIDS and Social Policy Journal,* called attention to the cohesion-producing element of anal (and oral) sex between gays. He observed that the exchange of semen has significant social meaning and is an important aspect of intimacy between gays. While the act of exchanging semen is independent of sex institutions, the institutions facilitated such exchange with a variety of partners and thus promoted social bonding and cohesion among gays.

The normative sex-positive orientation of gay subcultures was related to the spread of HIV in still another way: through the spread of STDs. The prevalence of STDs increases as polygamous behavior does. When populations differ in STDs, differences in polygamous behavior are assumed (Mann et al., 1992:174; Root-Bernstein, 1993:301). STDs also increase the risk of contracting HIV. (STDs are thus both indicators of polygamous behavior and risk factors in HIV.) Significantly, STDs were increasing by epidemic proportion in the gay population during the 1970s, just prior to the epidemic in AIDS (Sandholzer, 1983:3–5; Rompola and Handsfield, 1989). This may have had a socially symbolic function. Michael Callon (*Surviving AIDS*) reported on hearing Edmund White (co-author of *The Joy of Gay Sex*) state in a lecture that "gay men should wear their sexually transmitted disease like red badges of courage in a war against a sex-negative society" (Root-Bernstein, 1993:286). The symbolic significance of such a view for boundary maintenance is obvious. But this view also encouraged polygamous behavior and deterred gays from protecting themselves against contracting STDs and hence HIV. The positive social functions of the gay sex norms of the gay subcultures were accompanied by tragic health results.

Migration, Gay Subcultures, and Rural HIV-AIDS. Statistics on HIV-infected gays outside cities is limited, but a study by Abraham Verghese et al.

(1989) of HIV-infected gays treated by physicians in upper east Tennessee suggests an intriguing sociological pattern. Between 1985 and 1989, 69 percent of eighty-one HIV-infected patients were gay. Many had been reared in the region and moved to urban areas, where they were first diagnosed as HIV positive. Others lived in the region but had histories of travel to urban areas where AIDS was prevalent, suggesting that they had acquired their infections there. (In 1985–1986 there were only occasional cases of HIV-AIDS in the area, and tests of gays from gay meeting places [a tavern and a church in Johnson City] were all seronegative.) The findings thus suggested a link between urban gay subcultures and rural HIV-AIDS.

Rural gays and semirural gays went to cities, either to seek permanent employment (usually as adolescents) or to visit, attracted by "a sophisticated gay culture [that] allowed pursuit of a life that could have posed problems at home" (Verghese et al., 1989:1052). When they became infected, they returned home to die and to be cared for by their families and hence increased the number of HIV-infected gays in rural areas, towns, and cities.

Another connection between gay subcultures and HIV-AIDS in rural and semirural areas is suggested by this study, however. After returning to their roots, infected gays may have infected other gays (the gay tavern in Johnson City enabled gays to make sexual contacts). Hence, HIV-AIDS in rural areas, towns, and small cities may be linked to urban gay subcultures by the sexual activity of infected gays after they returned to their roots and not just by the fact of their return itself.

Recapitulation

Not all gays participated in the sexual activities associated with gay sex institutions or even in the general activities of the subcultures. Exactly what percentage of the participants in polygamous sex were infected will never be known. It is clear, however, that the high rate of HIV among gays was the result of sociosexual changes in the gay subcultures during the 1960s and 1970s as these subcultures became decidedly sex positive in orientation. The change, in turn, was not unrelated to changing social forces in the wider society. Homosexuality was becoming socially acceptable to more people, and societal attitudes with respect to sex in general were becoming more permissive; these changes allowed gays greater freedom of sexual expression.[18] In addition, gay sex institutions were more than responses to the desire for polygamous sex. They were also manifestations of the American cultural pattern of consumer capitalism in a gay-sex context. Beyond this, sex institutions and the polygamous sex that took place in them (and elsewhere) acquired social meaning, strengthened social bonds between gays, and symbolized social beliefs and attitudes that went beyond sexual economics and the simple search for sensuous pleasure. Therefore, the social epidemiology of the gay AIDS epidemic in the United States was based on polygamous sex among gays as a normative sociosexual pattern intensified by gay liberation and reflective of features of the broader society. The biological microbe HIV did not cause the gay AIDS epidemic by itself.

Drugs and the Drug Subculture

The association of drug use and HIV stems primarily from injecting drug users (IDUs) sharing needles containing the HIV-contaminated blood of a user. IDUs are thus at high risk of contracting HIV.[19] The drugs that have historically been most associated with drug injection are the opiates, most commonly heroin and morphine. Although drug injection is at an acknowledged high level today (the number of IDUs is unknown), it was at a low level as recently as 1960 (Inciardi, 1992:80).

Prior to 1960 the only source of nationwide information on drug addicts was the list maintained by the federal Bureau of Narcotic and Dangerous Drugs (BNDD), which included persons who were reported to BNDD as addicts by local police departments. In 1960 the list contained 45,391 names of addicts (almost all heroin) who had been reported the previous five years. The numbers increased steadily throughout the 1960s: 57,199 in 1965, 62,045 in 1967, and 68,088 in 1969 (Winslow, 1968:220; Richards and Carroll, 1970:1036; Inciardi, 1992:80). Some question the validity of the BNDD statistics, contending that the number of addicts was higher. For example, in 1969 the New York City registry, which was based on reports by medical and other social agencies as well as the Police Department, listed 52,104 addicts for New York City alone. A nationwide projection gives an estimate of 108,941 (Richards and Carroll, 1970:1037). Estimates for 1967 based on more complex analysis and correction factors gave a virtually identical figure (108,424) for heroin addicts (Inciardi, 1992:80).[20] Regardless of the source, official statistics reveal that from 1960 to 1969 the number of IDUs increased 50–100 percent, depending on the figures used. The number increased even more dramatically in the next few years. In 1977, based on data obtained from a variety of sources (e.g., hospital emergency room visits, heroin-related deaths), the National Institute of Drug Abuse estimated that the number of heroin users nationwide in 1977 was between 396,000 and 510,000 (Inciardi, 1992:81). In addition, injection of cocaine increased. Thus, in the 1960s and 1970s drug injection escalated. It paralleled the increase in sexual activity in the gay population.

And just as polygamous sex evolved within the gay subculture, sharing needles, or "works," evolved within the drug subculture. As drug use grew, "needle sharing [became] a prominent aspect of the subculture of the street drug scene" (Inciardi, 1992:190). It was not uncommon for users to share works among themselves, thus engendering the spread of HIV. The following comments of a user illustrate the problem: "People don't clean their works before they shoot dope, they clean them afterward, and they clean them out of the same cup of water that everyone is using. So, while somebody is rinsing their syringe out in a cup of water, another person is pulling water out into their spoon to cook their dope in" (Inciardi, 1992:188). Since HIV can survive in water for a period of time, the danger of needle sharing, even when needles are rinsed, is obvious.

Sharing stems in part from convenience. When wanting to shoot up, a user may not have any works in his or her possession. But sharing may be important socially as well. It may serve as "a symbol of friendship and trust," and for sexual partners it can strengthen the emotional bond between them. In addition, mixing blood in drug use may symbolize brotherhood (Inciardi, 1992:191; see also Des Jarlais et al., 1986:119).

The institution called the "shooting gallery" seems to be the most significant factor in drug-related transmission of HIV. Since there are legal restrictions on the sale of needles, with many states requiring a doctor's prescription, as drug use grew in the 1960s, drug users and/or dealers opened galleries in basements, abandoned buildings, private apartments, and back rooms of storefronts, where they rent works to users (Friedman et al., 1990; Inciardi, 1992:191–192). Because the works may not be sterilized after each use, an HIV-infected addict may pass the infection on to other patrons of the gallery. The drug injector is now sharing works, not just with friends and partners but also with anyone else who comes along, and HIV gets spread among individuals who have no personal relationship with one another.

For many IDUs, the gallery is not a desirable place to do drugs (Hanson et al., 1985:42–43; Inciardi, 1992:190–191). Users must pay a charge and risk their health. At the same time, however, the gallery solves important problems for users: "how to get off the street quickly to avoid arrest for possession of drugs, where to obtain a set of works with which to administer the drugs, and where to find a safe place to" inject the drug (Inciardo, 1992:191). Consequently, many IDUs are constrained to patronize the galleries: "For many injecting drug users, ... the use of shooting galleries is routine and commonplace. Moreover, there are repeated occasions in the lives of all injecting users, including the most hygienically fastidious types, when galleries become necessary. If they have no works of their own, or if friends or other running partners have no works, then a neighborhood gallery is the only recourse" {Inciardi, 1992:192). Studies indicate that drug injectors travel frequently and inject drugs outside their community of residence (Des Jarlais and Friedman, 1994:84), in which case they "gravitate toward the galleries [because of] the heightened risk of arrest when carrying drugs and drug paraphernalia over long stretches" (Inciardi, 1992:192).

Additional aspects of what James Inciardi (1992:191) called "the functional niche" of galleries in the drug subculture pertain to their social functions for home, employment, and social relations. Galleries preclude the necessity of keeping works at home, thus reducing conflicts between the IDU and family members who disapprove of drug use (Des Jarlais and Friedman, 1994:84), or of shooting up at work and jeopardizing employment. And some drug users even prefer the galleries. One informant reported that he and his partner "usually go to a street house ... where you get high and socialize" (Hanson et al., 1985:43; Des Jarlais et al., 1986:119). As galleries perform these social functions, they increase the spread of HIV.

The danger of galleries in spreading HIV is demonstrated in a study of a sample of works from major shooting galleries in Miami: 10 percent of the works were found to be positive for HIV (Inciardi, 1992:193). Also, studies show that in the Northeast, particularly in New York City and in cities with close geographic connections to it and northern New Jersey, where the shooting gallery custom appears to be most common, HIV infection rates among IDUs are much higher than in other areas of the country (Curran et al., 1988:612). It seems that the subcultural institution of the galleries, not simply the sharing of works with partners or friends, contributes to HIV-AIDS.[21]

As with polygamous sex and gay subcultures, drug use and the drug subculture in the United States are not unrelated to general societal forces. Rates of drug use are especially high among low-income persons and those from racial minorities. The reasons for this are complex, but a lack of opportunity for occupational and economic successes and a feeling of deprivation are certainly central.[22] Drugs can make a person feel better even if she or he is a failure in terms of the social standards against which people are judged.

Race, Ethnicity, Class, and HIV-AIDS

Until recently, a common view held that HIV-AIDS is a disease of the white middle class (Fumento, 1990:129–144). With the wider recognition of the drug use connection to HIV-AIDS, this view seems to have lost its currency.[23] Nevertheless, even today, with the exception of famous sports personalities such as Ervin "Magic" Johnson and Arthur Ashe, African Americans and Hispanics are rarely interviewed on television about AIDS—as sufferers of the disease, as lovers of sufferers, or as advocates for public policy with respect to AIDS. Condom commercials to promote prevention typically portray the potential sufferers as members of the white middle class

TABLE 1.2   AIDS Rate by Race-Ethnicity and Sex, for 1993 (number per 100,000)[a]

| Race-Ethnicity | Adults/Adolescents | | Children |
	Males	Females	<13 Years
White, not Hispanic	57.3	5.0	0.4
African American[b]	266.2	73.1	7.2
Hispanic	145.9	32.2	3.6

[a]Figures reflect the expanded definition of AIDS used in 1993 and reporting delays.
[b]The CDC classification is black, not Hispanic.
SOURCE: CDC (1994a:15).

TABLE 1.3   African-American[a] and Hispanic Cases, Reported Through December 31, 1993[b]

| Exposure Category | Number of Cases | | | Percentage of All Cases | |
	Total	African American	Hispanic	African American	Hispanic
All categories	355,936	112,002	60,008	31.5	16.9
Male homosexual/bisexual	193,652	36,446	23,146	18.8	12.0
Injecting drug user	87,259	44,700	23,833	51.2	27.3
Male homosexual and injecting drug user	23,360	6,762	3,458	28.9	14.8
Heterosexual who has had contact with injecting drug user	12,688	6,688	3,168	52.7	25.0

[a]The CDC classification is black, not Hispanic.
[b]Figures reflect reporting delays.
SOURCE: CDC (1994a:8–10).

(and as heterosexual). However, African Americans and Hispanics are far more apt to have HIV-AIDS than is the majority white non-Hispanic population.

Table 1.2 gives the number of AIDS cases reported for 1993 for white Americans, African Americans, and Hispanics. For males, the rate is almost five times higher for African Americans than for whites and more than two times higher for Hispanics. Differences for children are even greater.

Table 1.3 gives the percentage by risk category of all adult/adolescent AIDS cases that are African American, Hispanic, or white. Since African Americans constitute about 12 percent of the adult population and Hispanics about 9 percent, percentages greater than these indicate an excess of these two groups in each risk category. For total cases, African Americans account for 31.5 percent of all AIDS cases and Hispanics, 16.9 percent. Each minority group has an excess for every risk category, though African Americans more so than Hispanics. African Americans account for 18.8 percent of the male homosexuals/bisexuals, whereas Hispanics account for 12.0 percent. More than 50 percent of the IDUs are African American, and 27.3 percent are Hispanic. Therefore, African Americans have more than four times their proportionate share in the IDU category, and Hispanics have about three times their share. These comparisons indicate that differences by ethnic group are due far more to drug injection than to gay sex. This is clear in the comparisons of percentages for the male homosexual/bisexual category with percentages for the male homosexual/bisexual *and* IDU category. Whereas African Americans and Hispanics account for 18.8 percent and 12.0 percent of the former, they account for 28.9 percent and 14.8 percent of the latter.

Shooting galleries may be significant in the racial-ethnic differences. Most galleries are located in inner-city neighborhoods, where a disproportionately high number of the residents are African American or Hispanic. Data are limited, but they do indicate that African-American and Hispanic IDUs share needles in shooting galleries more than white IDUs do (Friedman et al., 1990:93-94; Fumento, 1990:133).

Regardless of the specific causative factors, the findings for African Americans follow a pattern. For almost every disease and cause of death, African Americans have higher rates than the rest of society (Woolhandler et al., 1985; Schwartz et al., 1990; NCHS, 1991:80–82). The higher rates for the inner cities (or at least Harlem) are jarring (McCord and Freeman, 1990). For example, deaths related to drug dependency are 283 times that for the rest of the nation. There appears to be no *one* factor that accounts for these differences; many environmental and behavioral risk factors are involved. Lack of opportunity and hopelessness are certainly important, and for HIV-AIDS the shooting gallery phenomenon and needle sharing are particularly significant. It is possible that racial-ethnic differences in the quality of medical care and access to care, which may affect the onset and hence diagnosis of AIDS in persons infected with HIV, contribute to racial-ethnic differences in AIDS. Polygamous sexual relations may also be significant and are examined in Chapter 4.

There seem to be no firm statistics linking income directly to HIV-AIDS, though evidence suggests that HIV-AIDS is higher in the lower class independent of ethnicity (Fumento, 1990:134–144; Johnston and Hopkins, 1990:136–137; Schneider, 1992; Jonsen and Stryker, 1993:9). Virtually every disease is higher in the lower class, regardless of how class is measured (income, occupation, education, or some combination) (Antonovsky, 1972; Syme and Berkman, 1976; D. Williams, 1990). HIV-AIDS is probably no exception.

Conclusion

Although HIV is apparently a necessary and sufficient condition for AIDS, social forces were necessary for the AIDS epidemic. Without increases in gay sex and drug use in the 1960–1970 period, the evolution of certain sociosexual norms and institutions within the gay subcultures, and the evolution of needle sharing and shooting galleries within the drug subculture, the AIDS epidemic would not have appeared as it did in the United States. And since the gay and drug subcultures and changes in them were related to broader social forces, it is clear that social factors played a significant part in the etiology of the AIDS epidemic in the gay and IDU populations. Other sectors of the population (lower social classes, African Americans, and Hispanics) have rates higher than the overall population because the high-risk behaviors associated with the two major high-risk groups, especially IDUs, are more prevalent among members of these sectors than in the general population.

Neither the risk nor the mode(s) of transmission for people outside the high-risk groups, specifically non-IDU heterosexuals, was addressed in this chapter. For several years many people have been concerned that the dominant mode of transmission in the United States would be through sexual intercourse between non-IDU heterosexuals. Heterosexual HIV-AIDS is examined in Chapter 4, as are the trends for heterosexuals compared with the trends for gays and IDUs.

NOTES

1. Analysts do not agree on the exact features of these subcultures (Plummer, 1975:154–174). For this reason as well as the variance in subcultures from setting to setting, some contend there are a variety of subcultures, not a single subculture. I use the term *subcultures*.

2. Nevertheless, in a survey of male homosexuals in San Francisco in the 1970s, Bell and Weinberg (1978:420, 424, 426) reported that more than 25 percent of respondents had been arrested (one to eighty-seven times), 6 percent had had the police demand money illegally, and 16 percent had been threatened with exposure "in order to get something of value."

3. The same process was occurring in Europe and Canada (Gregersen, 1983:176; on Great Britain, see Weeks, 1990:185–206), though the decriminalization of homosexuality went further in England and Canada than in the United States,where many oppressive laws have remained on the books.

4. The rural to urban migration of males with a gay orientation is revealed in Edward Laumann, et al.'s (1994:303) national survey of sexual practices of 18–59 year olds: 9.2 percent of male respondents from the twelve largest cities identify themselves as homosexual, 7.8 percent in the next eighty-eight cities do so, and only 1.3 percent from rural areas do.

5. The 1970s were volatile years in the United States, and several factors other than sexual permissiveness contributed to greater acceptance of homosexuals. In particular, the civil rights and women's liberation movements were gaining strength, and these movements legitimized claims for gay rights. Also, toleration for the behavior

and lifestyles of alienated groups (hippies, beatniks, and opponents of the Vietnam War) was extended to homosexuals.

6. Some of the more creative and unusual forms (to heterosexuals anyway) are sadomasochistic practices, which can include a range of sexual activities in which a partner derives pleasure from inflicting or incurring pain (Muchmore and Hanson, 1991:112–117); "fisting" and "punching" (inserting one's arm up another's anus and punching with the fist) (Kleinberg, 1989:157–196); and the "sling" (in which one man straps himself into a device that suspends him in midair, while another, or several others, performs anal sex on him) (Kinsella, 1989:175).

7. Although this study was not based on a representative sample of the population, there is no reason to believe it was biased toward heterosexual or homosexual couples.

8. Even though answers to questions about number of sexual partners are fraught with problems of reliability and validity (Coxon, 1988:129–133), there is no reason to believe that these problems vary in seriousness according to the sexual orientation of the respondent (answers were anonymous).

9. Bateson and Goldsby (1988:43) also stated, "It sometimes seemed as if the 1970s style gay sex was an enactment of a male fantasy common to heterosexuals as ... uncommitted, impersonal, profligate sex."

10. Weeks (1990:233) noted that in gay novels such as Larry Kramer's *Faggots* and Andrew Holleran's *Dancer from the Dance*, "A new social purity movement was focusing on the moral danger of 'public sex,' that is, an explicitly sexual gay openness."

11. However, Kleinberg's (1980) analysis was in the spirit of symbolic interaction, though his focus was on deeper psychological motives, as portrayed in Freudian psychology.

12. Gay liberation meant different things to different gays. For many of them, sex was not central; occupational security and freedom from police harassment were. Many older gays who had developed stable relationships with other men and had become accepted in their jobs did not change their lives but were simply more comfortable with them. For many others, however, the link between gay liberation and sexual freedom was much stronger.

13. In addition, the social bonds that sexual activity and sex institutions nourished may have blunted for gays the general impersonal force of an urban industrial society from which many people (not just gays) felt alienated (Altman, 1982:104).

14. Note that the casual polygamous sex of the 1970s and early 1980s did not occur to the same extent among heterosexuals. Fumento (1990:233) stated, "The sort of promiscuity that characterized the homosexual communities of the United States in the later 1970s and early 1980s, and which still continues [in 1990] among many, is a creation uniquely homosexual. It may be that many a heterosexual male would, if he could, go to a place where he could have free sex with any number of beautiful women already disrobed and lying in wait. The fact is that he can't." Altman (1982: 17) observed that the gay baths "have no real counterpart" for heterosexuals or for homosexual women. That these patterns differentiated gay subcultures from the dominant heterosexual culture and established normative boundaries between them may have been one of the forces that sustained the gay subcultures.

15. For many gays, the association of gay pride with sexual freedom raises an interesting dilemma, namely, the contradictory claims that gays are a minority with a subculture that transcends sex, on the one hand, and that the only major difference between homosexuals and heterosexuals is sexual orientation, on the other. "Precisely because the affirmation of being gay is the affirmation of sexual desire, there is something radical about the gay movement that all the attempts of those who would claim respectability for us cannot dispell. Indeed, the very strengthening of the sense of gay identity leads both to claims that we are another minority and to an awareness of the fact that we organize our everyday lives in radical opposition to the sexual norms of this society. The contradiction underlies the complaint of Vito Russo that, 'I want what seems like a complete contradiction. I want society to cease viewing gays as defined solely by our sexuality, and at the same time I want the freedom to be as unabashedly sexual as I wish'" (Altman, 1982:211).

16. Kleinberg (1980:145, 157–196) believed that many gays were adopting the wider culture's image of masculinity and "eroticizing the values of straight society that have tyrannized their own lives." He also argued that polygamous sex and the macho and sadomasochistic forms that gay sex sometimes took were mirrors (that is, symbols) of masculine power and the masculine-dominated American culture. Sexual freedom was a mirage. As practiced by many gays, sex neither rejected the values of the wider society nor liberated gays. Sex bound them to the values of the wider society instead. The attempt to establish a normative boundary between gays and the rest of society may in fact have failed at a deeper psychological level.

17. The type and not just level of activity seems to have changed, with more sadomasochistic sex, fisting, and, in particular, anal intercourse. Bell and Weinberg (1978:111) suggested that older men are more likely than younger men to engage in fellatio, and Altman (1982:178) stated that "older American male homosexuals agree that there [was] a marked rise in anal as against oral sex and mutual masturbation" during the 1970s.

18. Although these changes contributed to the AIDS epidemic, they no doubt had positive health effects as well. The removal of homosexuality as a form of psychiatric pathology relieved gays of the stigma associated with mental illness. Beyond this, since homosexuality was becoming more acceptable to society, gays did not feel constrained to conceal their identities so much, which reduced stress and mental tension. Many gays undoubtedly felt better about themselves.

19. Two qualifying comments are in order. First, all addictive drugs, especially heroin, may have immunosuppressive effects, and this holds regardless of the route by which the drugs are ingested (sniffing, smoking, swallowing, needle injecting) (Root-Bernstein, 1993:120–128). Immunosuppression may lead to opportunistic infection. The problem is compounded by the adulteration of drugs with sugar, talc, and other substances, which may themselves suppress the immune system (Root-Bernstein, 1993:124–125). Second, drug users who inject in a muscle or just under the skin, not just those who inject into a blood vessel, also risk infection if they share needles (Des Jarlais and Friedman, 1994). Consequently, some experts (Don Des Jarlais and Friedman, 1994) argue "injecting drug user" (IDU) is a better term than "intravenous drug user" (IVDU). I use IDU with the caveat that some statistics are for IVDUs.

20. The BNDD figures were undoubtedly underestimates, but the number of addicts in the 1960s was small enough that legal authorities knew most of them. Writing in 1974, Raymond Glasscote et al. (p. 16) stated, "If one assumes ... that most addicts, because of the many illegal transactions in which they are regularly involved to maintain their supply of drugs, will come to official attention within any one five-year period, then the additional number (beyond the official record) will not be great." When official statistics included data from medical and other agencies along with those from legal agencies, such statistics may not have been far off.

21. For example, cities such as San Antonio, Baltimore, Denver, and metropolitan areas in southern California may have higher rates of needle sharing among IDUs than does New York City, but HIV is far less prevalent in those places. Only 2 percent of San Antonio users were infected with HIV, though 99 percent reported sharing needles, in comparison to a 61 percent infection rate in New York City, where 70 percent reported needle sharing and where shooting galleries are more part of the drug scene (Lange et al., 1988).

22. For the classic statement, see Merton (1938).

23. I had students in a lower-division undergraduate class complete a questionnaire in September 1991 and January 1993. In 1991 the percentage of students who thought AIDS was more prevalent among whites than African Americans was 86 percent. This declined in 1993, but 55 percent still got it wrong.

2. The Origin of HIV

The origin of HIV is a mystery. No one knows where it came from. Several hypotheses have been advanced, however, and some are reviewed in this chapter. One postulates that HIV originated with a nonhuman, and another posits that advances in medicine in the 1960–1970 period were instrumental in the disease's origin. Of particular sociological interest is the hypothesis that social changes in the gay and drug subcultures may have been significant. The origin of microorganisms is a matter of biological evolution and normally not a topic sociologists address. However, the origin of an infectious agent is always the result of a complex interaction among agent, host, and environment. Since the environment includes social factors, changes in social conditions may have been significant in the origin of HIV.

A few words about the notion of social changes: Sociologists view social phenomena as the result of some general social dynamic, as in the framework of Karl Marx. According to Marx, class conflict is the driving force behind social phenomena. My focus here, however, is on a biological phenomenon. I am investigating how very specific changes in the environment may have influenced the origin of that phenomenon, taking into account certain characteristics of the agent and the agent-host relationship. In no sense am I viewing HIV as a manifestation of some general social dynamic. I simply examine how social changes may have influenced the origin of HIV within the agent-host-environment framework. Partly because of the popularity of the animal origin hypothesis and partly to draw the contrast between this hypothesis and ones that emphasize changes in the environment, I review the animal origins hypothesis first.

The Nonhuman Origin Hypothesis

Humans share a number of diseases with other animals. For example, the plague bacillus infects rats and humans alike. Fleas that suck the blood of infected rats are vectors for this disease, transmitting the agent to humans as they jump from their rodent hosts to human hosts. Other microbes, including HIV, are specific to humans.[1] However, nonhumans may be the origin of these microbes.

According to Cockburn (1977:86–88), modern evolutionary theory assumes that all human infections descended from prehuman ancestors, and since humans and other animals are descended from a common source, many infectious diseases found in humans through history have also been present in other animals. Over time microbes mutated; some found the human host especially to their liking and could not survive on or in any other animal. They thus became specific to humans.

In other instances humans are infected with a new disease that is transmitted by a nonhuman contemporary in what is called a cross-species transfer. Nonhumans carry many microbes that cannot normally be transmitted to humans, but occasionally one mutates in the nonhuman host and succeeds or mutates after the cross-species transfer takes place. (Microbes reproduce very quickly, with a new generation coming along every few minutes, so they mutate very rapidly.) Regardless, if the microbe can then "be transmitted from man to man, then the stage would be set for the evolution of a new specifically human pathogen" (Cockburn, 1977:88). Cockburn believed that many common infectious diseases originated this way from domesticated animals during the early agricultural period. The smallpox virus, which is specific to humans, is similar to a range of viruses in domesticated animals, the closest being the cowpox virus, and smallpox may be a mutated version of one of them (Cockburn, 1977:91). Some believe that HIV is also a mutated version of a nonhuman virus.

According to one theory, a nonhuman HIV precursor may have been transmitted to humans via the animal blood that Haitian priests drink during voodoo ceremonies. The microbe then mutated into HIV, which, according to this theory, the priests transmitted to others through male homosexual contact (Moore and Le Baron, 1986). Most experts no longer take this hypothesis seriously.

The most well-known and accepted hypothesis about the animal origin of HIV postulates that HIV originated in Africa, where HIV-AIDS is so prevalent (de Cock, 1984; Gallo, 1988:55–56; Gallo and Montagnier, 1988; Gilks, 1991; Anderson and May, 1992:58). AIDS may have been first identified in the United States because the medical surveillance for detecting disease is superior to the surveillance systems in other places and not because HIV first appeared in the United States. The African origin hypothesis pivots primarily around three lines of evidence and reasoning.

The first evidentiary/reasoning line holds that the ancestor of HIV originated with a virus from African primates, probably the simian immunodeficiency virus (SIV) of the green monkey, which "somehow entered human beings, initiating a series of mutations," eventually resulting in HIV (Gallo, 1988:56). Estimates of when HIV may have evolved from SIV vary greatly from forty years to a few million (Sharp and Li, 1988), though most believe HIV is a relatively new microbe. The apparent codiscoverers of HIV, Robert

Gallo and Luc Montagnier (1988),[2] estimated it is at least 20 years old but no older than 100 years. Roy Anderson et al. (1991:586) believed the evidence indicates 140–160 years, and most estimates seem to be less than 300 years.

Some speculate that the HIV precursor was transmitted to humans by monkey bites or by people eating uncooked parts of monkeys, such as the brain. However, since no one is known to have been infected by saliva, and HIV is not enterically transmitted, these ideas are speculative. Monkey blood may have entered the human bloodstream when a monkey was slaughtered (for eating or sacrifice). Some have mentioned a cultural practice, said to exist among some African groups, in which monkey blood is injected into the pubic area, thighs, and back prior to having sex in the belief that this will heighten erotic experience (Shannon, 1991:24–25). (If this practice actually exists, it could have provided an efficient route of transmission.) Charles Gilks (1991) suggested that SIV was transferred to Americans in malarial experiments in which monkey blood was used. But regardless of the route, after being transmitted to humans, the virus is assumed to have mutated into HIV (Gallo, 1988:56; Anderson and May, 1992:58–59). Comparisons of HIVs (HIV-1 and HIV-2) and SIVs from several monkey species indicate significant homologies between them. Genetically, the green monkey SIV is a cousin to HIV-1 (Essex and Kanki, 1988) and even closer to HIV-2.

Nevertheless, the evolutionary relationships between SIVs and HIVs are far from clear (Grmek, 1989:145). One virologist believed the differences are too great for HIV to have originated from green monkeys "in recent times, as has been predicted by many people" (Mulder, 1988b; Fukasawa et al., 1988). A question of the direction of transmission has been raised—"the assumption of human to monkey transfer cannot be rejected out of hand" (Penny, 1988:494). Questions about the mechanisms of cross-species transfer are not answered (Gilks, 1991:262). The wide divergence of some estimates of the age of HIV raises even more questions. And the authenticity of certain comparisons of SIVs and HIVs has even been questioned (Kestler et al., 1988; Mulder, 1988a).

In short, the evidence and evolutionary theory are insufficient to conclude, with Roy Anderson and Robert May (1992:58, emphasis added), among others, that "the AIDS virus almost *certainly* evolved in Africa" (see also Walker, 1991:54). (Anderson and May apparently recognized this when they added that the homologies only suggest an African origin.) To the contrary, one reviewer concluded there is "no concrete evidence" for the African primate origin (Williams, 1992:8) and another believed the evidence disproves the green monkey hypothesis altogether (Sabatier, 1989:35).

According to Gallo and Montagnier (1988:9), in a second line of reasoning, the virus has been "present in small, isolated groups in central Africa or elsewhere for many years" (but apparently less than one hundred years). As these groups made contact with the outside world when they migrated to urban centers, HIV spread through the population and, via international travel, from Africa to other parts of the world.

Evidence for this is lacking. Instead, Gallo (1988:56) simply declared, "It appears that after remaining localized for some time, the virus began spreading to the rest of central Africa during the early 1970s. Later in the decade it reached Haiti and may have reached Europe and the Americas from there." Infectious diseases are indeed spread through migration and rapid urbanization, but in the absence of any evidence, the claim that isolated groups *"no doubt* brought HIV with them" when they migrated to urban centers (Gallo and Montagnier, 1988:9, emphasis added) is too conclusive. (It is just as reasonable to argue that HIV first appeared in urban areas in Africa and then found its way into rural areas.) Also, if Africa were the origin, HIV would have probably begun to spread in northern and southern Africa before it arrived in the United States. This was not the case, however, and HIV-AIDS is still not widespread in northern Africa.

The third evidentiary/reasoning line is based on medical evidence. Serological tests of frozen blood samples from patients revealed that HIV or a similar virus was probably present in Zaire as early as 1959 and that it may have existed in other African regions in the 1970s (Getchell et al., 1987; Grmek, 1989:134–137). Gallo (1988:56) stated that serological analysis of frozen blood serum from the 1960s and 1970s revealed no evidence of HIV "anywhere except a small region of central Africa."

The presence of HIV or a similar virus in Zaire in 1959 and the 1970s does seem probable, but later tests of blood samples using the Western Blot technique revealed that the technique (ELISA) used in the original test was unreliable and produced many false positives (false indications of the presence of HIV) (Grmek, 1989:135). Also, for some unknown reason Africans have uncommonly high rates of false positives (Grmek, 1989:134–137). And some test results for samples after 1970 were simply contradictory (Grmek, 1989: 178–179).

In addition, serological analyses of frozen blood samples indicate that HIV has existed in places other than Africa for as long as it has existed on that continent. One analysis proved that it existed among drug addicts in Manhattan in 1975–1976 (Des Jarlais et al., 1989) and Washington, D.C., in 1971–1972 (Moore et al., 1985). A patient who died in 1969 in a St. Louis hospital was definitely infected with HIV (Garry et al., 1988), and tests for an Englishman who died in 1959 and three Norwegians (father, mother, and daughter) who died in the early 1970s showed the same finding (Root-Bernstein, 1993:13). It is certain, therefore, that HIV existed in the United States and the West for at least a decade or more before the 1980s and possibly before it existed in Africa.

In addition to serological evidence, evidence based on retrospective clinical descriptions of patients who have died has been presented to support the African origin hypothesis. Descriptions of African patients in the years prior to the AIDS epidemic appear to show a pattern of opportunistic infectious diseases similar to the pattern of diseases characteristic of AIDS (Grmek, 1989:19–30, 114, 131, 134). However, all the clinical descriptions may not conform to the AIDS pattern as closely as originally believed, and certainly AIDS did not exist in Africa in epidemic form prior to the 1970s (Grmek, 1989:148, 172). In addition, retrospective analyses of American patients reveal clinical descriptions of patients who died in the 1930s and 1940s from infections associated with AIDS (Root-Bernstein, 1993:2–6; see also Grmek, 1989:119–123); the evidence for deaths in 1952 and 1969 is especially strong (Witte et al., 1984; Grmek, 1989:119–123). Unfortunately, in most cases blood samples were not available for serological analysis that would verify or refute the presence of HIV. Nevertheless, a number of specialists believe retrospective clinical evidence shows that AIDS-related infections existed in sporadic or episodic form in the United States well before the 1980s (Colebunders et al., 1984; Katner and Pankey, 1987; Garry et al., 1988: 2087; Grmek, 1989:120–137; Root-Bernstein, 1993:2–21), and they may have existed for at least a century in the Western world (Katner and Pankey, 1987; Root-Bernstein, 1993:2–21). Limited outbreaks of opportunistic infections caused by HIV may have occurred in the distant past even though the cluster diseases in AIDS were not recognized then as a distinct syndrome (Grmek, 1989:158–161).

Note also that the first Africans to be diagnosed with AIDS were middle- and upper-class persons who had gone to Europe for medical care. Wealthier Africans commonly go to Europe for vacation, and some might have contracted HIV through sexual contact and brought it back to Africa (of course, such persons may have introduced it to Europe). Indeed, evidence has been presented that HIV was introduced *into Africa* from a Euro-American origin (Katner and Pankey, 1987). In 1992 A. Olufemi Williams (p. 6) concluded that evidence "is heavily in favor" of this view. It is far from certain, therefore, that HIV originated in Africa.

Therefore, while it is conceivable that HIV was imported into the United States and other parts of the world from Africa,[3] it is also conceivable that AIDS was imported into Africa from the United States or that it emerged in both places at about the same time (Grmek, 1989:119–126, 171–182). Nevertheless, the belief in the African origin of HIV persists among many scientists. It is not clear whether this is because of the evidence or because of something else. (In Chapter 7 I suggest the reason is something else.)

Finally, SIV may have existed for many centuries so that, as French physician and medical historian Mirko D. Grmek (1989:146) stated, "there was ample opportunity for the virus to breach the barrier between monkey and man" before the 1970s. But "why then did such interspecies transmission not take place in some distant past?" This question implies that environmental changes in the 1970s contributed to the emergence of HIV. Among these changes, according to Grmek, advances in the medical treatment of infectious diseases may have been crucial.

Medical Intervention and Pathocenosis

In *Mirage of Health,* Rene Dubos (1959) introduced the proposition that social conditions, including medical intervention, that reduce the prevalence and mortality of a disease (or set of diseases) may cause other diseases to increase. For example, conditions leading to a decline in infectious diseases led to longer life expectancy, and diseases associated with older age, such as heart disease and cancer, increased. In some instances, as with infectious diseases, medical intervention may also make a disease harder to treat. Tuberculosis and malaria, which were major killers worldwide until the 1950s, are examples. Drugs developed in the post–World War II years killed the tubercle bacillus and the malarial parasites, and the death rates from tuberculosis and malaria declined sharply.[4] Many medical authorities were optimistic that tuberculosis and malaria would soon be under control worldwide, and this was in fact accomplished to a considerable degree by the 1970s. However, since infectious microbes mutate rapidly, a strain may evolve that is beyond the killer range of the drug, and the disease may then become resistant to treatment. Unfortunately, this has happened. Drug-resistant strains of the tubercle bacillus and malarial parasites now exist, and the anopheles mosquito, which is the vector for malaria, has developed resistance to insecticides.[5] Consequently, infectious disease experts fear that new epidemics of these diseases are just beginning, especially in Third World countries where social conditions are conducive to the spread of tuberculosis and malaria (WHO, 1992:15–16)[6] but also in the United States (Frieden et al., 1993; Specter, 1992).

In addition to contributing to drug-resistant microbes, drugs that kill certain microbes may give other microbes greater opportunities to proliferate. Grmek (1989) believed this happened with HIV. A basic aspect of the evolutionary theory of microorganisms is the notion of interspecific competition (Cockburn, 1961:1054), which Grmek (1989:158–161) extended with the concept of pathocenosis. Interspecific competition refers to different microorganisms sharing the same ecological niche and competing with one another for existence. Pathocenosis refers to an equilibrium in which different microbes are adapted to one another, and live in peaceful coexistence, but with some microbes suppressing others (Grmek, 1989:xi). If there are many infectious microbes, disease symptoms produced by one microbe may be concealed by the presence of other, more dominant symptoms produced by other microbes. This may explain why certain diseases are more prevalent in one population than in others. For example, populations with high rates of syphilis probably have low rates of yaws and vice versa (Cockburn, 1961: 1053–1054). Consequently, medical intervention to eradicate one infectious disease may cause another infectious disease to increase.

According to Grmek (1989:158), medical procedures that controlled and eradicated certain infectious microbes after World War II led to the "rupture in the pathocenosis, particularly the great fall off in the incidence of ... infectious disease." Before the rupture, HIV may have been suppressed by other microbes. With many microbes competing for nourishment, HIV's chances of surviving and proliferating may have been most limited, so its opportunity to infect large numbers of people and cause an epidemic would have been very low. Therefore, Grmek (1989:161) believed, the "dissemination [of HIV] was not possible before modern medicine's successes breached the bulwark that other common infectious disease had formed against it."

In particular, the eradication of smallpox worldwide in 1972 and the control of tuberculosis and malaria in the 1970s may have "awakened" HIV and given it opportunities to proliferate, thus triggering the AIDS epidemic (Grmek, 1989:158–161, 180–181). This is true for Africa no less than the United States because drugs had reduced the prevalence of these (and other) infectious diseases there also (Grmek, 1989:x–xi, 180).

Social Change and the Mutation of a Microbe

Another hypothesis emphasizes the role played by changes in social aspects of the environment, specifically changes in the American gay and drug subcultures during the 1960s and 1970s, which I reviewed in the last chapter, and sociosexual changes associated with massive urbanization in Africa during the same period, which I examine in the next chapter.

Many infectious diseases have evolved during periods of major changes in the social environment and behavior of populations. The transition from hunting-gathering to agricultural societies about ten thousand years ago was such a period (Cockburn, 1977; McKeown, 1979:45; Murdock, 1980:7). Since agents for many common infectious diseases, such as measles, can exist only by rapid transmission from host to host, they may not have existed prior to the growth and concentration of populations that accompanied agriculture (Cockburn, 1977:89). In addition, changes in customs and behavior, such as the emergence of extended and cohesive kinship systems, may have been significant. People also began living near domesticated animals, from which they may have contracted certain diseases[7] and through which lice, fleas, and other insects attracted to these animals acted as vectors of disease.

However, it was not until the emergence of cities that population thresholds were reached and adverse behaviors widespread enough for many infectious agents to emerge and survive. Also, old microbes may have become more virulent. Similarly, environmental changes may have led to the emergence of HIV as a new microbe or as a modified form of an already existing one. Before discussing how this could have happened, I review changes that occur in the agent and the agent-host relationship when the environment is constant, as posited in the natural history model of infectious disease. (This review also functions as background for the analysis of trends in AIDS in Chapter 4.)

The Natural History Model of Infectious Disease

Typically, in an unchanging environment and in the absence of human intervention (e.g., medical care), when an infectious agent first invades a population, it attacks a few persons, who get sick and sometimes die. Then the agent is transmitted to more hosts through host-to-host contact, and it multiplies rapidly. All the while the agent activates immune systems in the hosts to secrete immunocytes, allowing the hosts to fight back. Rather than being killed by the agent, the host may kill the agent. The immune response also usually gives protection against later attacks[8] (Burnet and White, 1972: 70–87).

All infectious diseases represent a conflict between the host and a tiny, foreign, but often virulent microorganism (Burnet and White, 1972:20-21). Individual hosts with strong resistance are most apt to survive. Over time through natural selection, the proportion of the host population with stronger genetic resistance to the agent increases. Sometimes natural selection operates very rapidly (in evolutionary time) so that the proportion of the population with natural resistance increases substantially in just a few generations.[9] And the proportion developing immunity also increases.

At the same time, a selection process takes place on the side of the agent. If the agent is too virulent, it kills the host before finding another host on which to feed and reproduce.[10] Consequently, to survive, infectious agents must usually mutate in the direction of becoming weaker over time.[11] Mutation occurs much faster in the agent than in the host, with new generations a matter of a few minutes rather than about twenty years as with humans.[12] At the level of the population (rather than the individual), host and microorganism eventually reach a mutual accommodation, or equilibrium point. This is evidenced by a more or less constant death rate from the disease.

According to the natural history model, then, infectious disease rates ebb and flow depending on the virulence of the agent, the resistance of the population, and its size (a larger number of hosts gives the microorganism more opportunities [Burnet and White, 1972:10]). When an agent is introduced to a virgin population, the disease and death rates increase rapidly. Subsequently, natural selection and the development of immunity lead to a decline in the disease rate until an equilibrium is reached.[13]

But such a process occurs only in a constant environment, including one with no medical intervention, such as the introduction of a vaccine (Burnet and White, 1972:10–21). Among humans a more or less constant environment has existed in all but a small fraction of history. Such an environment is approximated today only in populations in remote regions of the world. George Murdock (1952:9) described the double evolutionary process in such populations in the following way:

> Human beings gradually develop a relative immunity through a process of natural selection which eliminates the most susceptible strains in each generation. The disease microorganisms undergo an opposite evolutionary development which favors the less virulent strains; the more lethal strains kill their carriers and thus tend to be eliminated. In time, as a result of this dual process, the endemic disease of a region becomes less dangerous to its inhabitants and the latter become less susceptible to the disease.

Host resistance does not eliminate the agent, however. Because of the greater natural resistance, prevalence may actually *increase*. The virulence of the agent decreases, and infections become milder (subclinical). The deaths that do occur are less sudden, so the length of time between onset of disease and death increases. This gives the microorganism a better chance to reproduce and, along with its progeny, to move to other hosts (via air, water, food, vector, touch, or blood exchange, depending on the agent's mode of transmission). In this way the microorganism continues to survive and infect hosts as the resistance of the host population increases (Burnet and White, 1972:82, 84, 163).

Therefore, in the natural history model of infectious disease, a disease starts with a few deaths, evolves to an epidemic stage in which there are many deaths, and then moves to an endemic stage in which the death rate is much lower, though it may still be high (Dubos and Dubos, 1987:187).[14] The progress of the disease resembles a bell-shaped curve, following the principle of Farr's law.[15] In the endemic stage (the right portion of the curve), much of the population beyond childhood has been infected and thus naturally immunized, and it is among children that morbidity and mortality are usually high. For this reason endemic infectious diseases are frequently referred to as childhood diseases. Then as effective vaccines are developed, the diseases become rare and, as with smallpox, may disappear.

Social Change and HIV

A particular environment that gives a particular microbe access to the tissues, organs, or secretions of its hosts is necessary before a microbe can exist. Therefore, changes in the environment that affect the agent's access to hosts have significant consequences for the agent's evolution and survival. In the case of HIV, the environment must give the agent access to the blood of human hosts. Changes in the behavior of many gays and IDUs allowed HIV to spread rapidly through the gay and IDU populations. Could these behavioral changes have also led to the origin of HIV?

Note that, even though the tendency is for a microbe to mutate downward, it may also mutate upward and become more virulent. But if it is too virulent and kills the host quickly after infection, the microbe will become extinct because it dies with the host. This, however, assumes a constant environment, as in the natural history model. If the environment changes and opportunities for person-to-person transmission increase, the agent-host relationship may also change, and a formerly relatively benign microbe that mutates into a more virulent, even lethal, form may thrive. Some of the agents of common infectious diseases may have turned more virulent with the development of agriculture or urbanization and increases in person-to-person transmission. It is possible that HIV turned more virulent in the years just prior to the AIDS epidemic.

HIV may be a very old virus, existing for decades, even centuries, but for most of this period it may have been relatively benign (Ewald, 1994:125–143, 132). Even if it had been lethal, it may not have killed until thirty or forty years after infection rather than a few months or years, as is usually the case today. In fact, under the social conditions that existed for most of human history, HIV would not have survived unless it had been relatively benign. For example, in a predominantly monogamous and drug-free society, a lethal HIV would have died when the partner hosts died because it would not have been passed on to persons outside the monogamous relationship or from IDU to IDU. Under such conditions only a relatively benign HIV would have survived. Highly virulent forms would have killed the host in a short period before the microbes could have been passed on to other hosts (Ewald, 1994:125–143).[16]

The situation changed under conditions of rapid blood exchange, such as that which began in the 1960s and 1970s among many American gays and IDUs (and many men and women in Africa). With the rapid exchange of blood in the population, an HIV that killed in a few months or years could easily have survived. As sexual partner changes and needle sharing soared, by the time the original carrier host had died, he (or she) had already passed HIV to other hosts (in some instances, many hosts). Death of the original host was of little or no consequence for the survivability of HIV.

Therefore, changes in sexual and drug use patterns may have interacted with the mutation of HIV to contribute to a more virulent HIV. (The changes may have also interacted with medical intervention since, without the rupture of the pathocenosis, even a very virulent HIV may have been suppressed by other microbes.) This is not to say that social changes caused a more virulent HIV or that lethal mutants of HIV that killed the host did not exist prior to the 1970s. A more virulent HIV was caused by the natural process for microorganisms to mutate rapidly, upward and downward. HIV mutates very rapidly reproducing billions of copies of itself shortly after entering the bloodstream of the host (Wei, et al., 1995; Ho et al., 1995), and in the past only the less virulent strains may have survived. Grmek (1989:xi) postulated that "it [HIV] had once been controlled by natural selection favoring less virulent strains. Social factors enlarged its routes of transmission and allowed it to break through a sort of critical threshold that had previously limited its expansion." Hence, there was an explosive increase in HIV-AIDS in the 1980s.

Deaths from AIDS earlier may have been rare because HIV was more benign. Most persons infected with HIV would have died from other infectious agents that kill faster, or other causes, before the opportunistic infections common in AIDS appeared. Also, rates of infectious diseases were so high in most of history that opportunistic infections associated with AIDS may have been masked by symptoms associated with other, more prevalent infectious diseases. And if AIDS-related opportunistic infections did appear, the array of diseases common to AIDS may have appeared so infrequently that it was not recognized and identified as a separate syndrome of diseases. As with many "new" diseases in history, AIDS may not really be a new disease but an old disease that is suddenly recognized by medicine (Grmek, 1989:99–109; see also Katner and Pankey, 1987:1071). With the control of other infectious diseases as well as the emergence of a more virulent form of HIV, a syndrome of symptoms known as AIDS and affecting large numbers of people was identified by medicine.

It is impossible to know if a relatively benign form of HIV has existed for centuries. Evidence does suggest, however, that a benign form of HIV exists in the world today. Apparently, some persons have been infected with HIV for up to fourteen years without getting AIDS (*AIDS Alert,* 7, 1992:180–181), and 5 percent of the estimated 1 million Americans infected with HIV may never get AIDS (Gorman, 1993). If a more benign HIV were prevalent in the past, the percentage of persons who were infected with HIV but did not get AIDS may have been much higher. (HIV could not have been identified before the 1970s because techniques for isolating retroviruses were not developed until then.) However, as social changes occurred that increased the rate of blood exchange, HIV may have become more virulent. It was then transmitted rapidly from host to host, giving birth to the AIDS epidemic (Ewald, 1994:125–143).

It follows, therefore, that declines in sexual partner changes and needle sharing would lead to the proliferation of a more benign HIV. With less rapid blood exchange, an HIV that kills quickly could not compete for survival as well against a less virulent HIV. As we see in Chapter 4, sexual partner changes and needle sharing have declined among American gays and IDUs. Significantly, physiologist Robert Root-Bernstein (1993) observed that the time between HIV infection and onset of AIDS has increased over time in the United States but not in Africa. For example, in the United States in 1986 it was less than two years, but by 1992 it was estimated to be between ten and fifteen years (Root-Bernstein, 1993:55–56). Root-Bernstein wondered, therefore, if HIV is becoming less virulent, as does evolutionary biologist Paul Ewald (1994:144–150). If so, it would be consistent with the hypothesis that social changes were causal factors in the origin of a most virulent HIV.

Conclusion

Different hypotheses about the origin of HIV are not necessarily incompatible. Factors stipulated in different hypotheses may have played a role in the emergence of HIV-1 (and HIV-2). Humans may have been infected with SIV or a similar virus that was originally a relatively benign microbe. HIV may have become more virulent with the medical rupture of the pathocenosis as well as with behavioral changes that increased the exchange of blood. The American behavioral changes implicated in the AIDS epidemic were anchored in general social changes with respect to sex and drug use and in changes in social norms and institutions in the gay and drug subcultures. As with the emergence of new infectious microbes during the historical transition to agriculture and later to urbanization, the emergence of a lethal HIV may have been causally linked to these changes. If this is the case, the implications are ominous indeed. Social factors that are instrumental in the emergence of new microbes may not be limited to major historical transitions in simple societies of the past, such as a change from simple hunting-gathering to agricultural society and the movement from rural to urban life, both of which played out over the course of hundreds of years. Social transitions in modern industrial societies that occur in a much shorter period may also work to produce new and deadly infectious diseases. (For discussions of the ominous potential for the emergence of devastating infectious diseases, see Garrett, 1992, and Preston, 1994.)

Nevertheless, HIV-AIDS exists in societies, particularly Africa, that resemble the simple societies that existed in the West—and indeed throughout the world—in prior history. Significantly, rapid social changes were occurring in Africa at the same time changes were occurring in the gay and drug subcultures in the West, particularly the United States. In another way social factors rather than primate-to-human transmission may have been the crucial factors in why a lethal form of HIV appeared in Africa at about the same time it appeared in the United States and why it has also become so prevalent in Africa. The African pattern of HIV-AIDS is examined in the next chapter.

NOTES

1. Research has demonstrated that through injection captive chimpanzees and macaques can be infected with HIV, but the virus does not cause AIDS (Root-Bernstein, 1993:97–98). The reasons are not clear but could include the fact that the laboratory primates are not malnourished, addicted to drugs, or inoculated with semen, among other things (Root-Bernstein, 1993:369–370).

2. Gallo and Montagnier are the "apparent" codiscoverers because credit for who first isolated HIV is still disputed (Hilts, 1992, 1993; *Nature,* 361 [January 7, 1993]: 1, 3). The possibility that Gallo used a virus specimen of Montagnier's has been well publicized. Others contend that credit should be shared by a number of individuals (Gluckman, 1993).

3. But it is a long step from the statement that this is conceivable and the assertion that "there is no doubt that [AIDS spread] from its original home base in rural, central Africa" (Walker, 1991:54).

4. Actually, the decline in tuberculosis began about 1850 with changes in social conditions. No one knows when the tubercle bacillus emerged, and it may be thousands of years old. But since it cannot survive in ultraviolet light, its emergence as a major killer was associated with dark and poorly ventilated working and housing conditions as well as with crowding, which facilitated person-to-person transmission. These conditions were especially widespread in the early industrial city in the West. As conditions improved, the death rate from tuberculosis (as well as other infectious diseases) began a continuous decline (Eversley, 1965:57; McKeown, 1979: 45–65; Dubos and Dubos, 1987:231; Evans, 1987: 183–184).

5. Three decades ago Dubos (1965:374–375) warned about trying to eradicate infectious diseases and called attention to how the tubercle bacillus, malarial parasites, and anopheles mosquito might (and did) respond.

6. For a general technical analysis of the emergence of drug-resistant strains of infectious microbes, see Fisher (1994). For a good nontechnical discussion, see Begley (1994).

7. In 1976, the number of infectious microbes that humans currently share with certain domestic animals are as follows: poultry, twenty-six; horses, thirty-five; pigs,

forty-two; sheep and goats, forty-six; cattle, fifty; and dogs, sixty-five (McNeill, 1976:51).

8. For some diseases, one infection confers immunity for life, whereas others require repeated infections (Burnet and White, 1972:70–87, 131). And for diseases such as influenza and the common cold, there is no lifelong immunity regardless of the number of times a person is infected, as almost everyone knows.

9. For example, with respect to tuberculosis, "Study of [the inhabitants of Mauritius, which was settled in 1859] seems to indicate that it takes something over a hundred years after its first contact with tuberculosis for a race to develop a resistance against the disease equivalent to that of a European population" (Burnett and White, 1972:19).

10. Strictly speaking, the virulence of a microorganism is relative to the resistance of the host (McKeown, 1979:45; Ewald, 1994:9). The same microorganism that causes mostly mild illness in one population may have devastating results when introduced to a population with low resistance.

11. In this way "nature prefers that neither host nor [microorganism] should be too hard on the other" (Burnet and White, 1972:82). In general terms, when a relationship between a host and a microorganism exists, the survival of the microorganism is best served "not by destruction of the host, but by the development of a balanced condition in which sufficient of the substance of the host is consumed to allow the [microorganism's] growth and multiplication, but not sufficient to kill the host" (Burnet and White, 1972:29). Nature's rule for the relationship between agent and host seems to be "to live and let live."

12. Infectious agents vary in the mutation process, known as antigenic drift. The influenza virus is especially prone to mutate. The host population may develop immunity to a particular influenza virus, but in response the virus mutates to a partially new virus, which enables it to return to the same population in epidemic form two or three years later. Consequently, vaccines against influenza are almost always one epidemic behind (Burnet and White, 1972:210–212).

13. The disease rate might still fluctuate. The balance is an uneasy one, "more often swinging widely above and below the equilibrium point than remaining nearly stable, and liable to be forced to a totally different equilibrium by the introduction of some new organism into the environment" (Burnet and White, 1972:10).

14. Although it is conventional to distinguish between epidemic and endemic infectious diseases, the distinction oversimplifies the diversity among them (Burnet and White, 1972:118).

15. The law is named after William Farr, who first observed the bell-shaped trend for a cattle disease in Great Britain in 1893, Second Report of the Registrar-General of England and Wales (Bailey, 1957). The waves of prevalence for measles and diphtheria in South Australia in the first quarter of the century followed this pattern (Burnet and White, 1972:128), as did the progression of the disease myxomatosis among Australian rabbits in the 1950s (Burnet and White, 1972:139–142).

16. Ewald's analysis is more complicated than this suggests, involving the idea of evolutionary fitness and costs and benefits for the agent (HIV). The discussion here is sufficient for our purposes, however.

3. AIDS in Africa

Statistics show that since 1985, AIDS has been increasing faster in Africa than in any other region of the world (Mann et al., 1992:893–901). Surveys indicate that as many as 5 percent of the populations of Uganda, Rwanda, and Ivory Coast are infected. More than 20 percent of pregnant women in some urban areas are infected (Mann et al., 1992:41–47, 65), and extrapolation to the general population in one city (Kigali) gives an estimated *annual incidence* of 3–5 percent (Bucyendore et al., 1993). The International AIDS Center of the Harvard School of Public Health estimated that in 1992 more than 8 million Africans were infected, which would be about 65 percent of all cases worldwide (Mann et al., 1992:89–90). HIV-AIDS is about evenly distributed between males and females (Mann et al., 1992:76).

Several factors account for the pattern of high rates and balanced sex distribution. Poor nutrition and many infectious diseases compromise immune systems and possibly make people susceptible to HIV. Medical technology to screen donor blood for HIV and disposable hypodermics are quite limited. HIV-contaminated needles may be reused without being properly sterilized (Mann et al., 1992:433–434; Root-Bernstein, 1993:301–309).

In addition, STDs are exceedingly prevalent in Africa. For example, in a review of STDs in developing countries, Robert Brunham and Alan Ronald (1991:61) concluded that in some African countries STDs are one of the top five diseases for persons seeking health services. STDs are especially high for persons (men and women) infected with HIV (Allen et al., 1991:1660; Plummer et al., 1991:236; Plourde et al., 1992:89–90; Dallabetta et al., 1993:40). An epidemic of STDs appeared in the years preceding the AIDS epidemic in Africa (Arya and Bennet, 1976; Osoba, 1981; Mann et al., 1992:167), just as it did among American gays. One study in the early 1980s revealed that as many as 20 percent of Zimbabwe's urban population had an STD (Ungar, 1989:331). Another study showed that 10 percent of Ugandans had gonococcal infections in 1981; in comparison, only 0.4 percent of Americans and Europeans had these infections, and differences of similar magnitude for syphilis and other STDs were reported (Root-Bernstein, 1993:165, 301–303). Given the presence of HIV, the high rate of STDs assures that HIV will be widely transmitted in heterosexual intercourse, which may account for 90 percent of HIV infections (Williams, 1992:46).

But high rates of STDs do not act alone. Polygamous behavior spreads STDs and hence HIV, whereas monogamous behavior limits the spread. Most experts agree that polygamous behavior is a major factor in African HIV-AIDS,[1] and from a sociological point of view, it is the most relevant factor. It is also the focus of this chapter.

That STDs are so widespread is indirect evidence that polygamous behavior is also widespread.[2] Ethnographic studies leave no doubt that having multiple sexual partners is a common cultural practice in many groups in Africa (Caldwell et al., 1989:205–216; see also Southall, 1961:52; Gregersen, 1983:190; Hrdy, 1987; Larson, 1989; Bledsoe, 1990). For this reason many Westerners claim Africans are "promiscuous." This view is ethnocentric. Sexual behavior varies widely across societies (Davenport, 1977; Gregersen, 1983; Becker, 1984), and there is simply no universal cultural standard against which sexual practice can be judged as promiscuous and excessive (or repressive); what is appropriate in one society may be deviant in others. Sociologically, if the customs of a particular society approve polygamous behavior, such behavior is normal and appropriate by the standards of that society. To call it promiscuous simply reflects the view of persons who belong to sex-negative societies in which monogamous relations are the normative ideal and having multiple partners is viewed as deviant and immoral. Such moralizing does nothing to enhance our understanding of the practice. Analysis based on the cross-cultural perspective does.

The Cross-cultural Perspective and Sex

The central idea in the cross-cultural perspective is that behavior patterns that exist in one society but not in others or in varying degrees in different societies are the result of differences in the way societies structure and give meaning to behavior. This is true for sexual behavior no less than other types. Eroticism and, for heterosexual sex, reproduction are universal. But although the biological dynamics of sex are universal because the biology of sex does not vary with society, the social dynamics—how society structures the way sex is expressed and gives it social meaning—are not universal. Therefore, to understand why polygamous behavior is so common in Africa (and a major reason for the pattern of HIV-AIDS in Africa), we must understand why sexual expression is structured this way in African societies, or "tribes," and the social meaning sex has for members of most of these societies.

First, a word on the term *tribe*: Although it is used by most scholars who study African societies, the term was actually introduced by European colonialists, who used it pejoratively because they considered Africans to be "backward" and "primitive" (Shillington, 1989:357–358; Oliver, 1991: 242). Although its present-day meaning is not always clear, in general a tribe is an amalgam or cluster of clans, each of which consists of any number of subclans and extended families, so the term overlaps with kinship (Cockcroft, 1990:22; Oliver, 1991:242). The exact number of tribes in Africa is unknown, though anthropologists, sociologists, and historians agree that there are thousands and that virtually everyone in Africa belongs to one.[3]

These societies are what anthropologists and sociologists call preliterate or nonliterate; tribes are traditionally organized around simple agriculture or hunting and gathering activities and reside in one or more villages in the countryside. Certain cultural features are common to most African tribal groups,[4] including the social meaning of sex and the way it is expressed (for a review, see Caldwell et al., 1989; see also Southall, 1961:46–56; Molnos, 1968:46–64; Hrdy, 1987; Larson, 1989). Commonalities in the social dynamics of sex derive from (1) the traditional marriage institution and kinship ties, (2) cultural norms and beliefs about sexual expression (sexual culture), and (3) gender stratification.[5] The descriptions that follow are for rural tribal societies, even though HIV is more serious in urban areas, because sexual practices in towns and cities are patterned on rural customs. In addition, the rates of HIV-AIDS in rural Africa are low only when compared to rates in urban Africa. In comparison to most places in the world, the prevalence of HIV-AIDS in many rural areas in Africa is very high.

Marriage and Kinship

Polygyny

Traditionally, in most African societies polygamy has been the preferred form of marriage. Polygyny is still widespread, though polyandry is (and traditionally has been) rare (Gregersen, 1983:190; see also Southall, 1961:52; Molnos, 1968:50–51; Caldwell et al., 1989:201; Bledsoe, 1990:117). In certain regions in Europe and Asia, polygamous (mostly polygynous) marriage is also normatively approved, but only about 3–4 percent of marriages are in this form, whereas according to the World Fertility Survey, up to 30–50 percent of all marriages in Africa are polygamous (Caldwell et al., 1989:201). Consequently, the proportion of all women involved in a polygynous marriage at some stage during their lives is very high. Since multiple wives increase the spread of STDs in a population, polygyny obviously contributes to the high HIV-AIDS rate as well as the balanced rate between males and females.

Patrilineage

Typically, after marriage the couple lives embedded in a compound or adjacent huts usually belonging to the husband's extended family, subclan, or clan. This makes for cohesive kinship ties, which are valued more than marital ties. Children are usually descended patrilineally and belong to the husband's kinship unit.[6] They are valued as economic assets (to perform field labor and take care of parents and other relatives in old age) (Molnos, 1968: 50; Lamb, 1987:33–34; Ungar, 1989:184). Children also increase the numerical strength of clan and tribe. And a man's personal status within the clan-tribe rises as his progeny increases; traditionally, "the key measure of a man's wealth [has been] the number of dependents in his household" (Henn, 1984:5). Patrilineage thus gives men strong social incentives to acquire many wives (Southall, 1961:52; Caldwell et al., 1989:202).

It also promotes polygamous behavior outside marrriage. Wives are valued largely for their potential as "baby machines" (Lamb, 1987:39). The respect they receive in the clan-tribe depend on the number of children they bear. Children are social and economic assets to women no less than to men. Consequently, the physical and emotional aspects of sex in marriage are subordinate to childbearing (Molnos, 1968:58, 79). This makes for weak conjugal bonds (Caldwell et al., 1989:188–189, 200; see also Radcliffe-Brown, 1950:51–54; Larson, 1989:722; Bledsoe, 1990:117; O'Connor, 1991:51), so that extramarital sex is common, normal, and even expected, though more so for men than women (Caldwell et al., 1989:212). And the fact that children born from such unions belong to the husband and his kinship group is an incentive for men to engage in extramarital affairs. Thus, since patrilineage encourages men to acquire wives and to engage in polygamous nonmarital behavior, it is a major etiological factor in the African pattern of HIV-AIDS.

Sexual Culture

Sexual culture refers to the cultural beliefs, attitudes, and norms regarding sex. In contrast to Americans, who usually view sex morally and think that people who have multiple partners (even if unmarried) are immoral and unfaithful, most Africans do not judge sexual behavior in such terms at all. They experience little guilt about sex, and they enter into sex more casually and have more sexual partners than Westerners do. The cultural beliefs and norms that do bear most directly on sex are the transactional element in sexual relations, a masculine sexual ideology, and sex-positive beliefs.

The Transactional Element in Sexual Relations

In general, Africans view sex as an ordinary activity, much like work (Caldwell et al., 1989:194, 209, 218). Traditional sexual ethics are similar to those that regulate other services, namely, the ethic of exchange (Caldwell et al., 1989:203). Sexual relations are characterized by a "transactional element" (Caldwell et al., 1989:202–205), which is especially explicit in the traditional marriage.

Marriage is primarily an arrangement between kinship groups rather than individuals (Radcliffe-Brown, 1950:41–54; Little, 1971:17–20, 1974:4–8; La Fontaine, 1974:112). In return for loss of the daughter's labor as well as for her sexual favors and the children she will produce for the husband and his clan, the wife's family receives a bride-price (traditionally in the form of cattle).[7] The transaction is negotiated by family elders who have little, if any, concern for the wishes and passion of the couple (Lamb, 1987:37). (Indeed, in some instances marriages are arranged early in the couple's life and sometimes before birth.) This approach to marriage contributes to weak conjugal bonds, so that divorce, separation, and desertion are common (Caldwell et al., 1989:201; Larson, 1989:720; see also Pankhurst and Jacobs, 1988).

In extramarital and premarital affairs, men are expected to give women money and gifts as an expresssion of affection, respect, and gratitude (Larson, 1989:723; Caldwell et al., 1989:203; see also Shoumatoff, 1988: 155). And for women, such affairs are important sources of income. Extramarital sex is less common for women than premarital sex (Larson, 1989: 721), though a wife sometimes has several lovers, serially or concurrently (Obbo, 1980:151). This (or the threat thereof) may give her leverage over the husband and thus access to his economic resources (Caldwell et al., 1989:204). (The tactic may well backfire, however, especially if the husband has several wives.)

In general, then, in most sexual relations—whether casual liaisons, premarital relations, extramarital affairs, or marriage—"there is an economic core," with women "exchanging sexual favours and often also reproductive potential for economic benefits" (Barnett and Blaikie, 1992:77). This exchange is explicitly acknowledged and normatively accepted.[8] In some groups mothers may actually encourage their daughters to trade sexual favors for money and gifts as a way to provide for themselves (Caldwell et al., 1989:203–204).

Although many Westerners have difficulty seeing how this arrangement differs from prostitution, Western anthropologists who study African societies disagree on how prostitution should even be defined in the African context (Molnos, 1968:79; Little, 1973:84; Caldwell et al., 1989:218–219; Dirasse, 1991:10). The usual definition of prostitution holds that a prostitute is a woman whose income is derived more or less exclusively from payment for brief impersonal encounters with all comers, most of whom are strangers, in which no services or activities beyond the sex act are involved. (Many Westerners use "prostitute" more loosely to refer to all women who use sex to elicit money and other material favors from men.) By this definition, prostitution in Africa appears to have been most limited; in fact, prior to colonization in most groups prostitutes as a category of women were not even recognized (Gregersen, 1983:15; Hrdy, 1987:1112; Caldwell et al., 1989:220–221).[9] Even so, the transactional element in sex increases the spread of HIV, as the following example reveals.

In a study of lakeside trading villages in the Rakai district of Uganda, Tony Barnett and Piers Blaikie (1992:78) observed that women commonly support themselves through commodity trading. However, they also "set up independent households," with "one or more regular lovers who help them financially." These women are obviously involved in sexual transactions (financial help for sex) but they are not prostitutes. Although lovers may give them money, nonsexual activity is central to the relationship; sexual activity is simply integrated in a round of other activities that the partners share. In addition, such relationships are not the sole (or even primary) source of women's livelihood. And these relationships involve more than a single sexual encounter, the partners are not strangers, and a degree of affection may be assumed. Little (1973:81) observed the same pattern in African towns. Similar arrangements do exist in the West, of course, though they are less common and less open. More significantly, the arrangement in the West is almost always limited to one partner extending over a period of time. In contrast, in Africa "the rate of partner change can be assumed to be fairly rapid" (Barnett and Blaikie, 1992:78). Although many Americans would consider this immoral, even as prostitution, Africans do not; this arrangement is best viewed as part of the transactional cultural norm in sex rather than as either promiscuity or prostitution.[10] The implications for the transmission of HIV are clear. Barnett and Blaikie (1992:32, 69) reported that in the Rakai district, around 40 percent of men and women between twenty and thirty are seropositive for HIV.[11]

Masculine Sexual Ideology and the Status of Men

In most African societies a plurality of sexual partners is a male right (Southall, 1961:52; Molnos, 1968:66; Caldwell et al., 1989:202; Larson, 1989: 721; Barnett and Blaikie, 1992:77–78). This right is related to polygyny (if only as a rationalization for it) (Davenport, 1977:125). But it goes beyond polygyny since the right does not end with marriage. It is socially acceptable for a married man to have mistresses and "outside wives" (concubines) (Little, 1974b:17–18; Obbo, 1980:89; Larson, 1989:720). Men's extramarital relations are "taken for granted" and simply "expected of the normal man" (Caldwell et al., 1989:212). Indeed, sexual conquest and fatherhood are central to male identity, and children enhance a man's social status. This reinforces women's use of sex for material gain (Barnett and Blaikie, 1992:44, 77–78).

Masculine sexual ideology combines with the transactional element such that the more wealth a man has, the more sexual partners he can get. For example, a bride-price must be paid for a wife. Thus, traditionally "the key measure of a man's wealth [has been] the number of [wives and children] in his household" (Henn, 1984:5). Some chiefs are known to have hundreds of wives (Molnos, 1968:50). The association of number of female partners with male wealth suggests that HIV infection rates are higher among men with higher status than among men with lower status, a hypothesis I examine later.

Sexual Relations and a Sex-positive Culture

Most groups in Africa have sex-positive cultures. Sex is viewed as a part of courtship and a form of recreation, and relations between lovers are viewed as affairs between friends (Larson, 1989:723, 727). Despite the emphasis on sex for reproduction, *New Yorker* reporter Alex Shoumatoff (1988:154–155), who is married to a Rwandan, stated that most African societies "are unquestionably sex-positive." This is especially so for men, who tend to be "womanizers." Women "put up with it or participate in it depending on how much freedom they are allowed by their culture." (See also Barnett and Blaikie, 1992:77–78.) And by all accounts, as the existence of the transactional element in sex would indicate, in many groups women are allowed considerable freedom indeed (Molnos, 1968:58). Premarital sex for females is accepted (Molnos, 1968:58–59; Caldwell et al., 1989:195, 197, 203–205; Larson, 1989:727),[12] as is female adultery (Caldwell et al., 1989:197, 199, 212; Larson, 1989:723). According to Laketch Dirasse (1991:57), in at least one tribe (the Borana), men allow their wives "to have as many lovers as they want" (see also Bledsoe, 1990:123). Wife sharing is also reported for a number of societies, which permit or even require a wife to have sex with persons besides her husband, most frequently distant relatives of the husband's clan, sometimes as a form of hospitality to guests (Gregersen, 1983:190; Caldwell et al., 1989:213). In some groups a widow is inherited by one of her husband's brothers (levirate), and a woman may have sex with each brother to see which one would please her most in case her husband dies (Schuster, 1979:14).

In sum, for females as well as males, "fairly permissive ... sexual attitudes are found generally across sub-Saharan Africa" (Caldwell et al., 1989:222). Many scholars of African society have observed that a "wide range of all types of unstable and occasional [sexual] unions" are widespread in Africa (Molnos, 1968:79). Beyond polygamous relations, sex is simply "regarded ... positively [and as] normal and good for the health, and which, if not experienced, might well result in ill health" (Caldwell et al., 1989:209). In short, sex is viewed in sex-positive terms.

At the same time, sex is socially regulated. That the traditional African marriage is an economic arrangement between families limits the choices individuals have in mate selection. Family decisions are constrained by the custom of exogamy, and lovers usually must also be selected from outside the clan, subclan, or tribe (Davenport, 1977:125; Lamb, 1987:11). In other instances groups stipulate that the wife may have sex only with her husband's relatives or members of his age group (Gregersen, 1983:190; Caldwell et al., 1989:213). The nature of village life puts women under the surveillance of the husband's relatives and clan, and any deviation from the duties of wife and mother are apt to be quickly detected, as are deviations from restrictions on the tribal affiliation of sex partners. Even so, for most of Africa social norms permit and even encourage sex with multiple partners. Polygamous sexual relations are thus widespread for the married no less than the unmarried (Gregersen, 1983:186). This is the hallmark of a sex-positive culture. It also facilitates the spread of HIV.

Gender Stratification

Some form of gender stratification based on social (as distinct from biological) differences between males and females exists in virtually all societies. Males are usually defined as superior and are favored in status, privilege, and power. In most African societies male dominance is about as extreme as anywhere in the world (Obbo, 1980; Cutrufelli, 1983; Henn, 1984; O'Connor, 1991:27–28; for a description in one country [Mozambique], see Urdang, 1989). In some places "a husband can still forbid his wife to travel, trade, or work for wages," and when she does work, custom gives him the right to her earnings, even if he is living in another village with another wife (Henn, 1984:17). Several factors are central in male dominance.

Division of Labor. Most of Africa is still rural and dependent on agriculture, which is still very labor intensive (sickle and hoe). In most African groups the sexual division of labor is about what it was in precolonial times (Oliver,

1991:254), although there are differences between groups (Guyer, 1984; Davison, 1988). Typically, males clear and till the land, tend to livestock, and hunt, while women do most of the "stoop" and heavy labor (hoeing, planting, weeding, and harvesting) and produce about 80 percent of the food (Jacobson, 1993:67). Women also carry any surplus food to the market for sale, fetch water, gather firewood, cook, care for children, and tend to other household duties (Henn, 1984; Oliver, 1991:254; Jacobson, 1993:67–68). Women's burden and its contrast to that of men are captured in the following description.

> Drive down almost any country road in East Africa and you will see a procession of women padding along the shoulder, their backs parallel to the ground under the weight of huge piles of firewood or jars of water. The outdoor marketplaces—the most important source of economic activity in any village—are run and staffed exclusively by women. And the men? The elderly ones are apt to be sitting in the shade of the trees, smoking their pipes, drinking homemade beer, discussing their cattle—or saying nothing at all. The younger ones are either in school, in the city or in the local beer hall. (Lamb, 1987:38)

If anything, the woman's workday may be longer and harder than in the past (Henn, 1984) (for example, when the husband migrates to cities and leaves the wife solely responsible for crop production along with her other duties).

Women must obey their husbands. Obedience includes having as many children as their husbands want and providing for the children's care. An infertile woman is disgraced, and traditionally infertility is grounds for divorce. Since the wife's natal family may be required to repay the bride-price if she leaves the husband, is unable to have children, or otherwise fails to do as the husband commands, she is under pressure from her own kinship unit as well as the husband's to submit to his wishes and demands. Therefore, in most tribal societies "the traditionally decent women have been [and continue to be] those who have submitted to control by men" (Obbo, 1980: 151).

Control of Land. Traditionally, land has been the property of families and clans; it is allocated to men depending on household need. Husbands then provide their wives with plots to cultivate. Since land is the primary source of wealth in most of Africa,[13] it is a central aspect of gender stratification. Inconsistencies among traditional customs, state law patterned on European property law, and government land policies make for some confusion in landownership, and in some places women can and do own land (Davison, 1988a:10–12, 1988b; see also West, 1972; Barnett and Blaikie, 1992:12–13, 75–76, 79–81). In general, however, statutory law and government programs as well as custom make it hard or impossible for women to own land. For example, in land reform programs land titles are almost invariably given to men as heads of households rather than to women or jointly to husbands and wives (cowives) (Jacobson, 1993:71). Women's primary access to land is the plots their husbands give them to cultivate.

Even then, the husband may favor one wife over another in the allocation of plots. The wife's vulnerability is furthered by the possibility of divorce, desertion, or death. In some groups wives cannot leave their husbands for any reason, but husbands may (and do) divorce and desert their wives and children whenever they wish (Pankhurst and Jacobs, 1988), leaving the wife landless. If the husband dies, the land passes to the sons, thus keeping the land in the husband's clan.[14] In some instances the wife may have usu-fructory rights to the land (right to use but not own the land). Even so, the husband's male relatives or the wife's ex-husbands may try to dislodge her and appropriate the land for themselves in accordance with the custom of patrilineal ownership (Pankhurst and Jacobs, 1988:211–212).

Cash Crops and Food Security. Land may be used to grow cash crops as well as food staples for household consumption. The decision is the husband's, and he gets the cash from cash crop production, even though the wife (wives) does (do) most of the work (Davison, 1988a:13, 1988b:157). Even where women may legally acquire land, they are usually limited to growing staples. Cash crops require more capital for irrigation, fertilizers, pesticides, and hybrid seeds, and women rarely have the capital or the credit to purchase these goods (Jacobson, 1993:71–72). Since all or most of the food crop is consumed by the household, women have little opportunity to generate cash income. And if divorcées or widows are unable to retain the land, they usually must return to their brothers' families or fathers' compounds, where they work in the fields and households.

Thus, women in Africa are burdened with physically demanding work from dawn to dusk, they are responsible for producing and caring for many children, they are landless and poor, and their lives are dominated by men. As daughters, they perform field labor and household duties for their fathers or brothers. As wives, they perform field labor and produce children for their husbands and their clans and incur the economic insecurities inherent in a polygynous marriage and patrilineal control of land. As estranged wives or widows, they return to their natal family and clan, where they are under the domination of father or brothers again. In the African system of gender stratification, then, women have very little independence and freedom from male domination.[15] Because this stratification, along with the sexual culture, structures the sexual relations of women, it is a major factor in the social etiology of HIV-AIDS.

Gender Stratification, Sex, and HIV-AIDS. Gender stratification is so oppressive that Barnett and Blaikie (1992) argued that sexual favors and reproductive potential are about the only way women can gain access to land, cash, and other economic goods. Material favors gained from sex also lift some of the heavy work burden that women traditionally carry. The sex-positive culture and the transactional norm in sex give women the freedom to use sex for this end.

The significance of gender stratification in women's use of sex to gain material favors is not unique to Africa, of course. The difference is that African women are much more oppressed, their access to economic resources is far more limited, and the social acceptance of their use of sex for material ends is much more explicit than in most societies. And most important, since the use of sex is a major way women can gain independence, sex is a very significant *social* activity. The social meaning of sex is linked to women's freedom from male domination[16] and relief from a physically brutal workload. Unfortunately, it also raises the risk of HIV-AIDS.

In fact, Barnett and Blaikie (1992:163) believed that gender stratification may be the central factor in the spread of HIV in Africa. This spread is due in large part to the cultural practice whereby "a woman maximizes her chances for economic security by creating links to several men" (Bledsoe, 1990:119). But more than gender stratification is involved. In addition, the sexual culture gives women considerable sexual freedom and lowers restraints on polygamous behavior. As Barnett and Blaikie (1992:78) stated, "In communities where people's attitudes [are] fairly relaxed by the public standards of many other cultures," women seek to escape male oppression by gaining "access to economic resources through a range of sexual relationships with men," from selling sex for cash, to being "kept women," to entering into various types of marriage.

The interaction of gender stratification with sexual culture is part of the causal chain of the African pattern of HIV-AIDS. Beyond this, since customary and statutory law supports the sexual division of labor and male control of land and cash, African legal culture is involved in the social etiology of HIV-AIDS.

Urbanization, Sexual Relations, and HIV-AIDS

About 70–75 percent of the population in Africa still live in village settings (O'Connor, 1991:111), but this is changing rapidly. From colonization to the post–World War II years, urbanization was slow, but as independence came and the European colonialists left in the 1950s and 1960s, urbanization accelerated. For example, Kinshasa, Zaire, which had a population of about ten thousand in 1900, still had only three hundred thousand in the 1960s; by 1990 it had a population of about 4 million (O'Connor, 1991:44–46). There are eleven cities with a population of 1 million or more in Africa, and among all cities in the world with populations of 2 million or more, the two with the highest growth rates (Lagos and Kinshasa) are in this region (U.S. Bureau of the Census, 1991:errata sheet). Overall, urbanization in Africa is increasing at a rate of about 6 percent a year, by far the highest in the world (Linden, 1993). And as in other parts of the world, HIV-AIDS in Africa is predominantly an urban phenomenon (Piot et al., 1992:15; Mann et al., 1992:76–77).

The rate of HIV-AIDS is higher in urban areas because, among other reasons, the reporting systems in rural areas are even less adequate than those in the towns and cities. Nevertheless, the difference between urban and rural areas is too great to dismiss (Anderson et al., 1991:584; Mann et al., 1992: 35, 42–43, 76–78; Williams, 1992:6). In addition, general population surveys in Rwanda and Uganda show much higher rates for urban dwellers (Mann et al., 1992:42–43). In 1989 the Rwandan HIV Seroprevalence Study Group reported that HIV seropositivity rates were about thirteen times higher for urban areas (Mann et al., 1992:181). More generally, in 1987 in the cities of Uganda, Rwanda, Zambia, Congo, Ivory Coast, Malawi, Central African Republic, and Zaire, from 7.1 percent (Zaire) to 24.1 percent (Uganda) of fifteen- to forty-nine-year-olds were estimated to be infected; percentages for rural areas in those countries were far lower (e.g., only 0.7 percent in Zaire) (Barnett and Blaikie, 1992:27). This comparison is consistent with the fact that most infectious disease rates are higher in urban areas.

More is involved than urbanization, however; few cities in other parts of the world have rates as high as African cities. For example, in only one American city was the reported number of AIDS cases more than 1 percent of the population in 1992 (it was 1.32 percent for San Francisco [CDC, 1993a:8]). The high rate of HIV-AIDS in Africa is due in large part to the high rate of STDs. But it is also the result of urbanization occurring in societies where the practice of polygamous behavior is embedded in cultural norms and societal institutions.

Of course, when Africans migrate to urban areas, some erosion of traditional customs occurs (O'Connor, 1983:109–111), and some analysts believe this includes norms and institutions regulating sex (Mann et al., 1992: 180). However, the hold of tradition on urban sexual relations is still strong. Just as age-old political customs influence political actions and organization in urban areas (Cockcroft, 1990), traditional sexual customs exert influence on sexual relations in urban areas. This may be best seen by examining how urban sexual relations are affected by the way Africans adapt features of tribal society to urban environments.

Sex as Transaction, Gender Stratification, and the Sexual Relations of Women

Economic opportunities are better for women in urban areas, including more sexual strategies for gaining access to the economic resources of men. Consequently, a diversification and expansion of the sexual relations of women have taken place.

Prostitutes. By all accounts, prostitution is widespread in African cities. Although it is illegal in many cities, as in much of the West, authorities in Africa also tend to turn their heads. More significantly, even though some groups do not approve of women accepting money for sex (Little, 1973:76–101; Dirasse, 1991:54–58), there is little ostracism of the practice (Little, 1973:90; White, 1984:65; Wipper, 1984:79; Caldwell et al., 1989:220; Dirasse, 1991:124).[17] Much of the ostracism that does exist is directed at the fact that prostitutes are single, unattached, and not destined for marriage, that is, not under the control of men, as all decent women traditionally have been.

The first surge of prostitution came during the colonial period with the migration of men to mines and plantations, usually in connection with labor contracts with European owners. Some women followed and established camps outside the work areas and serviced workers as prostitutes, though many prostitutes were from groups indigenous to the work areas (Ardener, 1961:93; Du Bois, 1967:11, n. 3; Little, 1973:97–98; La Fontaine, 1974). An increase in STD rates followed (DeLancey, 1978; Hunt, 1989). This process continues today and is one way HIV and STDs get transmitted (Hunt, 1989:356).

Migration from rural areas accelerated with independence (Southall, 1961), and prostitution increased. No one knows the exact number of urban prostitutes, but by all accounts it is very large. A sample of household heads in Addis Ababa in 1973 revealed that 8 percent of female heads of households were prostitutes. When prostitutes who were not household heads (e.g., "streetwalkers") were included, it was estimated that 25 percent of adult women were prostitutes.[18] Overall, prostitution was "by far the largest occupational category for women" in the "informal" labor sector of Addis Ababa (Dirasse, 1991:xi, xiii, 1, 37, 75–105).[19] According to Luise White (1984:64–65), a historian of African women and prostitutes, prostitution is one of the four main roles to have emerged for women in urban Africa (the other three are housewives, sellers of cooked food, and brewers of illegal liquor). Since prostitution is often combined with the other roles, most frequently with brewing, the number of prostitutes is very large indeed. Just as the concentration of gays in San Francisco, New York City, and other American cities was associated with high STD rates prior to the HIV-AIDS in the

United States, the rapid growth of urbanization and the concentration of prostitutes in towns and cities in Africa were associated with high STD rates in the 1970s prior to the AIDS epidemic in Africa (Meheus et al., 1974; D'Costa et al., 1985). For example, of the sixty prostitutes interviewed at length in the 1973 household survey in Addis Ababa, 95 percent said they had contracted gonorrhea at least twice, and 63 percent had contracted syphilis at least once (Dirasse, 1991:67).[20]

By the 1980s rates of HIV-AIDS for prostitutes had soared. In samples of prostitutes from twenty-two African countries circa 1990, infection rates were more than 30 percent in ten countries, and in many cities rates approached 50 percent (Mann et al., 1992:52–54). Other surveys in cities in Rwanda, Kenya, and Zaire showed prevalence rates for prostitutes of up to 88 percent (Piot et al., 1988:574; see also Kreiss et al., 1986; Grmek, 1989: 177; Hunt, 1989; Plummer et al., 1991; Piot et al., 1992:16).[21] In comparison, percentages for prostitutes in the United States and Europe are much lower (though rates for IDU prostitutes are much higher than for those who are not IDUs). In some places the percentage is extremely low, and in Nevada, where prostitution is legal and prostitutes receive regular medical examinations, no cases have been reported at all (Darrow, 1991:93; Root-Bernstein, 1993:39–43). In addition, the percentage of African prostitutes who have HIV has increased over time and parallels the increase of HIV in the overall population, at least in Nairobi: 5 percent in 1982, 12 percent in 1983, 22 percent in 1984, 54 percent in 1985, 65 percent in 1986, and 83 percent in 1987 (Grmek, 1989:177). In contrast, one study showed that the percentage (4.5 percent) of non-IDU call girls in New York City who were infected with HIV did not increase at all from 1982 to 1989 (Root-Bernstein, 1993:41).

The customers of African prostitutes seem also to be at high risk for contracting HIV. In a sample of men recruited from an STD clinic in Nairobi, 89 percent of those who were infected reported having had frequent contact with prostitutes (versus 74 percent who had not had frequent contact) (Simonsen et al., 1988:275). Exact comparisons for the United States are not available, but the customers of prostitutes in the United States may have an HIV rate no higher than 1 percent (Wallace, 1989). Therefore, in contrast to the United States, African prostitutes constitute a major reservoir of HIV (Fumento, 1990:120).

The large number of prostitutes in African cities is obvious reason for alarm. But more alarming is how prostitution is so interwoven with social forces. Several factors are involved. The male-female ratio in many African cities is greater than one (Robertson, 1984:41; Larson, 1989:720), and some contend the imbalance is one reason prostitution is so widespread (Ardener, 1961:93–94; Southall, 1961:47–48; Molnos, 1968:73; Little, 1973:76, 80; Caldwell et al., 1989:217–218). However, a number of urban areas have more women than men (Larson, 1989:720), including Addis Ababa, which has many prostitutes (Dirasse, 1991:1). Poverty is also a factor. With no job skills and not much or no formal education, women have limited opportunities for gainful employment in cities, and this may lead women into prostitution (Schoepf, 1992:263). One author claimed that "financial factors" account for 85 percent of African prostitutes (Williams, 1992:341), though this would not account for the social acceptance of prostitution. At least as important as the sex ratio and poverty are the cultural conception of sex as transaction and the system of gender stratification, as women adapt them to the peculiarities of the job structure of African cities.

African cities are unlike cities in the West and elsewhere in that urbanization is occurring without industrialization (Gugler and Flanagan, 1978). Most cities have little manufacturing or heavy industry, so wage-sector jobs are scarce (Iliffe, 1987:164–192). Jobs for women are especially limited since women have less education than men[22] and most have no work experience beyond working in the fields and trading in the food market. Even if they do qualify for the few jobs available, they commonly encounter gender discrimination (e.g., Zaire's cities have about as many women as men, but women constitute only 4 percent of formally employed workers) (Schoepf, 1992:263).

Consequently, women (as well as many men) turn to petty trade in goods and services (e.g., hawking and vending), legal and illegal (Gugler and Flanagan, 1978:138–144; O'Connor, 1983:144–150, 1991:114; White, 1983). Most jobs are strikingly similar to the economic roles women perform in tribal society, where women are duty bound to provide services to men (sex, children, and domestic and field work) and trade sex within and outside marriage for economic gain. White (1984:64) remarked, "What were women [in cities] to do? To earn money, they became independent suppliers of those domestic services that made life tolerable to men living in cramped quarters on low wages. They sold sex, companionship, bath water, beer, [cooked] food (greatly in demand by men with no previous cooking experience), and sometimes a dinner for two." Thus, as in rural settings, women's major economic role is to service men. This includes the provision of sex, as the large number of prostitutes makes clear.

In contrast to the West, where prostitute-client relations are viewed as qualitatively different from other sexual relations, in Africa "gradations in the commercial component of sex" are recognized (Caldwell et al., 1989: 220), with prostitution simply at one end of a transactional continuum. The normative acceptance of this continuum simply makes trading in sex as acceptable as trading in other services, with which it is frequently combined (e.g., provision of food and lodging). For example, Dirasse (1991:37) stated that in Addis Ababa prostitution has "become a standardized normative behavioral pattern." African culture simply guides women into prostitution much more easily than Western culture does. According to some reports, women "become prostitutes as reasonably and as self-righteously as they would have become typists or telephone girls" (Wipper, 1984:79; see also Little, 1973:84). To a large extent, then, prostitution is the adaptation of the transactional element in sex to urban settings.

It is also women's adaption of gender stratification to urban areas. Men remain dominant in urban areas, but prostitution allows women to extract economic resources from them and thus escape the most oppressive features of male dominance, just as women's use of sex allows them to gain a measure of freedom in rural settings. Because the money earned belongs to the prostitute, who does not have to share it with a man (unless she is married), prostitution allows women more economic independence than they could possibly gain in traditional tribal settings, and many women migrate to urban areas for the explicit purpose of becoming prostitutes (Little, 1973:84, 87). Thus, in a 1961 review of the effect of urbanization in Africa, Aidan Southall (p. 51) stated that the economic independence of women (a major source of which is prostitution) was one of the "most striking characteristics of African towns in contrast to rural areas." Tragically, however, this independence has come at a very high cost, as the high rates for HIV-AIDS among prostitutes show.

Therefore, to characterize prostitution in Africa as a threat to public health, as many medical reports and publications do, is certainly valid: The number of prostitutes is very large, and the rate of HIV-AIDS among them is extremely high. But prostitution is the product of demographic, economic, and gender-role forces, especially traditional tribal social forces as they are expressed in African cities. These are the real threat to public health, not prostitution itself, since prostitution is not likely to decline until the social forces that produce it decline. To attribute the high rates of HIV-AIDS primarily to prostitution oversimplifies greatly.

Furthermore, gradations in the commercial component of sex mean that all women who use sex to improve their economic prospects are not prostitutes in the narrow sense. As John Caldwell et al. (1989:218) noted, prostitution accounts for "a very small part of sexual relations in Africa, even those relations with a transactional component." Similarly, Daniel Hrdy (1987:1113) stated, "It is unlikely that female promiscuity is confined to 'professional' prostitutes, especially in urban areas." Urban women, single and married, develop a variety of sexual-economic relations with men that the idea of prostitute-client relationship simply does not capture (Molnos, 1968:72–92; Little, 1973:76–129). Such relations have significant implications for HIV-AIDS.

Single Women. In contrast to prostitutes, who provide brief sexual favors and usually accept all comers for a uniform fee,[23] other women provide sex for a man over a period of time, are more selective in whom they have sex with, and are apt to negotiate over the fee received, which may be in kind rather than money (e.g., clothes, housing, access to fancy automobiles). These women include "free women" (*femmes libres* in the French-speaking regions), who emerged with the growth of cities after independence (Davidson, 1955:132–135). Women migrated to towns and cities for various reasons (and continue to do so), but as with prostitutes, "emancipation" (escape from tribal oppression and burdensome physical work) was (is) a major reason (Obbo, 1980; Hanna and Hanna, 1981:51–53). In the city women may become independent of husbands and male kin and are not obligated to share their earnings—hence the term *free women* (Little, 1971:23, 1974:18; La Fontaine, 1974; Obbo, 1980:153; Schoepf, 1992:264). The term applies in particular to attractive women who develop a certain elegance and coquetry, have a taste for fashion and expensive clothes, and derive their livelihood from sex but are very discriminating in their choice of men, with whom they maintain a relationship for weeks or months. That relationship represents a form of concubinage, mistresshood, or outside wifery (Davidson, 1955:132; La Fontaine, 1974:94–98; see also Little, 1973:113–117; White, 1983; Iliffe, 1987:183–185; Shoumatoff, 1988:169; Cockcroft, 1990:77–79).[24] They accept only the more wealthy, powerful, charming, and handsome men, whose standards of behavior they approve and whom they accompany to socials and outings. Men give them money and gifts or provide for their housing and maintenance in return for sexual favors that are usually granted regularly over a period of time. Most free women work out of hotels, nightclubs, and other establishments frequented by businessmen, professionals, and tourists at night, though some are also employed in offices and shops or trade in other services or commodities during the day. Free women frequently maintain a relationship with several men either concurrently or sequentially.

Most people view free women as traders and accord them a higher standing than ordinary prostitutes.[25] Free women have been considered part of the African urban petty bourgeoisie for over half a century (White, 1983; see also Little, 1973:116–117; Schoepf, 1992). In places such as Kinshasa, for a free woman to have many successful men as lovers is a mark of success, just as having many mistresses or wives is a mark of success for a man (La Fontaine, 1974:98). Since the material favors she receives are hers and need not be shared with a husband, a free woman achieves an independence that women in oppressive tribal villages can only dream about (Cockcroft, 1990:78–79). Free women thus "represent a deliberate act of feminine emancipation" (Davidson, 1955:132). Even so, since their livelihood revolves around the management of sexual relations in return for housing, clothes, cars, money, and entertainment, the relationship is in accord with the cultural norm of sex as transaction. Quite simply, it is an extension of women's traditional strategy of using sex to gain access to land, crops, and cash.

Other women trade in sex but less consistently than either ordinary prostitutes or free women. Some seek occasional sex partners (*pneus de rechange,* or "spare tires") to make ends meet, as during periods of unemployment or during the summer when a university student exchanges sexual services for money much as an American student works as a waitress (Little, 1973:84–85; Schoepf, 1992:263). In an environment that offers few jobs and that favors men for those jobs, the traditional transactional element in sex makes it a reasonable and socially acceptable way to get through hard times (Little, 1973:84–85). Sexual practices that present high risks for contracting HIV are clearly not limited to prostitution.

Indeed, free women may be a major reservoir of HIV.[26] A study of a sample of *femmes libres* in a town in Rwanda in the early 1970s revealed that 51 percent had gonorrhea (Meheus et al., 1974). Two studies of Nairobi prostitutes in the early 1980s may have included free women. One reported that 50 percent of prostitutes working out of bars in 1981 had an STD (D'Costa et al., 1985); the other reported that prostitutes working out of the bar of a tourist hotel had an HIV infection rate of 26 percent (Kreiss et al., 1986).[27] (Note that these statistics are for infection rates at one point in time and are lower than those reported in Dirasse's 1973 study in Addis Ababa, which asked if the prostitute had *ever* had gonorrhea or syphilis.) Studies of HIV among prostitutes have probably included some free women and women who engage in sex intermittently for payment.[28]

Statistics for unmarried women, for whom the HIV rate is very high, most certainly include free women. (In the 1950s it was estimated that 25 percent of all women in Elizabethville and Léopoldville were *femmes libres* [Davidson, 1955:132].) Results of two studies, one of women in Nairobi attending an STD clinic and one for childbearing women attending prenatal or pediatric clinics in Kigali, are presented in Table 3.1. Although the rates for the unmarried are not as high as studies have reported for prostitutes, they are still alarmingly high. (The Nairobi study reported a rate of 52 percent for prostitutes, but women of all marital statuses were included in the category [Plourde et al., 1992:87].) Brunham and Ronald (1991:73) reported that in many urban regions sexually active men and women had an HIV infection rate greater than 20 percent and that the same was true for women who sought prenatal care.

How much these rates are due to free women, other women who exchange sex intermittently for material gain, and prostitutes is impossible to know. But since the number of sexually active unmarried women is much larger than the number of prostitutes, the problem of HIV-AIDS in Africa is much greater than the figures on prostitutes indicate. And this is not all. Even for

TABLE 3.1 Percentage of Women Attending STD Clinic (Nairobi) or Prenatal or Pediatric Clinic (Kigali) Testing HIV Positive

Exposure Category	Nairobi	Kigali
Prostitute[a]	52	N/A
Divorced/separated/widowed	34	55
Single	18	48
Married	8	22
Common law	N/A	35
Cohabiting, monogamous	N/A	24
Cohabiting, not sure if partner is monogamous	N/A	25
Cohabiting, nonmonogamous	N/A	38

[a]Prostitute category may include married and formerly married; marital status overlaps with cohabiting status.

SOURCE: For Nairobi, Plourde et al. (1992); for Kigali, Allen et al. (1991).

women who have steady partners—married women and cohabitors—the HIV rate is very high.

Married and Cohabiting Women. Table 3.1 shows that the HIV-infection rate for married women is 8 percent in the Nairobi study and 22–35 percent in the Kigali study; for cohabiting women (for Kigali only), it is 24–38 percent. No doubt one reason for the high rates is that wives and cohabitors, like single women, have sex with several men to gain a certain measure of economic independence. Southall (1961:55) observed that it was acceptable for urban wives to add partners "in order to raise money and gifts," which went to her "and not to the male provider." This social pattern may ease the constraints of male domination, but it is not without great costs in STDs, including HIV infection rates, as figures in Table 3.1 indicate.

Polygyny, Masculine Sexual Ideology, and the Sexual Relations of Men

The way women adapt the transactional element in sex and gender stratification to urban life obviously affects the sexual relations of men in urban areas. However, their relations are more than a mirror image of women's relations. They are best understood in terms of the way men have adapted polygyny and the masculine sexual ideology to urban life.

Although polygyny is more common in tribal settings, it is also widespread in urban areas (Larson, 1989; Bledsoe, 1990; Schoepf, 1992:266). It produces lots of children for men, which enhances their status even in urban areas (Lamb, 1987:39; Bledsoe, 1990:123), where the masculine sexual ideology is still strong. Recent reviews and research (Caldwell et al., 1989:202; Barnett and Blaikie, 1992:77–78) affirm Southall's (1961:52) conclusion in his earlier review of the effects of urbanization: "Most Africans still consider that sexual access to a plurality of women is a male right."

At the same time, urban life poses problems for men. Women and children are not the economic assets they are in crop production; the maintenance of several wives and their children is simply beyond the financial reach of most men (Bledsoe, 1990). In addition, the strong patrilineal kinship ties that support polygyny are weakened (Southall, 1961:31–45). The arrangement by which families live as parts of extended families in village compounds is economically prohibitive for most men, and necessary housing is otherwise difficult, if not impossible, to arrange in urban areas (even if extended families migrate en masse) (Southall, 1961:52; Cockcroft, 1990:89). Consequently, urbanization puts polygynous marriages under considerable stress (Southall, 1961:31–45; Caldwell et al., 1989:205; Bledsoe, 1990:120).

Despite this, Southall (1961:52) concluded that polgyny was still thriving in 1961; the traditional norms and values about polygyny had just "found expression in new form." By all accounts, the situation was unchanged in the 1980s. Polygynous marriage has been replaced by various forms of "informal polygyny": serial monogamy, *deuxieme bureaus* ("second offices"), outside wives, polyandrous motherhood, longer-term girlfriends, and *femmes libres* (Larson, 1989:720; Caldwell et al., 1989:202, 214; Bledsoe, 1990:120; Schoepf, 1992:266).[29] In towns and cities men are still attracted to women primarily for sex—"the only hold many women have [for their husbands] appears to be the attraction of their sexual services" (Southall, 1961:55). Consequently, when wives do not satisfy their husband's sexual desires, the husbands may add partners. For example, postpartum sex taboos, which continue to be observed in urban areas, may last up to two years, and husbands may seek sexual pleasure from other women during that period (Southall, 1961:55). Consequently, HIV infection rates for married men are probably relatively high, just as they are for married women. The evidence is limited, but two studies of attendees at an STD clinic in Nairobi suggested that rates are actually higher for married men than for unmarried men (Piot et al., 1987:1110; Simonsen et al., 1988:275), and the results of a serologic survey revealed that the rate for married men (and married women) is unusually high.[30]

It may be that the extramarital activity of husbands more than that of wives accounts for the relatively high infection rates for married women and common-law wives (see Table 3.1). Differences between women according to cohabitation status (which cross-cuts the married/unmarried distinction) for the Kigali study are suggestive. Childbearing women who cohabit with polygamous partners have a higher HIV infection rate than women who cohabit with monogamous partners. But note that 24 percent of the women in a monogamous relationship are infected. Many women who have a steady partner may actually be part of multiple partner networks with the husband at the center. Another finding from the Kigali study (not reported in Table 3.1) bears on this suggestion. Although 86 percent of women report being married or in a common-law union, only 34 percent report having a monogamous relationship (Allen et al., 1991:1659–1660). Obviously, their steady partners have sexual relations with other women.

It would come as no suprise, therefore, to find high rates of HIV among women who *say* they have monogamous sexual relationships, which is what Table 3.1 shows. Thus, the risk to women is not just (or even) their own polygamous sexual activity. A more important risk may be the polygamous activity of the men with whom they live (as wives or cohabitors). Indeed, Jonathan Mann et al. (1992:345, 348) reported HIV is spreading to monogamous African women, whose "only risk factor [is in] being powerless to influence their husband's behavior." And because the husband's behavior is anchored in the institution of polygyny and the sexual masculine ideology, until these change, the sexual activity of men is not apt to change. And HIV will continue to spread.

Socioeconomic Status, Sexual Relations, and HIV-AIDS. Just as men of higher status have more sexual partners in tribal society, higher-status men in urban areas probably have more sexual partners. Men may have a right to a plurality of sexual partners, but sex is a transaction and thus not free, so that men with higher income can afford more women. It has been suggested, therefore, that polygamous behavior is especially common among men in the middle and upper classes (Hrdy, 1987:1112). One observer stated:

> It is no secret that in many of the [high-HIV-]affected African countries, prosperous upper- and middle-class men, among others, tend to have many sexual liaisons at the same time whether or not they are married. Indeed, among the elite of Zaire and Rwanda, it is commonly joked that men often take a long time to arrive home from work because they must make a stop at their *deuxieme bureau,* or "second office." Some confide that their schedule becomes especially complicated when they have to fit in occasional visits to their *troiseme* (third) or *quartrieme* (fourth) as well. (Ungar, 1989:475)

Therefore, HIV infection may be higher for men of higher socioeconomic status. Several lines of evidence indicate that it is.

The diagnosis of AIDS among Africans was first made for professional men in Europe (Williams, 1992:7). Only the well-to-do can afford to go to Europe for medical care, and according to an informed French medical historian, the number of African AIDS patients seeking medical care in Europe began to increase around 1982 (Grmek, 1989:177). One study of men attending a STD clinic in Nairobi asked about travel and found that men who traveled to neighboring countries (and hence had the money to do so) were more apt to be HIV positive than men who did not (Simonsen et al., 1988: 277). (Barnett and Blaikie [1989:26] believed that the concentration of wealthier and higher-status men in urban areas is one reason urban HIV rates are so high in African cities.) Childbearing women in the Kigala study were more apt to be infected if their primary partner had an annual income of $10,000 or more (Allen et al., 1991:1661). Another study showed that pregnant women attending an antenatal clinic in Malawi were more apt to be infected if their husbands were of higher socioeconomic status (had eight years or more of education) (Dallabetta et al., 1993). Thus, although evidence is limited, it strongly suggests that higher-status men are more apt than lower-status men to be involved in a network of sexual relations. Accordingly, such men and the women to whom they are formally married may have higher rates of HIV-AIDS than their lower-class counterparts.[31]

Continuity and Discontinuity in Sexual Relations

Some authors emphasize that sexual relations in urban areas are extensions of tribal customs (Larson, 1989), whereas others remark on the discontinuity (Grmek, 1989:176). Both are correct. The foregoing discussion emphasized continuities. Of course, gender stratification is not as oppressive, and the transactional cultural custom affords women more economic independence in urban areas (Caldwell et al., 1989:217–218, 222–223). At the same time, economic factors restrain the number of wives men can accumulate. Nevertheless, the forces of gender stratification and the transactional element, on the one hand, and the forces of polygyny and masculine sexual ideology, on the other, complement each other in urban settings as they do in tribal settings. Greater emancipation from men and economic security, when viewed from women's perspective, are the continuation of polygyny (if only informally) and masculine sexual ideology when viewed from men's perspective. The sexual behavior of men and women in urban areas represents continuity with tradition rather than a sharp break with it (Larson, 1989).

Nevertheless, discontinuity is also evident. For over a century sociologists have written about various pathologies of urbanization, particularly anomie. Traditional rules that regulate individual conduct weaken, and crime, deviance, and various forms of personal and social disorganization increase. (For the classic statement, see Wirth, 1938.) Anomie is also a factor in HIV-AIDS in African cities.

Factors in a tribal setting limiting sex outside marriage include population size, the day-to-day routine of life in the village compound, and, for women, the restraints imposed by husbands and the close surveillance by their kin. In contrast, urban areas offer women more opportunities to earn money, including a wide range of sexual relationships. Williams (1992:1) observed that this represents a break with tradition since in rural areas sexual relations "are still regulated ... to a large extent by culture and religion."

Southall (1961:53) was more specific. He noted that as women move "out of traditional contexts [they] simply assert themselves in a practical manner, rejecting in their own lives the traditionally held male standards of women, choosing their own mates and supporting themselves independently." That is, women "demand for themselves the same standards of sexual behavior as they see practiced by most men." If men "obtain sexual access to numerous women, both before and after marriage, women as a whole see no reason to refrain themselves from complementary behaviour." (See also Caldwell et al., 1989:217.) (Observe the parallel with the demand by gay men for sexual freedom arising out of the gay liberation movement.) Urban sexual relations represent a weakening of tribal customs and a break with tradition.

Central to the process of deregulating sex is the way sexual partners are selected. In tribal society the selection of a marriage mate is typically a family decision (unless the man has the resources to pay the bride-price himself) made under tight tribal and village controls. The controls are weaker in urban areas. There are more "free marriages," and partner selection is "more a matter of personal choice than of family dictate" (Bledsoe, 1990:118; see also Caldwell et al., 1989:200). For example, free women are discriminating in their choice of sex partners. Grmek (1989:176) puts it this way:

> [With urbanization] a system of "free partners" replaced traditional polygamy. Since time immemorial there had been a great deal of flexibility in African sexual customs. Long-lasting unions had been unusual; in a lifetime women and men alike had multiple partners. But sex life had nonetheless been regulated in a way that, if it corresponded to no strict Christian moral code, was still no less constraining and hence considerably limited the genital transmission of pathogenic organisms. ... Liberated from the yoke of behavioral expectations imposed by the traditions of small village groups, the inhabitants of the big cities abandoned themselves heartily to elaborate sexual play. Urban prostitution, and still more the emergence of new categories of "free women" and single males, promoted a multiplicity of partners.

This discontinuity occurred in the overall context of what some Africanists call the detribalization process.

One aspect of detribalization is the erosion of tribal beliefs and customs, even as many urban Africans continue to identify strongly with clan and tribe (O'Connor, 1983:76, 103–109, 1991:57; Cockcroft, 1990:21–35, 89, 99–103). Another aspect is the weakening of intraclan and tribal ties caused by interaction with people outside the clan in the workplace, neighborhood, trade unions, cooperatives, occupational associations, and other groups. Social relations may depend more on common interest than common descent

(Little, 1965; see also Southall, 1961:31, 32, 35, 40, 41–45; Cockcroft, 1990:89–90), even though social ties to clan or tribe may continue to some extent in urban areas through clan and tribal segregation (Little, 1974:49–53; Lamb, 1987:31; Cockcroft, 1990:89, 99).

Similarly, tribal affiliation as a criterion in mate selection is less important. It is true that "feeling against inter-tribal marriage is frequently strong." But "less notice is taken when the relationships between persons of different tribes are extramarital," in which the criteria of physical attraction and social skills (flirting, charm) rather than tribal affiliation dominate (Little, 1973:77). The selection of sexual partners is individualized, and a laissez-faire attitude about sexual relations and cohabitation emerges (Little, 1974: 18). Sexual relations are detribalized to a large extent, and family-clan-tribal control over mate selection declines, as is the case with free women.

This change is significant for the transmission of HIV (as well as other STDs). If sexual partners, regardless of number, were all intratribal or at least limited to certain tribes, HIV-AIDS would be limited to one tribe or to a few. However, with an increase in the tribal mixing of sexual partners, the potential for HIV to be transmitted to many tribes also increases:

> Population movements [including rural to urban movements] in Africa contribute to the "sexual mixing" of various African groups and may be related to the spread of AIDS. ... It is probably significant that AIDS cases seem to have been present in large numbers in Africa only since the 1970s—a time frame that correlates with the intensification of urbanization and population shifts [and hence sexual mixing]. (Hrdy, 1987:1112–1113)

Urban practices of sexual behavior and of sexual relations thus represent both continuity and discontinuity with traditional tribal practices.

Both increase sexual activity. Traditional sexual relations have been extended (continuity), while restraints on partner selection have eased, and alternate forms of sexual relations have been added (discontinuity). All analysts agree that a wide range of loose, casual, and transitory sexual liaisons intertwined with economic motives characterize African cities, even though cities do vary in this regard (Iliffe, 1987:183–184). When urbanization accelerated in the African sex-positive culture, sexual activity also accelerated. As Shoumatoff (1988:155) observed, urbanization has been "a tremendous liberator of sexual activity," so that African cities are even more sex positive than traditional rural villages. In terms of the risks of contracting and spreading HIV-AIDS, the heterosexual sex-positive culture of African cities is not unlike the urban gay sex-positive subcultures in the United States in the 1970s and 1980s.

From Urban to Rural

As noted in the last chapter, one aspect of the urban-rural HIV-AIDS connection in America concerned gays who had been infected in urban areas, presumably through networks in the gay subcultures, returning to their rural roots to be cared for by kin. They might have also infected rural gays. The urban-rural connection is much different in Africa.

Even though sexual practices are more tightly regulated in village settings, polygamous behavior is still customary, so a high rate of HIV-AIDS would be expected in rural areas. Thus, a 1989–1990 serologic survey of fifteen villages in rural Uganda found that 8.2 percent of adults were HIV positive (and almost as many had had another STD in the previous six months) (Wagner et al., 1993), and HIV-associated mortality for the villages accounted for 89 percent of the deaths for persons twenty-five to thirty-four years old (Mulder et al., 1994). HIV-AIDS in rural areas has also increased in recent years (Anderson and May, 1992:581; Mann et al., 1992:35, 78–79; Williams, 1992:6; Piot et al., 1992:15). In areas such as the Rakai district in rural Uganda, the rate is as high as in the capital, Kampala (Mann et al., 1992:78). Significantly, a study of this district highlights gender stratification and masculine sexual ideology as major factors in the etiology of HIV-AIDS (Barnett and Blaikie, 1992:73–85).

But another factor is also at work. Urbanization includes the establishment of routes of transport that connect cities and towns with remote areas. Travel along these routes has taken HIV into these regions (Mann et al., 1992:78–79), sometimes by persons who return to their rural tribal roots to visit (Williams, 1992:1, 8). Then rural customs take over. "In the more remote villages, more traditional relationships based on beer-drinking and sex seem to be the norm, but it was not until AIDS had been introduced by travelling men, often of a higher educational status with cash to spend, that these traditional networks took the infection further into rural areas" (Barnett and Blaikie, 1992:78). Thus, although the high rates of HIV-AIDS in urban areas are due largely to the rural tribal traditions that emigrants brought to urban areas, the high rates of HIV-AIDS in rural areas are largely the result of people from urban areas taking the virus to rural areas where these traditions are still strong. The rural-urban connection in the transmission of HIV-AIDS has come full circle.

What About Homosexuality?

In the early 1980s some African leaders denied the prevalence of AIDS in Africa, saying the disease was an affliction of homosexuals and drug users, neither of which, they argued, existed in significant numbers in Africa. The claim about drug users is undoubtedly true; there is too little wealth in most African populations to attract much drug traffic. Differences between African and industrial nations in homosexuality may be much smaller, however.

Although some medical experts believe that in certain African countries, such as Kenya, homosexuality is uncommon (Kreiss et al., 1986:417), anthropological evidence suggests that homosexuality exists in certain regions (Gregerson, 1983:195–197; Serwadda et al., 1985). It may also exist in migrant labor camps and South African mines (Ungar, 1989:475). Williams (1992:8) contended, however, that it has not been observed or reported "as commonly accepted behavior" in these settings, though it may be common in prisons.

Insofar as there is a genetic component in homosexuality, and some evidence suggests there may be (Bailey and Pillard, 1991; LeVay, 1991; Hamer et al., 1993),[32] the component is probably as prevalent among Africans as other populations. But gay *subcultures* are not as prevalent. David Greenberg (1988:14) observed that anthropological and historical research shows that gay subcultures do not exist in nonliterate societies, such as the tribal societies in Africa. This, in turn, is related to the cultural conception of and societal reaction to homosexuality. In most African societies homosexuals are severely ostracized (Lamb, 1987:37; Chirimuuta and Chirimuuta, 1987: 103; Grmek, 1989:175). For example, in a 1992 debate by delegates to an assembly of United Methodists about accepting homosexuals in the church, a delegate from Zaire opposed such acceptance, stating, "We do not want our culture contaminated by what we believe to be a disease" (Waddle, 1992:D-1).

It is understandable, therefore, that African homosexuals would take great care to conceal their homosexual orientation, just as American homosexuals did (outside the gay subcultures) prior to gay liberation. Designated open meeting places for gays (bars, discos, bathhouses), not to speak of gay marriages, are virtually or entirely nonexistent in most African countries today. Men have sex with other men in more clandestine settings. But African men are obliged by their kinship unit to marry, sometimes to more than one woman, and to produce many children. As a result, men who engage in homosexual liaisons are apt to be bisexual (Padian and Pickering, 1986). After having sex with a male partner in an urban area, the man goes home to his wife or wives, with whom he also has sex. (The same pattern is suggested for Haiti, where homosexuality is also severely ostracized [Pape et al., 1983: 949].) A custom whose intent is to eradicate the "disease" of homosexuality may serve to facilitate the spread of HIV.

The Age of HIV and Social Forces

The foregoing makes clear that the pattern of HIV-AIDS in Africa, no less than the pattern in the United States, is interwoven with social forces. The patterns are different, of course, but this is because the cultural norms and social institutions that regulate sex are different. Nevertheless, some scientists reject this position. They assume that Africa is the origin of HIV and argue that the African pattern results because "the epidemic is simply further advanced" there (Anderson and May, 1992:59). As the last chapter showed, it is far from certain that HIV is more advanced in Africa. Furthermore, HIV may have emerged in Africa the way it may have emerged in the United States: by the interaction between a more virulent HIV mutant and the heightened sexual activity in the 1960–1970 period. In addition, it is a simple fact that polygamous sexual practices with deep historical roots in cultural tradition are widespread in African societies. So even if HIV *were* older in Africa, social forces and not the age of HIV would have caused the African pattern to be what it is.

Beyond this, an older HIV in itself would not account for some of the most significant aspects of African HIV-AIDS: differences between prostitutes and other women and between married and unmarried women as well as the relatively high rates for married women, the fact that HIV infection rates are probably higher among persons of higher socioeconomic status, and differences in urban and rural rates and the recent increase in the latter. Social factors account for these differences and affirm the validity of the cross-cultural perspective for examining differences between societies in the prevalence and sex distribution of HIV-AIDS.

Conclusion

The transmission of HIV among gays depends on the prevalence of certain types of high-risk behavior, namely, anal intercourse with multiple sexual partners in which body fluids are exchanged. Transmission in Africa also depends on the exchange of body fluids, but in penile-vaginal sex in which multiple partners are common. In each instance, therefore, the environment—the behavior of the host population—is largely responsible for the high prevalence of HIV-AIDS and its distribution between males and females.

But to focus on behavior gives an incomplete picture of the social etiology of HIV-AIDS. Polygamous behavior is an expression of cultural norms and social institutions. Among male homosexuals in the United States, such behavior is socially structured and given social meaning by social institutions and other aspects of the gay subculture that are related, in turn, to aspects of the broader society. Among heterosexuals in Africa, polygamous behavior is structured and given social meaning by the social institutions, cultural norms and beliefs, and gender stratification of the wider tribal culture. In both instances high-risk behavior is embedded in social forces. Such forces are therefore cofactors with HIV in the etiology of the AIDS epidemic on both continents.

NOTES

1. Research in the mid-1980s showed that a sample of African men with AIDS had had more regular sexual partners per year than African men who did not have AIDS (Clumeck et al., 1985:182), and longitudinal observations of high-risk groups in Zaire, such as prostitutes and men with STDs, "demonstrated rapid dissemination of HIV infection among individuals with multiple sex partners" (Piot et al., 1992:16). Reviews of studies based on samples of various populations of women (e.g., women attending STD clinics, childbearing women attending prenatal and pediatric clinics) indicate that having multiple sexual partners is a risk factor for HIV among women (Piot et al., 1992:17; Williams, 1992:5; for individual studies, see Allen et al., 1991; Plourde et al., 1992; Dallabetta et al., 1993). And case-controlled comparisons between HIV-positive and HIV-negative men and women matched for age and village of residence show that HIV-positive men and women have significantly more sex partners (Malamba et al., 1994).

2. As noted in Chapter 2, a high rate of STDs is an indicator of polygamous behavior (Mann et al., 1992:174; Root-Bernstein, 1993:301).

3. Anthony O'Connor (1983:57) stated, "In countries such as Brazil or India the term 'tribe' normally applies only to small groups who make up, collectively, a minor proportion of the national population: in most African countries it applies to almost everyone." In addition, individuals identify far more strongly with these units than with nation-states, which are simply artificial entities in the minds of most Africans (Cockcroft, 1990:31–35, 84–96; see also Lamb, 1987:11; O'Connor, 1991:57; Oliver, 1991:148). The boundaries of African nation-states are partitions drawn by the European colonists that divided the continent among themselves, which Roland Oliver (1991:184) called "a ruthless act of political amalgamation, whereby something of the order of ten thousand units was reduced to a mere forty" (see also Shillington, 1989:302–317, 333).

4. The colonialists emphasized that groups were divided by culture rather than recognizing that different groups had many cultural features in common. There was a strategy here. It impeded the development of African unity and facilitated the governing of indigenous peoples (Shillington, 1989:357–358). However, differences between groups derived (and continue to derive) primarily from kinship and clan rather than from culture (Oliver, 1991:185). Intertribal conflicts were (and are) primarily struggles between kinship systems and clans for political power or economic advan-

tage rather than struggles for cultural dominance (Shillington, 1989:357; Oliver, 1991:185).

This is not to deny the presence of cultural differences. For example, many tribes today have their own distinctive language or dialect. There may be 200 tribes and seventy-five different languages in Zaire (Lamb, 1987:11, 14), and 395 groups with "mutually unintelligible languages" are said to have been identified in Nigeria (Ungar, 1989:123). According to one estimate, all of Africa today "is inhabited by 2,000 tribes or ethnic groups, most of which have a specific language or dialect" (Lamb, 1987:xiii; see also Okri, 1991:58; O'Connor, 1983:57).

5. Other similarities in culture include submergence of individual identity and wishes to those of family, clan, and tribe; extended postpartum period; emphasis on tradition and custom rather than statutory law; ancestor worship; belief in animism and the idea that spirits permeate the natural and social orders; and belief in sorcery, magic, and witchcraft, especially about disease (Mair, 1974; Caldwell et al., 1989: 188; Cockcroft, 1990; Okri, 1991). Lawrence Cockcroft (1990:64, 21–35) argued that there is a common political culture in Africa that reflects "a consistent African philosophy or set of philosophies" with historical roots to the precolonial period.

6. Other forms of lineage do exist. In fact, Lucy Mair (1974:6–7, 41–46, 62, 65) stated that, although the majority of Africans are patrilineal, many of the societies (most of which have very small populations) are matrilineal, and a few have a double descent system.

7. Children's value for kinship-clan-tribe is reflected in the way bride-price is paid in some groups. An installment is paid up on marriage; the rest is paid when children are produced (children belong to the mother's kin until the second payment is received) (Davenport, 1977:140).

8. Like most generalizations, there are exceptions to this rule. Some groups disapprove of women taking money for sex even on occasion (Little, 1973:82–83). On tribal and ethnic differences in approving the acceptance of money for sex, see Little (1973:76–101) and Dirasse (1991:54–58).

9. In a comprehensive social history of prostitution, Vern and Bonnie Bullough (1987:13) devoted only one page to prostitution in Africa. They stated that prostitution is rare in societies that grant women a great deal of sexual freedom. Prostitutes have existed in some tribal societies, however. They existed in Addis Ababa when it was still rural and dominated by the traditional culture prior to Italian occupation (Dirasse, 1991:21–27). And in some Congo tribal societies husbands could force their wives to sell their services to strangers (Bullough and Bullough, 1987:13).

10. The extent to which the transactional element in sex is socially accepted and how it differs from prostitution may be seen from the following example. When divorcées or widows return to their natal families, relatives may expect them to pay for their upkeep by obtaining income from sex as well as by working in the fields and doing housework. Some anthropologists believe this shows that prostitution is an age-old custom in Africa (Fortes, 1978:22). However, Caldwell et al. (1989:218–219), among others, contended that this argument confuses prostitution with the transactional element in sex. Kin do not see the women as different but accept and integrate them in everyday activities of the household and village, like other women. In fact, the women "would have been mean-spirited to their relatives if they [did] not ... [seek] material assistance through sex for their upkeep" (Caldwell et al., 1989:218).

11. To deplore the high rate of HIV-AIDS is not the same as saying the practice is promiscuous. To call it promiscuous is to make a moral judgment, and such a judgment does not explain the practice, or even reveal the practice's tragic consequences for HIV-AIDS.

12. However, some groups strongly oppose premarital sex by females (Caldwell et al., 1989:198). Many Westerners believe that clitorectomy, which is practiced by a number of groups in Somalia, Ethiopia, Sudan, and Nigeria (Gregersen, 1983:106–107; Ahmed, 1991:115–117; Okafor, 1991:139), is intended to reduce the premarital sexual activity of females. However, it is not clear that this is the intent, or even the consequence, of the practice (Molnos, 1968:59–60; Gregersen, 1983:107). Some analysts believe the real purpose of the practice is social control. Mutilating and humiliating females keep them docile and subordinate to men (Cutrufelli, 1983:137).

13. For example, 60 percent of Buganda's gross domestic product comes from the agriculture-forestry-fishing sector. As Henry West (p. 3) wrote in 1972, land "is, and must for the foreseeable future remain, the primary source of wealth."

14. Marriages are exogamous, and a woman retains the clan of her birth. Since she normally returns to her clan if her husband dies, if she could inherit her husband's land, it would become the property of her clan, and the husband's clan would be the loser. (On Buganda, see West, 1972:108.)

15. According to some writers, the idea that African women are oppressed should be balanced by the fact that wives are valued and respected as mothers and members of a production unit (which is symbolized in the bride-price), have the security of being part of the husband's extended kinship system and being taken care of during old age, and are given considerable sexual freedom (Molnos, 1968:46–64; Sudarkasa, 1987).

16. Significantly, some societies that ostracize prostitutes do so because their sexual activity gives them independence, and it is their independence, not their sexual activity per se, that makes them deviant. Margaret Strobel (1984:99) observed that sexual freedom is central to the entire issue of equality between the sexes, which most African societies strongly oppose.

17. For example, in a study of prostitutes in Abidjan of Ivory Coast, Victor Du Bois (1967:8) stated, "African prostitutes lead remarkably bourgeois lives, which are not too dissimilar from those of their neighbors. Many of them have children; they are good mothers and consider themselves devout Christians. Certainly they do not look upon themselves as pariahs." Indeed, "a prostitute having [an automobile, expensive clothes, and money] will command far more respect from her neighbors than the more moral but less glamourous girl who has none of them."

18. In addition, in this study certain women whose sexual behavior involved a transactional element were not classified as prostitutes (Dirasse, 1991:1–15).

19. The informal sector consists of jobs that are generally not recognized by the government through regulation, taxation, minimum wage, etc.

20. Since the figures are for a sample of prostitutes from a household survey that excluded prostitutes who were streetwalkers, the figures for all prostitutes might have been higher.

21. It is not always clear how a prostitute is defined in these studies. Subjects have been women who were recruited from a "special prostitute research clinic" (Piot et

al., 1987), prostitutes who practiced "from their homes" (Plummer et al., 1991), and prostitutes from "an economically depressed neighborhood" and "from the bar of a tourist hotel" (Kreiss et al., 1986). Whether the definition of prostitute is based on an American definition or an African definition, which is a narrower definition, is not clear. As I noted, many African sexual relations involve a transactional element that many Westerners would consider forms of prostitution but that Africans do not.

22. The overall illiteracy rate in Africa is said to be about 75 percent, and only 11 percent of school-age children are in school (Lamb, 1987:21). The situation is worse for females, whose literacy in 1980 was only 61 percent that of males, and enrollment in primary and secondary school was 75 percent that of males (Sivard, 1985:23). The sexual difference is greater in rural areas, where girls are responsible for assisting their mothers in the field, fetching water and firewood, and caring for younger siblings.

23. Sometimes the fee is negotiated, but it is generally the same depending on the attractiveness and age of the prostitute (it may be as low as fifty cents per encounter for some prostitutes) (Kreiss et al., 1986:414). In some instances fees are set by associations of prostitutes (Du Bois, 1967:6–7; Little, 1973:100).

24. Lusakans refer to a similar category of women as "pleasure girls" and "fun girls" (Schuster, 1979:146–147). Dirasse's (1991:45–46) category, "free lance consorts" in Addis Ababa, seems to be similar to free women.

25. For discussions of the distinctions Africans make among different types of women who earn money from sex, see Little (1973:76–129), La Fontaine (1974), White (1983), and Schoepf (1992:266).

26. For discussion of the possible role of *femmes libres* in transmitting HIV, see Shoumatoff (1988:139–140, 167–172) and Grmek (1989:175–177, 179).

27. As high as these rates are, they are lower than the 70 percent for a sample of prostitutes from a poor residential district (apparently "street prostitutes") (D'Costa et al., 1985) and 64 percent for prostitutes from an economically depressed neighborhood (Kreiss et al., 1986).

28. Caldwell et al. (1989:218) stated, "If a prostitute is a female who sells sex commercially, charging standard rates on the spot on each occasion, dealing for the most part with strangers and making no emotional commitment, and operating from group commercial premises or a brothel that is primarily used for this purpose, then many of the women tested at clinics treating sexually transmitted diseases and described as 'prostitutes' in reports are probably not being accurately named."

29. In many instances the outside wives are legal wives who, along with their children, are marginalized by the husband; they are simply ignored and not recognized by the man, who allows them to fend for themselves (Bledsoe, 1990).

30. This survey, for fifteen rural Ugandan districts, showed that HIV seropositivity was 19.4 percent for thirteen- to twenty-four-year-old married men, much higher than for nonmarried men, though the number of cases was small. The infection rate for young married women was also high (17.3 percent). For men and women twenty-five and older, the rates for the married were lower than for the single and divorced (but not the widowed), though rates were still high for married persons (8.7 percent for men and 7.3 percent for women) (Nunn et al., 1993:83).

31. This could be due partially to higher-status men and women having better access to medical care (STD clinics and for women, prenatal and pediatric clinics) and therefore being diagnosed.

32. For a debate on the scientific evidence for a genetic component in homosexuality, see LeVay and Hamer (1994) and Byne (1994).

4. Trends in HIV-AIDS and Preventive Behavior

To this point I have examined the transmission and possible origin of HIV from three different sociological perspectives. In this chapter I deal with another aspect of HIV-AIDS—the rate of increase in AIDS in the United States over time—from the social behavior perspective. This perspective holds that when individuals are confronted with alternative courses of action, they choose the course that promises the most reward, benefit, or satisfaction.[1] Thus, according to this view, when people perceive that certain types of behavior reduce their chances of contracting an infectious disease, an increase in preventive behavior would be expected and would be reflected in the trend or rate of increase for the disease. The social behavior approach also maintains that in selecting one course of action over others, people are influenced by the cultural context. In particular, they are guided by social norms as they assess different courses of action, and with specific respect to disease, they are guided by norms of preventive behavior.

These two tenets of the social behavior perspective account for the overall trend in AIDS in the United States. They also account for racial differences in the trend and explain why, contrary to the predictions of many experts, a heterosexual epidemic of HIV-AIDS has not occurred and is not likely to do so. At the same time, they help explain why the heterosexual epidemic in Africa will probably continue.

The Trend for Total Rates in the United States

A few years ago many projections for AIDS in the United States were frightening in the extreme, with millions of cases being projected in the very near future (Fumento, 1990:302–303). Those making the projections included extremists, of course, but also esteemed scientists and experts in virology, infectious disease, and sexual behavior, whom Fumento (1990:349–363) called the "doctors of doom." For example, on April 19, 1987, noted Harvard geologist, biologist, and science historian Stephen Gould wrote in the

TABLE 4.1   AIDS Diagnoses and Deaths Thirteen Years and Older, as Reported Through December 31, 1992[a]

Year	Diagnoses	Annual Percentage Increase	Deaths	Annual Percentage Increase
Pre-1981	81		30	
1981	295	264	126	320
1982	1,093	271	441	250
1983	2,935	168	1,458	231
1984	5,956	103	3,372	131
1985	11,227	88	6,706	99
1986	18,267	63	11,669	74
1987	27,313	50	15,568	33
1988	33,578	23	20,043	29
1989	38,878	16	26,763	34
1990	40,298	4	28,683	7
1991	41,871	4	31,381	9

[a]Figures reflect reporting delays.
SOURCE: CDC (1993a:17).

New York Times Magazine about the "exponential spread of AIDS," in which AIDS "may carry off a quarter or more of us" (Gould, 1987:33). Alarmist projections are significant aspects of the societal reactions to the AIDS epidemic and are examined in later chapters. Here, I simply show that everyone making doomsday projections missed the mark by a very wide margin.

Nevertheless, the number of AIDS cases *has* grown rapidly. The CDC (1993a:17) has reported that 376 persons had been diagnosed as having AIDS and that 156 persons were known to have died from AIDS through 1981. Twelve years later, as of December 31, 1993, 315,390 diagnoses and 194,334 deaths had been reported (CDC, 1993b:12). By 1992 HIV-AIDS was the leading cause of death for males twenty-five to forty-four years old and the fourth leading cause for females in this age range (CDC, 1993d). Nevertheless, these rates do not even remotely approach some of the catastrophic projections being made just a few years ago.

Table 4.1 gives the number of reported new AIDS cases and deaths by year through 1991 for persons thirteen years of age and older. The numbers are for the years in which diagnosis and death occurred, not the years when they were reported. (About 20 percent of diagnoses were reported in the year after the diagnosis had been made [CDC, 1992:17].)

The annual percentage increase in diagnosis and deaths has declined over the course of the epidemic. For example, prior to 1981 there were 30 deaths; in 1981 there were 126, an increase of more than 300 percent. The percentage increase almost consistently decreased each succeeding year, and the same was true for diagnoses. From 1989 to 1990 deaths increased only 7.2

FIGURE 4.1   AIDS Diagnoses Through 1991 (Thirteen years and older)

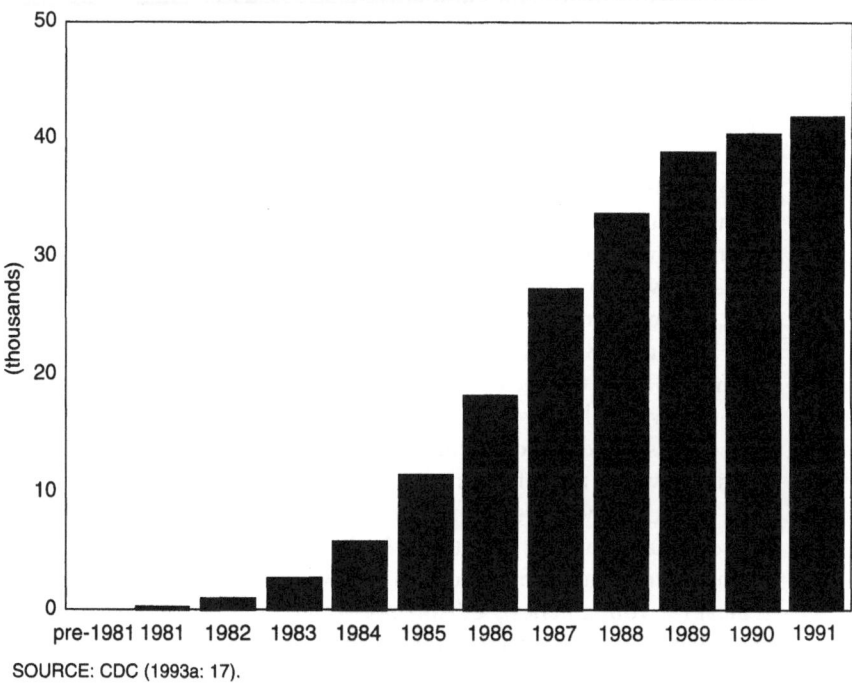

SOURCE: CDC (1993a: 17).

percent, and diagnoses increased only 3.7 percent. Numbers reported for the latest years are not complete because of reporting delays, so the decline in these years was probably less than the figures in Table 4.1 indicate. However, the slowdown in the increase extends over several years and may be seen graphically in Figure 4.1, which is for the diagnosed cases.

Table 4.1 is for total cases, not for the rate, such as the number per one hundred thousand. The increase in the rate has slowed more than the cases. To calculate the rate, the number of cases is divided by the total population and then multiplied by one hundred thousand. Since the population increased each year, the denominator is larger in later years, thereby reducing the rate relative to the total cases. And since changes in the definition of AIDS in 1985 and 1987 broadened the criteria for AIDS (CDC, 1990a:21), some of the increase in the number of cases reported in later years was simply definitional. Therefore, despite the reporting delays (especially for 1990 and 1991), the rate of increase for AIDS has slowed even more than that shown in Table 4.1. HIV-AIDS will not reach the astronomical level that some projected just a few years ago.

However, the human tragedy of this epidemic is not to be minimized; there have been many deaths, and many more will occur. In addition, even with reporting delays, the cumulative diagnosed cases in the three years from 1989 through 1992 still increased 106 percent and deaths increased 112 percent (CDC, 1993b:12). But, the point is that the rate of increase has decreased. From 1981 to 1984 the cumulative cases increased 2,875 percent (from 376 to 10,360 cases) but 1,470 percent from 1982 to 1985, 505 percent from 1983 to 1986, 648 percent from 1984 to 1987, and 220 percent from 1988 to 1991.[2] If the annual increase in the early 1980s had continued, the accumulative number of cases at the end of 1992 would have been far greater. The doctors of doom were obviously wrong.

Just how wrong is revealed in the only seroprevalence survey done based on a random sample of households in the United States; conducted by the NCHS from 1988 to 1991, the survey was reported on December 13, 1993 (Altman, 1993). On the basis of this survey, only about 550,000 eighteen- to fifty-nine-year-olds may be infected. However, because the survey was for households, it excluded people living in prisons, hospitals, and other institutions for whom the infection rate is higher than for the rest of the population. Also, many IDUs, from whom it was difficult to obtain a sample of blood, were probably excluded. And since a disproportionate number of young males refused to participate (a lower response rate to health surveys is typical for young males), a disproportionate number of gays may have been excluded. With these factors taken into account, the investigators believed that the actual number of infections may be closer to 1 million than to 500,000.[3] They estimated that the percentage risk of eighteen- to fifty-nine-year-olds having HIV is between 0.21 and 0.72 percent. Even 0.72 percent is far below the doomsday projections.

Why the Doomsday Projections Were Wrong

The trend may have been influenced to some extent by new drugs such as Zidovudine (AZT). AZT is an antiviral drug designed to suppress HIV and hence delay the onset of some AIDS symptoms. However, it works only for some patients for a limited period of time, and its overall benefits in delaying the development of AIDS and of extending life are questionable (Aboulker and Swart, 1993; Bartlett, 1993; Cooper et al., 1993; Maddox, 1994). The slowing trend may have also been influenced by saturation effects (percentages of people who have died from AIDS) for gays and IDUs, which reduced the number of them over time who could transmit the virus through high-risk behavior.[4] Conceivably, also, natural history processes were at work. The trend in Figure 4.1 does resemble the left portion of the bell-shaped curve that describes the course of an epidemic according to the natural history model. Dennis Bregman and Alexander Langmuir (1990) suggested that the AIDS epidemic will follow this pattern, in accordance with Farr's law. This implies the development of immunological resistance to HIV and, in the long run, perhaps genetic selectivity. However, there is no evidence that resistance to HIV has strengthened, and it would take several generations for genetic selection to unfold. (Genetic selectivity is complicated by the fact that many who have AIDS are exclusively homosexual and so do not pass their genes on to a new generation.) Other criticisms have been made of Bregman and Langmuir's view (Gail and Brookmeyer, 1990; Morgan et al., 1990). The primary sociological criticism is that it omits the role of behavior in the trend, specifically the reduction of high-risk behavior by gays and IDUs, which the social behavior perspective predicts.

There are several variations on the social behavior perspective, but all view individuals as behaving to maximize their outcomes, variously defined in terms of reward, punishment, cost, reinforcement (positive and negative), utility, values, disutility, alternatives foregone, and opportunity cost (Shaw and Costanzo, 1982:23–108; Ritzer, 1988:369–399).[5] The perspective has its origin in psychology and economic theories, but the sociological version emphasizes that most rewards and punishments are linked to cultural values and the opinion of others. Equally significant, social norms always influence how people seek and avoid certain outcomes, whatever they are. Sociologists have applied this perspective to several areas, particularly to social interaction (social exchange) (for an early statement, see Homans, 1961; for a review, see Cook, 1987) and to deviant behavior (Akers, 1987). The perspective also applies to the way people behave to avoid contracting an infectious disease. In general, as scientific knowledge of the causes of a disease increases, people modify their behavior so as to avoid getting the disease, an unpleasant outcome.

A Lesson from the Past

After many centuries at very high levels, infectious diseases began continuous declines in the West around 1750 (Eversley, 1965:57; McKeown and Brown, 1965:306; McNeill, 1976; McKeown, 1979; see also Douglas, 1976:174). These declines were not caused by medical care because few, if any, effective medical treatments and preventives existed then (McKeown and Brown, 1965). Many factors were involved, but in general improvements in sanitation and better living and working conditions gave infectious microbes fewer opportunities to thrive, on the one hand, and improvements in nutrition raised the immunological resistance of the population, on the other. Since the changes were gradual, the declines in infectious diseases were gradual. Suddenly, however, shortly after the formulation of germ the-

FIGURE 4.2   Life Expectancy at Birth for Massachusetts Males 1850–1910

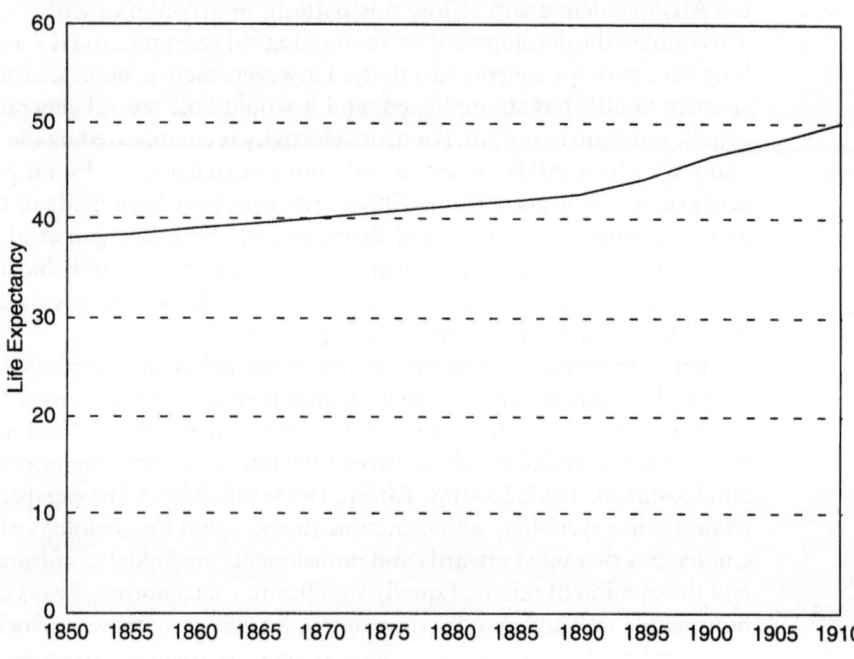

SOURCE: U.S. Bureau of the Census (1975:56).

ory in the early 1890s, mortality rates from infectious diseases began a sharp decline in the United States and other countries in the West.

Unfortunately, few data permit a comparison of rates of infectious diseases before and after germ theory was formalized. However, since most deaths were due to infectious diseases, trends in overall mortality and life expectancy reflect trends in infectious diseases. Thomas McKeown (1979:31) showed that mortality rates declined sharply in England and Wales in the 1890–1910 period, and Gordon Douglas (1976:161) revealed the same trend for Australian infant mortality, most of which was due to infectious diseases. Statistics on life expectancy at birth are consistent with the trend for mortality. Life expectancy for various years since 1850 is available for Massachusetts and is plotted for males from 1850 to 1909–1911 in Figure 4.2. Longevity increased gradually, from 38.3 years in 1850 to 42.5 years in 1890, for a gain of 11 percent. However, from 1890 to 1909–1911 life expectancy increased to 49.3 years, for a gain of 16 percent. In twenty years life expectancy increased about 50 percent more than it had during the forty-year period 1850–1890 (U.S. Bureau of the Census, 1975:56). The sharp change was not limited to Massachusetts or even the United States. Samuel Preston's (1976) statistical analysis of life expectancy for 165 national populations indicated that life expectancy increased significantly after the 1890s. The abruptness of the changes around 1900 strongly suggests that germ theory played a major role in these changes, which is what Preston concluded.

Germ theory led to the development of many drugs and vaccines, but substantial declines for most infectious diseases had already occurred before drugs for treating or preventing them had been developed (for the United States, see McKinlay and McKinlay, 1977). Most of the decline was due to changes in social behavior. In his study Preston (1976:82) concluded that germ theory led to "improved antiseptic practices, quarantines and segregation of infectious patients, and it gave impetus to the movements for cleaner food and water, better personal sanitation, and improved infant feeding." Once the causes of disease were identified, knowledge diffused quickly, and communities and individuals modified their behavior to prevent contracting infectious diseases. In terms of the social behavior perspective, the avoidance of disease was simply preferred to the contracting of it. On the surface such a statement is self-evident. However, more was involved than a desire to avoid disease. Cultural change also occurred.

With the ability to isolate specific microorganisms, scientists could use experimental laboratory methods to learn how to kill microorganisms that thrived in the community environment. Thus, for example, once it was discovered that chlorine killed the cholera bacillus, public officials could see that putting chlorine in public water supplies, which began in 1908 (Page, 1987:110), would produce significant benefits for individuals and the community. People realized that the benefits of less disease and fewer deaths outweighed the cost of taxes for water purification systems. Boards of health were established, existing ones were strengthened, and health regulations based on medical science were formulated. Scientific knowledge was incorporated in the political process and legal statutes (Rosenberg, 1962:213; Evans, 1987:495–496) and became part of the culture.

In general, then, people learned that changing certain habits to conform to norms based on science produced significant health benefits, as in boiling water to sterilize eating utensils, especially those used to feed infants. In other instances existing practices and habits were put on a scientific footing and given sharper focus. For example, quarantine, which had been practiced in the nineteenth century as well as during the Middle Ages and before to ostracize people who were diseased (McNeill, 1976:170; Murdock, 1980:18), was rationalized to prevent physical (as opposed to social and moral) contamination.[6] The situation was more complicated with sexually transmitted diseases, as historian Alan Brandt (1987) showed in *No Magic Bullet*. For example, although the causal agent of syphilis was identified and the delayed symptoms of syphilis were gradually recognized in the early part of the twentieth century (Lasagna, 1975:17), the way people viewed syphilis and other STDs was still mediated by moralism, stigma, and fear. Sex education was largely based on these attitudes (e.g., preachment about abstinence). Brandt (1988b:131, 1988a:369) believed that during the first half of the twentieth century education based on moralism and fear was generally ineffectual in directing sexual expression in the face of more powerful social and cultural attitudes. Since statistics on STDs are so fragmentary prior to World War II and the development of penicillin, which led to a sharp decline in these diseases, the effect of preventive sex education is difficult to assess. However, statistics are available for the military, and several points about them are worth noting.

Syphilis declined in the major armies of the West from 1860 to 1910. This could not have been due to an effective treatment, so it must have been due in large part to sex education (Lasagna, 1975:19). Since ways to kill the agent or impose barriers to avoid contact with it were not known because the agent had not been identified, education was probably based on moral preachments (e.g., for abstinence and against promiscuity) and fear. After the agent was identified and delayed symptoms were recognized, declines continued from 1910 to 1935 in the U.S. Army and Navy as well as in some states and municipalities (Parran, 1937:65–67). Brandt (1987:115–116) noted that chemical prophylaxis (application of a chemical to the genitals shortly after having sex) was the major factor in the decline of STDs during World War I. In addition, he observed that infection rates were kept low during World War II probably because of self-applied chemical treatments and the use of condoms (as many as 50 million condoms were sold or freely distributed to the troops each month) (Brandt, 1987:164). Instruction in and use of chemicals to kill STD agents and condoms to act as a barrier against them recognized that STDs are caused by infectious agents; hence these actions were based on science.

Therefore, even though moral attitudes and warnings may have impeded the effectiveness of preventive education among the troops, as Brandt contended, these attitudes did not altogether cancel out the effectiveness of science-based preventive efforts. And when chemical prophylaxis and condoms were not used, this may have been due as much to inconvenience costs as to resistance to moral preachment. (How general the preventive efforts were in civilian society cannot be determined, though attitudes and behavior in the military do reflect those of the wider society. Furthermore, members of the armed forces took preventive attitudes and behavior with them into civilian society when they were discharged.)

In general, then, as scientific knowledge of disease advanced, people learned more about the biological causes of disease, and they modified their behavior accordingly, though the choice between safe sexual behavior and risky sex behavior with respect to STDs undoubtedly posed a more difficult choice than that posed by so many other diseases. Therefore, germ theory was more than just another theory that guided scientific experiments. It guided community action and individual behavior, providing alternative ways to achieve better outcomes, namely, avoidance of disease and death. Scientific knowledge became social knowledge, a part of the culture. Preventive programs and behavior were accepted, and norms of preventive behavior were institutionalized in society. The same happened with HIV-AIDS, a fact that escaped the doomsayers.

Gays, IDUs, and Preventive Behavior for HIV-AIDS

Because of the prevalence of AIDS in the gay population, it was widely believed shortly after the epidemic began that the disease was somehow related to the sexual practices of male homosexuals. The exact mode of transmission was not known, but it was widely publicized that AIDS was transmitted through gay sex. Surveys indicated that as early as 1983 most gays in Chicago, New York, and San Francisco knew how AIDS was contracted, and interviews in 1984 revealed that many drug injectors in New York City and New Jersey knew that the cause of AIDS could be transmitted by sharing needles (Weitz, 1991:53). In an editorial about AIDS and "defensive living" in the June 21, 1985, issue of the *Journal of the American Medical Association,* Dr. George Lundberg expressed the hope that homosexuals would modify their sexual behavior. The closing of the bathhouses in New York City and San Francisco in 1985 eliminated settings in which much high-risk gay sex took place. To many gays, the closings symbolized a defeat in their struggle for social acceptance, a blow to gay pride, and a loss of the social relationships that bonded them to the gay community and the gay liberation movement. At the same time, the closings sent a clear message about what medical science believed: Certain types of sex that commonly took place in bathhouses were causally related to AIDS. In addition, as the scientific evidence about the mode of transmission emerged and was published in technical journals (Curran et al., 1985, 1988; Friedland et al., 1986; Sande, 1986; Friedland and Klein, 1987; Lifson, 1988), it was reported in the press and other media. Furthermore, medical authorities were reporting directly to the public through the media that HIV-AIDS could be prevented if homosexuals and IDUs changed certain habits (Fineberg, 1986; Lamb and Liebling, 1989). One can be sure gays and IDUs were paying close attention. Indeed, they had already started to change certain high-risk behaviors.

For example, a study of gay clients from an STD clinic in San Francisco showed that unprotected, receptive anal intercourse with nonsteady partners was twenty-seven times higher in 1978 than in 1986 (Stall et al., 1988: 878; Darrow, 1991:91–92). Answers to a San Francisco questionnaire administered to gays in 1983 indicated that for gays who had polygamous relations, unprotected, receptive anal intercourse had started to decline

(McKusick et al., 1985). Other studies in San Francisco, Chicago, New York City, and other areas in the United States indicated that the number of sex partners and the frequency of anal intercourse among gays decreased sharply during the 1980s and the use of condoms increased (CDC, 1985, 1991c; Riesenberg and Fishbein, 1986; Stevens et al., 1986; Becker and Joseph, 1988; Joseph, 1988; Stall et al., 1988; Fineberg, 1988; Winkelstein et al., 1988; Johnston and Hopkins, 1990:42; Sittitrai et al., 1990; Adib et al., 1991; Catania, Coates, Kegeles et al., 1992). European studies showed the same trend (Mann et al., 1992:382–383). By any standard the changes in behavior were absolutely dramatic. For example, in a cohort of 4,395 gays from New York City, the percentages engaging in sex with twenty or more nonsteady partners in the previous six months declined from 64 percent (1976–1980) to 46 percent (1981–1982) to 14 percent (1984); declines in receptive anal intercourse were from 80 percent to 73 percent to 46 percent (Stevens et al., 1986:2168). Ron Stall et al. (1988:878) referred to these changes as "the most profound modifications of personal health-related behaviors ever recorded" (see also Mann et al., 1992:381).[7]

Such changes were guided by an increase in knowledge about the way HIV is transmitted. In 1986 the surgeon general (U.S. Public Health Service, 1986a) along with the Institute of Medicine (1986) of the National Academy of Sciences issued reports recommending educational programs in safe sex. Such programs were too controversial for governments to sponsor, and the positive effect, if any, of those that were sponsored remains in doubt. But many volunteer community-based safe-sex educational programs already existed and were led by homosexuals (Goldsmith, 1985; Riesenberg and Fishbein, 1986), many of whom publicly repudiated certain sexual practices and the "fast-lane life" (Beauchamp, 1990:616). Even though systematic studies of the effects of these programs were not conducted, Bayer (1987: 226), among others, concluded that they "produced dramatic ... changes in the sexual behavior of gay men" (see also Langone, 1988:206–208; Lamb and Liebling, 1989; Patton, 1990a:41). In some communities public health departments developed partnerships with these grassroots organizations (Jonsen and Stryker, 1993:38). Since many of these programs were in operation in the early 1980s, a decline in high-risk gay sex began a few years before the annual increase in AIDS began to decline.

It was thus the gay community, with its cohesion and existing social institutions, that provided much of the preventive education. Sociologist and expert on gay subcultures Ken Plummer (1988:41–43) observed that as early as 1982 gays "had already made distinctions between high and low risk sex" and were "organized into a new culture of resistance" to prevent AIDS by advocating safe sex. Gay communities were socially equipped to do this. Padgug (1989:299–300) stated:

The speed with which gay self-help and political organization sprang up to meet the AIDS crisis, and the efficiency with which they achieved their aims, was a measure of the community's organizational and institutional sophistication. The gay community, and the so-called gay ghettos, had long since developed a wide variety of social, cultural, political and legal institutions—including a large number of newspapers and magazines—that could be enlisted in the fight against AIDS.

A social paradox thus unfolded: The gay subcultures, which were such a major factor in the etiology of the epidemic, were also a major factor in the slowing of it. In summarizing the role of the subcultures in Great Britain, Weeks (1990:246) wrote:

Here we can see an important paradox in the history of the epidemic. The spread of the HIV virus in the male gay community was obviously due in large part to the growth during the 1970s and early 1980s of the highly sexualized subcultures, where sexual contact was easy. ... But what on one level increased the risks of coming into contact with the virus, also provided the social infrastructure for coping with the epidemic. It seems likely that gay men in Britain began adopting safer sex before they had any direct personal knowledge of people falling sick with AIDS. The community had developed a sufficient maturity to generate its own forms of knowledge ... before outside agencies began to intervene.

Similarly, Patton (1990b:3) observed that "safer sex was above all a form of resistance developed by gay men acting in micro-networks linked by their own newspapers" (see also Patton, 1990a:17, 41).

Thus, gay communities developed their own knowledge of the cause of AIDS and later converted scientific knowledge into community knowledge. Gays did not wait for public health and other agencies to start programs that would educate gays in safer sex. Such programs, sponsored and implemented by nongays, would have been of questionable benefit anyway because of the moral attitude they would have conveyed about gay sex. Regardless, the changes in behavior were contrary to the stereotype that homosexuals would not modify their sexual behavior because they were so compulsively driven by sex.

Just as governments have been reluctant to sponsor programs on safe gay sex, they have been reluctant to sponsor programs in hygienic needle use. However, based on information from the media and the informal diffusion of knowledge in the drug subculture, drug injectors began to alter their behavior (illicitly purchasing sterilized needles, sharing needles less, and cleaning needles before use with bleach, hydrogen peroxide, or alcohol) before formal programs had even been proposed (Becker and Joseph, 1988:403–

404; Friedman et al., 1990:91–93; Des Jarlais and Friedman, 1994:85; Moss et al., 1994:225). Evidence reported by the CDC (1990c) showed a decline in risky drug practices for cohorts of IDUs in five cities from 1987 to 1989. In several cities annual increases in HIV seroprevalence began to level off in the late 1980s (in New York City it has been stable since 1983) (Des Jarlais and Friedman, 1994:85–86).

These findings were contrary to the stereotype that drug addicts were little concerned about their health, or if they were, their compulsive use of drugs deterred them from modifying their behavior. Even if IDUs did continue to shoot up, many of them chose safer alternatives when they shared "works" (Institute of Medicine, 1986:107; Friedman et al., 1990:93; Des Jarlais and Friedman, 1994:85–86).

Therefore, in general terms the response of gays and IDUs to knowledge about the way HIV is transmitted was not unlike the general public's response to knowledge generated by germ theory around 1900 about the way a variety of infectious agents are transmitted. Just as people started boiling water, avoiding infected persons, and engaging in other measures to avoid contracting or spreading cholera, typhoid, syphilis, and other infectious diseases years ago, gays and IDUs reduced high-risk behavior to avoid contracting HIV. Housewives boiling water in response to the warnings of general practitioners in 1907 may seem far removed from gays using condoms in 1987 in response to the counsel of gay bartenders. But from the perspective of social behavior, the processes were very much alike.

It is not surprising that preventive behavior increased, given the lethal nature of AIDS and the growing recognition that certain types of sex and drug use were high risk for contracting HIV. This proposition is self-evident today, but it was not just a few years ago, even among many scientists and medical professionals. Otherwise, many of the projections would not have been so far off the mark. Many analysts simply failed to realize that changes in behavior, not just a microbe and drugs, would influence the course of the epidemic.

Some extreme projections were based on what might be called the automatic pilot analogy. It was not uncommon to hear and read that AIDS was increasing at a "geometric rate," doubling every year (about what it was doing up to 1986), with projections of further increases to come. That people would alter their behavior to avoid infection and hence death was just not entertained. For example, in a book published in 1988 a physician simply declared that AIDS was a disease that increased geometrically and then stated that 250,000 people would die from AIDS in 1991 (Kurland, 1988: 55) (about 335,000 died) (CDC, 1994b:14). More sophisticated projection models were based on extrapolation (extending current trends into the future) combined with back calculation (working backward from the number of AIDS cases and taking into account the time it takes HIV to lead to AIDS).

Using this model in February 1990, the CDC (1990b) estimated that by the end of 1993, the cumulative cases of AIDS would be about 435,000 (390,000–480,000) new cases and about 312,500 (285,000 to 340,000) deaths. In fact, as of June 30, 1993, 315,390 cases and 194,334 deaths had been reported (with a much expanded definition for cases reported in 1993). These figures were better than automatic pilot projections but were still way off. One reason many projections were so far wrong was that analysts held stereotypical views of gays and IDUs and failed to recognize that many would change their behavior to reduce the risks of contracting a fatal disease.[8]

Erroneous projections were not due entirely to stereotypical ideas but derived also from a general misconception about American social behavior. Brandt (1988c:162) expressed pessimism about the future course of HIV-AIDS because he believed that sexual and drug use behavior do not conform very well to the "cultural logic" about American social behavior, which, Brandt argued, stipulates that people will modify their behavior if they are informed of the risks. This belief derives from an assumption "deeply ingrained" in American culture that behavior is "entirely voluntary." Brandt questioned the validity of this logic, at least with respect to sexual behavior and drug addiction.

Brandt's view, however, ignores another kind of logic underlying American social behavior—namely, that Americans more than many people weigh action that is emotionally driven or based on tradition and custom against action based on rational norms. They frequently choose the rational course. This applies to sexual behavior and drug use, even if less than to other types of behavior. As noted, many gays and IDUs have modified their behavior, and the increase in AIDS has slowed.

These changes simply cannot be explained by the biomedical model, which assumes that the epidemiology of AIDS and the slowdown in the rate of increase will be due to medical intervention (or processes of natural history). The social behavior perspective, however, does account for these changes. Certain types of practices associated with the gay and drug subcultures were cofactors with HIV in the AIDS epidemic, and by the same token changes in these practices led to the slowing of the epidemic.

How permanent these changes will be, especially for gays, is unknown. Because polygamous sexual behavior in gay subcultural settings was of more than erotic significance during the years of gay liberation and was socially meaningful and rewarding, producing a sense of gay pride and identity, social acceptance, and status, changes in high-risk sex may impede the achievement of the important socially rewarding outcomes that many gays derive in gay sex. Sex institutions may therefore return in some other form, such as "safe sex clubs."[9] Widespread relapses in preventive behavior by gays have been reported (Odets, 1994). Epidemiologists at the Center for AIDS Prevention Studies at the University of California at San Francisco fear a second wave of HIV infections has begun among gays in San Francisco. Indeed, statistics reported by the CDC (1994a:17) in June 1994 indicated that for all U.S. cases that had been reported through December 31, 1993, the percentage increase from 1991 to 1992 was greater than from 1990 to 1991. Evidence from gay therapists and gay focus groups,[10] as reported by *New York Times* reporter June Gross (1993), suggests that one factor in this is a desire gays have to be cohesive with the gay community. For some gays, AIDS has become a symbol of gay identity, or in the words of one gay, "the red badge of courage." Gross (1993:8) wrote in the *Times,*[11] "With homosexual identity and AIDS so interwoven, particularly in gay enclaves like the Castro [the gay community in San Francisco], some men said they were attracted to the idea of getting sick because it would deepen their sense of belonging." It is probable, however, that it is not contracting HIV per se but the way it is contracted that contributes to cohesion. Odets (1994:11), who noted that to gays the exchange of semen in anal intercourse is an aspect of social bonding, stated, "For a man who has suffered many losses personally or in broad identification with the gay community, contracting HIV [mostly through anal intercourse] is a way of sharing with those lost." If a second wave of the AIDS epidemic does occur, it may be due primarily to social factors associated with gay sex, just as the first wave was.

*Preventive Behavior and the Racial
Distribution of HIV-AIDS*

The slowdown in the epidemic has not been the same for all groups. In a 1993 report the National Research Council concluded "that the HIV-AIDS epidemic is settling into spatially and socially isolated groups" and concentrating "in socially marginalized groups" (Jonsen and Stryker, 1993:7). HIV-AIDS has always been marginalized, of course, because of its concentration in two ostracized groups. But, said the council, it has also increasingly become a disease of the poor, uneducated, and jobless.

Although few nationwide data exist for socioeconomic differences in HIV-AIDS, HIV-AIDS is disproportionately concentrated in racial-ethnic minorities in which large numbers of the poor, uneducated, and jobless are found; the rate is especially high for African Americans. African Americans have lagged behind white non-Hispanics and Hispanics in the slowing trend. Table 4.2 gives the percentage of AIDS cases by race-ethnicity from 1984 to 1992. As the table shows, the percentage of white Americans has continuously declined; of Hispanics, has remained more or less constant; and of African Americans, has continuously increased to 36.6 percent of all cases in 1992.

TABLE 4.2 Percentage of AIDS Cases Thirteen Years and Older by Race-Ethnicity[a]

Race-Ethnicity	1984	1986	1988	1990	1992
White, not Hispanic	61.8	60.1	56.1	54.2	49.5
	(2,678)[b]	(7,797)	(16,950)	(22,147)	(22,217)
African American[c]	24.9	25.3	29.2	31.3	36.6
	(1,095)	(3,281)	(8,813)	(12,794)	(15,505)
Hispanic	13.6	13.6	13.8	13.4	14.6
	(597)	(1,769)	(4,162)	(5,480)	(6,564)
Total cases	4,391	12,967	30,198	40,856	44,859

[a]Figures reflect reporting delays.
[b]Figures in parentheses are numbers of cases.
[c]The CDC classification is black, not Hispanic.
SOURCE: NCHS (1992:190, 1994:145).

Probably more ominous for African Americans are the results for group differences in HIV infection. In 1993 the CDC (1994a:22–23) began reporting HIV infection cases for states with confidential HIV infection reporting. Although states vary in HIV reporting procedures, for the twenty-six states that did report, 53.7 percent of all infections were for African Americans (there were no substantial differences by sex). Significantly, however, four states with large Hispanic populations (California, Florida, New York, and Texas) did not report, so the percentage for this group would not be meaningful. The omission of these states distorts the percentage for African Americans to some extent also (probably inflating it). But this omission would probably have no substantial effect on the African-American/white comparisons, and these show that of all such cases, 59 percent are African Americans (53 percent for males and 73 percent for females [CDC, 1994a:22–23]). Although the CDC (1994a:31) cautions that the HIV infection reports are probably not representative of all HIV infections, such results strongly suggest that the prevalence of HIV infections in the African-American population is extremely high relative to its prevalence in the white, non-Hispanic population. They also indicate that as HIV infections progress to AIDS, the percentage of AIDS cases in the African-American population will grow significantly beyond the 36.6 percent that existed in 1992.

The social behavior perspective on infectious disease anticipates this result. A number of factors are involved in the higher rate for African Americans, but significant among them is the fact that African Americans are the most segregated and rejected minority in the United States. As a result, they may not have been exposed to preventive educational efforts (formal and informal) as much as other groups. But a lack of knowledge is not the only or necessarily the most important factor. For example, a study of women attending a prenatal clinic found that almost all African-American women who were infected with HIV knew transmission could occur through sexual contact; yet they reported far more sexual partners than women who were not infected (Ellerbrock et al., 1992). Sad as this finding is, preventive behavior may be perceived as having less benefit to members of a very deprived minority, even if it would save their lives. Life is simply less rewarding, as the following comments of an IDU prostitute illustrate:

> Every day I risk my health, and my life for that matter, when I shoot up. Every time I go out to cop [buy drugs] I risk getting cut [stabbed] or even killed. Every time I'm strolling [walking the streets soliciting clients] at night, there are all kinds of crazies, geeks, thugs, and death freaks out there just waiting to carve up my ass. Now they say that if I use some dirty needle I can get sick, even die in a few years. So I care? I'm probably already dead. (Inciardi, 1992: 194)

The Trend for Heterosexuals

After the mode of HIV transmission had been identified, many analysts began predicting a heterosexual epidemic of HIV-AIDS. In examining this issue, I wish to distinguish among primary, secondary, and tertiary transmission (Fumento, 1990:78–83).

Primary, Secondary, and Tertiary Transmission

Primary transmission occurs when a member of a high-risk group infects another member of a high-risk group (through anal intercourse, sharing needles). Secondary transmission occurs when an infected member of a high-risk group passes HIV heterosexually to a member of a non-high-risk category, as when a male bisexual or IDU infects a female in sexual intercourse. Tertiary transmission occurs when a person who has been infected through secondary transmission infects a heterosexual through sexual intercourse (vaginal or anal). Most transmission of HIV is primary, occurring through gay-to-gay and IDU-to-IDU contact.

However, when it became known that HIV was transmitted through heterosexual intercourse in Africa, some concluded that this would be repeated in the United States. For example, the January 12, 1987, issue of *U.S. News & World Report* declared that AIDS was no longer a disease of certain high-risk groups but was "now a plague of the mainstream, finding fertile growth among heterosexuals" (McAuliffe et al., 1987:60); and six months later, on June 15, it warned that now *"everyone* is at risk" (Kramer, 1987:13; emphasis in original). In brief, HIV-AIDS was beginning to spread from high-risk groups to the rest of the population through secondary transmission and then between members of the rest of the population through tertiary transmission. (For an overall discussion, see Fumento, 1990.) The analogy of a domino effect was being suggested: gays to gays, IDUs to IDUs, bisexual men to women, IDUs to heterosexual sex partners, and heterosexual men and women to their sex partners.

The danger of domino effects and tertiary transmission was highlighted by the media (Fumento, 1990:78–83). For example, a segment of ABC's February 20, 1987, "20/20," entitled, "Now Sex Can Kill," stated that a bisexual man could infect a heterosexual women, who, in turn, could infect a heterosexual man who could infect any number of heterosexual partners. The use of the domino effect analogy was not limited to the popular media, however.

For example, in May 1992 scientists Anderson and May (p. 59; emphasis added), writing in *Scientific American,* argued that HIV-AIDS began with homosexuals and moved to drug addicts, among whom the epidemic had peaked, was now spreading to heterosexuals, and "pose[d] a serious threat to *most* sexually active adults." Similarly, William Johnston and Kevin Hopkins (1990:62) observed that except for exclusively homosexual males, all HIV-AIDS cases were heterosexuals, and they estimated that "at least 630,000 heterosexuals [were] infected with HIV as of the end of 1988." Whether heterosexuals had been infected through drugs or through some form of secondary transmission did not matter, they said. Many would still infect other heterosexuals through tertiary transmission—"no matter how they contracted the disease, [these people] can pass it on to other heterosexuals" (Johnston and Hopkins, 1990:61). According to this view, domino effects from primary to secondary to tertiary transmission had occurred on a wide scale, and HIV-AIDS was already "pervasive throughout the heterosexual community" (Johnston and Hopkins, 1990:63).

The NCHS seroprevalence survey for 1988–1991 refuted this assertion. And CDC data indicated that cases of secondary transmission from IDUs and male bisexuals were a very small percentage of all reported cases. Although 43 percent of all reported infected females thirteen years and older (through December 31, 1992) said they had had sexual contact with an IDU (1.8 percent of males), only 3.4 percent of all heterosexuals (male and female) reported sexual contact with an IDU. And some (perhaps most) of these transmissions may have been via needle sharing rather than sex. As for secondary transmission from bisexuals to females (through December 31, 1992), only 3 percent of all reported females (0.33 percent of all cases) had reported sexual contact with a bisexual male (CDC, 1993a:11). Thus, the frequency of secondary transmission through sexual intercourse is much less than many scientists and commentators have assumed.

And tertiary transmission is far less frequent. The CDC (1993a:9) reported that as of December 31, 1992, 16,254 heterosexual cases had been reported, which represented 7 percent of all AIDS cases thirteen years and older . When those who had sexual contact with IDUs are eliminated (possible secondary transmissions), only 3 percent of all cases are left. Then if persons who were born in a pattern II country (a high-risk category) are eliminated along with persons who had sexual contact with partners from other high-risk categories (birth in pattern II country, recipient of blood product, and, for females, bisexuals), only 1.3 percent of the cases (those classified as having "sex with HIV-infected person, risk not specified") were possibly infected through tertiary transmission. Based on 1990 census figures, this gives 11.8 cases of AIDS per 1 million persons from the fifteen- to forty-four-year-old age range (about the same for males and females). (Population figures are from U.S. Bureau of the Census, 1992:23.) Therefore, even though AIDS is a leading cause of death for all fifteen to forty-four-year-olds, the risk to heterosexuals who have no sexual contact with members of high-risk categories is extremely low, with tertiary transmissions constituting no more than 1.3 percent of all cases.

Moreover, tertiary transmission may be less than 1.3 percent because the category includes persons who are male homosexuals or IDUs but deny they are. Therefore, cases of apparent tertiary transmission may actually be cases of primary transmission. Root-Bernstein (1993:319–323) contended that if sufficient evidence were forthcoming for cases of apparent tertiary transmission (e.g., by more intensive follow-up interviews), the number would decline substantially. In addition, some of the cases may be persons who have had sex with IDUs or bisexuals (for females) but denied doing so; they may have been infected through secondary transmission. It is not uncommon for individuals to deny falsely that they or their mates engage in stigmatic and illegal behavior. Therefore, most cases of heterosexual tertiary transmission may be cases of primary and secondary transmission instead.[12]

In general, then, heterosexual transmission of HIV is extremely rare in the United States. When heterosexuals from high-risk categories as well as heterosexuals who have had sexual contact with members of high-risk categories are excluded, heterosexual transmission is rare indeed (Root-Bernstein, 1993:319–323). That the high proportion of female cases having sexual contact with IDUs were infected in sexual activity rather than in drug use is not clear. That penile-vaginal intercourse is *not* a serious risk factor for contracting HIV (in the absence of an STD) is clear. Most certainly, HIV-AIDS is not pervasive in the heterosexual population.

Has Heterosexual Transmission Increased?

Another issue is the trend of heterosexual AIDS. Some analysts note that the number of heterosexual cases since 1982 and the percentage of all cases that are heterosexual have increased. However, to conclude that this indicates the

TABLE 4.3 Percentage (Number) of All AIDS Cases Who Report Being Heterosexual and Having No Sexual Contact with an IDU, by Sex and Year, Thirteen Years and Older[a]

Year	Males	Females
1982	0.00 ( )	2.00 (10)
1983	0.05 (1)	4.96 (7)
1984	0.03 (1)	4.66 (13)
1985	0.16 (2)	5.93 (31)
1986	0.24 (19)	8.44 (84)
1987	0.36 (45)	8.99 (151)
1988	0.36 (99)	7.42 (226)
1989	0.45 (141)	9.41 (330)
1990	0.75 (283)	10.50 (503)
1991	1.10 (429)	12.67 (726)

[a]Figures reflect reporting delays and exclude persons born in a pattern II country.
SOURCE: NCHS (1989:84–87, 1991:112, 114); CDC (1991d:9, 1992:9, 1993a:9).

beginning of a heterosexual AIDS epidemic (Anderson and May, 1992) is premature, as Table 4.3 demonstrates.

The table shows that when persons who report having sexual contact with an IDU (which is by far the major potential source of secondary transmission) are excluded, annual increases in heterosexuals with AIDS have not been large or accelerating rapidly. (Note that figures for 1982–1988 and 1989–1991 are not based on the same precise categories. Figures from 1982 to 1988 [from the NCHS] include heterosexuals who have had sexual contact with certain high-risk categories, but figures for 1989–1991 [from the CDC] do not include this group.) For example, the number of males increased from 141 to 283 from 1989 to 1990, for an increase of 100 percent, but the increase from 1990 to 1991 was from 283 to 429, or 52 percent. The annual rate of increase is still high, and statistics for 1992 (as of June 1994 [CDC, 1994:8]) suggest it may have accelerated from 1991 to 1992. This is not clear because for 1992 the CDC included persons born in a pattern II country in the heterosexual category, whereas such persons are excluded in Table 4.3. Since about 14 percent of the heterosexual cases were born in a pattern II country in 1991 (CDC, 1993a:9), the increase in heterosexual cases from 1991 to 1992 may be largely an artifact of changes in the classification system. The general point is there is no evidence that HIV-AIDS has been exploding into the non–drug injecting heterosexual population the way many have assumed.

The trend through 1991 is presented graphically in Figure 4.3. A generally steep increase does appear for the latest years, which contrasts with the trend in Figure 4.1. The contrast is sometimes shown by placing a curve for total cases or for the two high-risk groups next to a curve for heterosexuals (usually including heterosexuals who were born in pattern II countries and who

FIGURE 4.3   Heterosexuals Diagnosed with AIDS Who Have Not Had Sex with IDUs
Through 1991

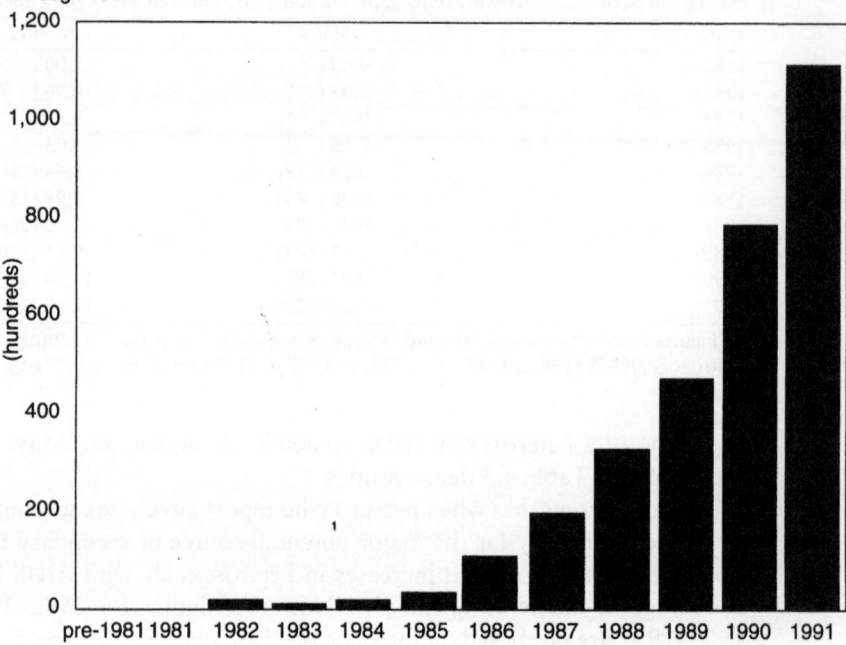

SOURCE: For 1982–1988, NCHS (1989: 84–87, 1991: 112, 114); for 1989–1990, CDC (1991d: 9,
1992a: 9, 1993a: 9); for 1991, CDC (1991d: 9, 1992: 9, 1993a: 9) and NCHS (1989: 84–87, 1991: 112,
114).

had sexual contact with persons from high-risk categories [CDC, 1991b:
360]). This highlights the fact that AIDS is increasing faster among heterosexuals than it is for total cases. But the contrast, alas, is not as great as the
comparison suggests because the scale for Figure 4.1 is one hundred times
that for Figure 4.3. When the trend in Figure 4.3 (for males and females) is
drawn to the scale of that used for total cases in Figure 4.1, a much different
picture emerges, as Figure 4.4 reveals. In comparison to the trend for total
cases, the trend for heterosexuals does not indicate that the increase is of epidemic proportion at all.[13]

At the same time, the trend from 1987 to 1991 resembles to some extent
the trend for all cases from 1981 to 1987. The number of reported cases due
to heterosexual contacts in 1992 was much higher than the total number of
cases reported in 1981, which increased rapidly in the following years. Nevertheless, even the *absolute* number of heterosexuals who were *apparently*
infected by sexual intercourse with non-IDU heterosexuals is still very low.
Although HIV-AIDS is moving into the overall population through secondary transmission and could conceivably be sustained through tertiary trans-

FIGURE 4.4   Total AIDS Cases and Heterosexual AIDS Cases Who Have Not Had Sex with IDUs Through 1991

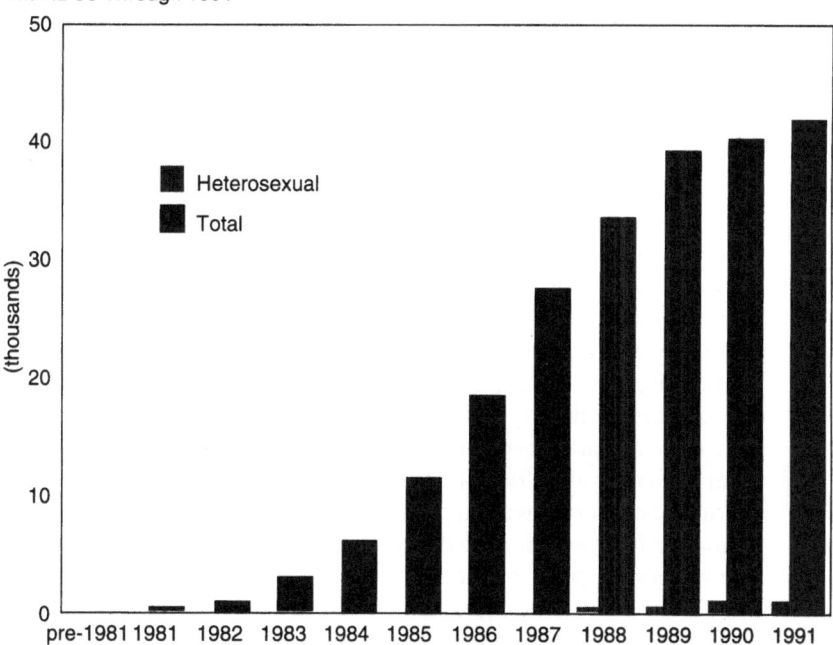

SOURCE: For 1982–1988, NCHS (1989: 84–87, 1991: 112, 114); for 1989–1991, CDC (1991d: 9, 1992: 9, 1993a: 9, 17) and NCHS (1989: 84–87, 1991: 112, 114).

mission, the number and the trend itself do not even suggest that we are in or on the threshold of an epidemic of heterosexual HIV-AIDS.

Therefore, statements that HIV is a serious threat to "most sexually active adults" (Anderson and May, 1992:59) are gross exaggerations. And claims that everyone is at risk or that "the heterosexual population is at risk" (Anderson, 1993:393) do not mean very much. True, the risks are not zero for anyone (neither is being struck by lightning); anyone could get infected if exposed. However, the chances of infection in male-female sexual intercourse are very low.

Why No Heterosexual Epidemic
Has Occurred or Is Likely To

There are several reasons for the lack of a heterosexual epidemic. One is that opportunities for secondary transmission from bisexuals are far less than some have assumed, and another is the difficulty of HIV being transmitted in penile-vaginal intercourse (tertiary transmission). (Both factors are discussed in the Appendix.) The role of the social environment, including normative sexual preference and preventive behavior, predicts that transmission of HIV among heterosexuals is low and will remain so.

The Social Environment and Normative Sexual Preference. By all accounts, polygamous behavior has increased since the sexual revolution of the 1960s, and having sex without being totally committed to a single partner appears not to be exactly rare in certain groups, such as teenagers and single adults. Adultery certainly exists. At the same time, monogamous relations are still the dominant norm by far.

In the most comprehensive national survey of American sexual practices yet conducted, Laumann et al. (1994:177) reported that only about 17 percent of eighteen- to fifty-nine-year-olds reported having had more than one sexual partner during the previous twelve months. Another survey found that only about 7 percent of adult heterosexuals had done so (Catania, Coates, Stall et al., 1992). Nationwide surveys consistently show that extramarital sex is very low: Laumann et al. (1994:177) found that only 5 percent of married persons reported having had a partner outside marriage in the twelve months prior to the interview, and Dolcini et al. (1993:210) found only 2.1 percent. Findings of other studies are similar: 0.5 percent of fifteen- to forty-four-year-old married women (and 3 percent of sexually active women) the previous three months (Kost and Forrest, 1992:248), 1.6 percent of cohabiting/married women eighteen to forty-nine living in twenty-three high-risk urban areas the previous twelve months (Grinstead et al., 1993:254), and 4 percent of married men twenty to thirty-nine in the previous eighteen months (Billy et al., 1993:56). In addition, Laumann et al. (1994:182) reported that many persons who had had more than one partner had had only one partner at a time. Another survey reported that when an outside relationship did occur (for cohabitors as well as for the married), it was apt to have been a "fling" or a onetime episode rather than a pattern (Blumstein and Schwartz, 1983:271–280).[14] It is clear, then, that, despite the loosening of sexual norms since about 1960, sex with single partners is still the dominant norm and the preferred choice for the overwhelming majority.

Several factors account for this social fact. In the first place, there is simply no general normative tradition of polygamous behavior in the United States.[15] People who have sex outside their primary relationship are regarded as deviants (as "cheaters"). Hence, affairs are apt to be costly in terms of guilt and social disapproval (e.g., ostracism, rejection by primary partner and others) if discovered. Many persons may dream of having multiple partners, but in the real world life gets complicated. Few people have the resources to manage a relationship with more than one partner while holding down a job, attending to various social commitments, and, for the married, assuming internal and external family responsibilities. The costs of time, energy, and (for men) money are high. And considerable care must be taken to prevent discovery (partners must "sneak around"). In short, for all but a few the costs of having multiple partners are too high a price for the pleasure that such affairs might yield. Monogamous heterosexual relations produce more satisfying outcomes than polygamous relations and are overwhelmingly preferred (Laumann et al., 1994:111–121, 546).

Consequently, even if HIV were efficiently transmitted in penile-vaginal intercourse (in the absence of STD), which appears not to be the case (see Appendix), the social preference for monogamy would contain the spread of HIV. Contrary to some alarmists, *most* sexually active adults are *not* in danger of contracting HIV, and a heterosexual AIDS epidemic is not likely. Polygamous relations through which HIV is spread in a population are simply not embedded in the social reward system of the United States and thus are not pervasive in the heterosexual population. To argue or imply that the trend of the HIV-AIDS epidemic in the United States will follow the African pattern (Johnston and Hopkins, 1990:69; Anderson and May, 1992) simply makes no sociological sense.[16]

Preventive Behavior. Sex is a powerful motive, of course. The doctors of doom imply it is so powerful that few people will change their sexual behavior even if they are aware that certain practices increase the risk of contracting HIV. In contrast, the social behavior perspective anticipates that preventive sexual behavior would increase. This, of course, is the aim of many safe-sex education programs. Although controversial, many safe-sex efforts in the schools and the media were launched in response to the AIDS epidemic. Even though few, if any, well-designed systematic, formal efforts have been made to evaluate the effectiveness of these programs, it would appear that safe-sex messages are getting through and that knowledge of the preventive measures that would reduce the risks of contracting HIV is generally quite high (Laumann et al., 1994:427–428). For example, one national survey found that condom use was higher among those who were at higher risk (had multiple partners), especially among young adults (Catania, Coates, Stall et al., 1992:1105). More compelling evidence comes from national surveys in the late 1980s and early 1990s in which respondents were asked specifically if they had changed their sexual behavior after the AIDS epidemic or after hearing about AIDS or in an attempt to avoid getting HIV-AIDS.

Laumann et al. (1994:434) found that nearly 30 percent reported making changes, and a nationwide survey by NCHS revealed that about 31 percent of sexually experienced unmarried women fifteen to forty-four reported one or more changes (Mosher and Pratt, 1993). Changes in several specific practices have been reported. As early as 1986, a Gallup poll found that 58 percent of respondents reported they or someone they knew was taking greater care in selecting sexual partners (Morganthau et al., 1986:33). In a *New York Times*/CBS survey, half the single adults younger than forty-five said fear of AIDS had caused them to change their sexual behavior, most frequently using condoms more and limiting the number of sexual partners (Kagay, 1991). A four-city survey of young urban adult heterosexuals found that nearly 50 percent reported changes, most commonly reducing the number of sexual partners and being more careful in partner selection (Melnick et al., 1993:584). It also found that heterosexuals who said they had a history of having anal sex, which is a risk factor for heterosexuals as well as gays, also reported more changes in sexual behavior, which suggests a decrease in anal sex (Melnick, 1993:585). And as the risk of anal sex is increasingly recognized, further decreases would be expected; this would be encouraged by the fact that few persons (1 percent of women and 4.1 percent of men) say they enjoy anal sex (Laumann et al., 1994:158; see also Root-Bernstein, 1993:316), and few engage in it on a regular basis (see Appendix). In addition, Laumann et al. (1994:198–199) found that men and women turning twenty during the period just prior to the AIDS epidemic were more apt than others to abstain from sex, which may be in response to the fear of contracting HIV. In a national survey of high school students, Roper Starch Worldwide reported that 83 percent of the students who said they abstained from sex gave fear of AIDS as a reason (Ingrassia, 1994:62). In sum, in surveys in which respondents are asked if AIDS has caused them to change their sexual behavior, a substantial proportion answer in the affirmative.

In addition, longitudinal studies that do not ask about behavioral changes and AIDS indicate that preventive behavior increased after the AIDS epidemic began. A study of seventeen- to nineteen-year-old single males in metropolitan areas shows that condom use at last intercourse had increased from 20 percent in 1979 to 58 percent in 1988 (Darrow, 1991:94). Surveys of college women in one university in 1975, 1986, and 1989 revealed that the use of condoms had increased from 12 percent, to 21 percent, to 41–51 percent (DeBuono et al., 1990). And a study in San Francisco revealed that IDUs had reduced their number of sexual partners from 1985 to 1990 (Moss et al., 1994:225), though other evidence indicates that condom use among IDUs may have increased only slightly, if at all (CDC, 1990b, 1990c, 1991d).

Finally, the social behavior perspective would expect secondary transmission to decline, and there is reason to believe that it has. Although no one can say what proportion of heterosexuals know the HIV risk identity of their sexual partners, as heterosexuals become increasingly aware that having sex with bisexuals and IDUs poses high risks of contracting HIV, efforts to avoid sexual contact with such persons would be expected to increase. In a 1988 NCHS survey of fifteen- to forty-four-year-old women, the changes that sexually experienced unmarried women most often reported to avoid getting

TABLE 4.4   Female AIDS Cases Who Report Sexual Contact with an IDU, 1990–1993[a]

Year	Number	Percentage[b]
1993[c]	2,833	45.3
1992	1,428	58.0
1991	1,291	59.1
1990	1,105	64.3

[a]Figures reflect reporting delays.

[b]Figures represent percentage of all females presumed to be infected through heterosexual intercourse.

[c]Figures are based on expanded definition of AIDS.

SOURCE: CDC (1992:9, 1993a:9, 1994a:8).

HIV were "Stopped having sex with more than one man" (16 percent) and "Stopped having sex with men I don't know well" (12 percent) (Mosher and Pratt, 1993:2). And the recent trend of reported AIDS cases for females may reflect women's increased selectivity of sexual partners. On the basis of CDC figures as reported by NCHS (1991:112), the percentage of all females who were presumed to be infected through heterosexual intercourse with an IDU was about 70 percent for each year from 1984 to 1988 (too few cases were reported for 1982 and 1983 to be meaningful). However, Table 4.4 shows that the percentage consistently declined from 1990 to 1993. (The numbers for the latest years reflect reporting delays and hence are underreports, but this would have no apparent effect on the percentages.) This finding suggests that women are indeed being more selective of their sexual partners and are avoiding IDUs more. Thus, many experts who predicted a heterosexual epidemic of HIV-AIDS, especially those postulating domino effects, ignored a basic sociological principle: When people view individuals and groups as threats or as somehow contaminated (physically or socially), they avoid contact with these groups. The cost of doing otherwise are too high relative to the rewards.

But if the rate of heterosexual transmission were to increase rapidly and heterosexuals knew persons who had contracted HIV through heterosexual transmission, the social behavior perspective anticipates further reductions in risky sexual practices and containment of the spread. Responses to the widely televised news in late 1991 that Ervin "Magic" Johnson had HIV are informative in this respect. Attendees at a Philadelphia STD clinic were asked if they had changed their sexual behavior after hearing about Johnson; 45 percent replied in the affirmative (were using condoms, had become monogamous or had reduced the number of sexual partners, or were more selective in choosing their partners) (Hollander, 1993). More convincing are the results of a study reported by the *New York Times* (January 19, 1993:A-7) and based on attendees at a Maryland STD clinic in which respondents were not asked if they knew about Johnson. Respondents reported significantly fewer sexual partners after the announcement than before.

In sum, evidence leaves little doubt that heterosexuals have been practicing safer sex to avoid contracting HIV,[17] which is exactly what the social behavior perspective would anticipate. Whether the overall increase in preventive behavior among heterosexuals is due more to formal safe-sex programs or to information gained from the media and other sources is not known, though the response to the Magic Johnson case indicates that changes do not depend on formal safe-sex instruction. Simply knowing the dangers of polygamous sex, anal intercourse, and having sex with members of high-risk groups is apparently sufficient to decrease these practices. The fact that knowledge about risks reinforces the rewards of monogamy (and the avoidance of anal sex) makes certain preventive measures easy to accept. A general heterosexual HIV-AIDS epidemic in the United States is not in the cards on sociological grounds.

Populations have generally responded to epidemics or potential epidemics in the past by changing behavior, and there is no reason to believe HIV-AIDS would be an exception, as considerable evidence has already shown. From the social behavior perspective, a major reason for the avoidance of risky sex behavior is that such avoidance is consistent with the rewards associated with dominant practices.[18] Note again that the investigators of the NCHS seroprevalence survey reported in December 1993 that only 550,000 of eighteen- to fifty-nine-year-olds (some of whom were no doubt from high-risk groups and therefore infected through primary infection) were infected with HIV. This undermines not only the projections of the doctors of doom in general but also the predictions of a heterosexual HIV-AIDS epidemic in particular. But this is exactly what the social behavior perspective anticipates.

The Racial Distribution of Heterosexual HIV-AIDS. Table 4.5 shows the percentage of heterosexual cases that are African American has been far in excess of their proportion of the population since 1984. (This high proportion appears not to be limited to urban areas and inner cities. Small communities [less than 50,000] with the highest HIV-AIDS rates for heterosexuals have disproportionately high African-American populations. For example, Belle Glade, Florida, where 77 percent of HIV-AIDS cases are heterosexuals, has a population that is more than 98 percent African American [Darrow, 1991:96–97].) That the percentage increased from 1984 to 1992 means that African Americans have not kept pace with the rest of the population in the declining rate of increase. More than this, Table 4.5 reveals that since 1990 the number of heterosexual cases who are African American (reported as blacks by NCHS) has exceeded that for all other groups combined.

TABLE 4.5 Percentage of Heterosexual Non-IDU AIDS Cases That Are African American[a]

Exposure Category	1984	1986	1988	1990	1992
All heterosexuals	41.1	47.9	48.4	53.4	57.9
	(56)[b]	(338)	(1,173)	(2,292)	(3,505)
Excluding those having had sex	42.9	41.2	37.2	46.6	54.3
with injecting drug user	(14)	(102)	(328)	(753)	(1,568)

[a]The CDC classification is black, not Hispanic. Figures exclude persons born in a pattern II country.
[b]Figures in parentheses are total number of cases.
SOURCE: NCHS (1992:190, 1994:145).

And racial differences in HIV-AIDS may be greater than the figures in Table 4.5 indicate. The table excludes persons born in pattern II countries, and almost all of these are classified as black (NCHS, 1994:145). Also, based on the twenty-six states for which HIV infection cases are available for 1993, the percentages of the two categories in Table 4.5 classified as African American (black) by the CDC (1994a:22–23) are 66.1 percent and 67.7 percent, with percentages higher for males than females (approximately 70 percent versus 60 percent for each category). Again, the differences are distorted to some extent by the exclusion of the four states with large Hispanic populations. But for African Americans and whites only, the ratio of African-American to white cases is about 3.7:1 for males and 2:1 for females (the ratio is the same for all heterosexuals and heterosexuals who have had sex with a drug injector) (CDC, 1994a:22–23). Since HIV infection occurs several years before the onset of AIDS, as HIV progresses to AIDS, heterosexual AIDS portends to be increasingly concentrated in the African-American population, continuing the trend shown in Table 4.5.

Several factors probably account for this. One is that, based on the responses of women, African Americans use condoms about half as frequently as white Americans (NCHS, 1989:52). In light of the poverty level of many African Americans, the cost of condoms may be too high relative to the perceived benefit. A higher rate of drug use among African Americans is almost certainly a factor, leading to a higher rate of secondary transmission from IDUs. Table 4.5 shows, however, that from 1988 to 1992 the percentage of African-American heterosexual AIDS cases who reported no sexual contact with IDUs also increased. The percentage of all heterosexuals (which includes heterosexuals who had sexual contacts with IDUs) who are African American also increased.[19] These statistics suggest that high-risk sexual behavior is more prevalent among African Americans. Several lines of evidence indicate that this is the case.

Survey data indicate a higher rate of polygamous behavior for African Americans—sex at an earlier age, more premarital and extramarital sex, and sex with more partners (Weinberg and Williams, 1988; Kost and Forrest,

1992:246, 248; Dolcini et al., 1993:210; Billy et al., 1993:54, 56; Lauritsen, 1994:868–869; Laumann et al., 1994:177). Survey findings for racial differences are not altogether consistent for women (Kost and Forrest, 1992:248, 249; Grinstead et al., 1993:254), but an African-American teenage pregnancy rate that is about three times higher than that for white girls and a rate of unmarried mothers that is about four times higher (NCHS, 1989:47) suggest that polygamous behavior is more common among African-American girls and women. In addition, rates of STDs, which are markers for polygamous behavior, are many times higher for African Americans. According to data reported by investigators from the CDC, in 1988 the rate of syphilis was forty-five times higher and gonorrhea about thirty-four times higher for African-American non-Hispanics than for white non-Hispanics (Moran et al., 1989), and in 1990 and 1991 the rate of syphilis was about *sixty* times higher (Webster and Rolfs, 1993:15).[20] (In light of these results, the 3.7:1 and 2:1 ratios for HIV are not surprising.)

How much these differences are due to education, knowledge of the consequences of sexuality, or normative environments is impossible to say. However, that the racial difference in syphilis is still substantial even after a number of risk factors (e.g., education, income) are controlled for (Hahn et al., 1989), and that African Americans have more permissive attitudes about premarital and extramarital sex than the rest of the population (Weinberg and Williams, 1988:200, 207–208), indicate that polygamous behavior and hence a sex-positive orientation are normative for African Americans more than for the rest of the population. That the proportion of women who have never been married and have children out of wedlock has been comparatively high for African Americans throughout the twentieth century also suggests a sex-positive tradition in which polygamous behavior is more socially accepted in this population (Preston et al., 1992; Morgan et al., 1993).[21] Some sociologists believe that this tradition is largely due to the cultural heritage of polygynous patterns in West Africa, the ancestral home of most African Americans (Sudarkasa, 1981; Preston et al., 1992; Morgan et al., 1993; Ruggles, 1994). Even so, to the extent that this is the case, the pattern is probably reinforced by sex-positive norms rooted in the poverty, drug subculture, and welfare dependence of the underclass, a disproportionate number of which consists of African Americans (on the original concept of the underclass, see Wilson, 1978). Normative differences in polygamous sex may be due as much or more to socioeconomic factors than to historicocultural factors. (Note that a high proportion of residents of Belle Glade, Florida, are farmworkers, the most economically and educationally deprived occupational group in the country [Rushing, 1972].) Certainly, more than a cultural legacy is involved since certain factors contributing to the persistence of high rates in Africa do not apply to the African-American pattern.

The Trend of HIV-AIDS in Africa

In contrast to the United States, the epidemic in Africa is not slowing down. The International AIDS Center of the Harvard School of Public Health, which estimated that about 8 million Africans were infected in 1992, projects that between 21 and 34 million will be infected by the year 2000 (Mann et al., 1992:105, 107). There are several reasons for the high number (Barnett and Blaikie, 1992:74–81), three of which are especially relevant to the social behavior perspective. These are widespread poverty, beliefs and attitudes about reproduction, and beliefs about the causes of infectious diseases.

Poverty and Preventive Behavior

In most African countries per capita income is less than $400 a year. In Kenya, Zaire, and Uganda, where rates of HIV-AIDS are especially high, per capita income is $290, $230, and $170, respectively (Ungar, 1989:521–542). Most household budgets have no room for condoms. In addition, poor living conditions make condoms inconvenient to use. "Crowded living conditions, the lack of running water and the cost of condoms themselves all represent obstacles to their easy acceptance" (Barnett and Blaikie, 1992: 162). To people as poor as most Africans, the rewards of condom use are simply not perceived to be high enough relative to the economic and inconvenience costs.

Sex, Reproduction, and Preventive Behavior

Reductions in fertility and polygamous behavior are hard to change because both are important to male and female sexual identity, gender superiority for men, and respect and economic freedom for women. Children are also economic and social assets, and reduction in reproduction would "deprive parents of hands needed to till the field today and care for the elderly tomorrow" (Lamb, 1987:17). Use of condoms may be resisted simply because the risks of infection may be worth the rewards of having children. In many instances reproduction may be the primary hold a woman has on a man. Therefore, "women married to potentially infected men may be willing to risk infection in order to have children" (Larson, 1989:728).[22]

Because of the cultural significance of reproduction in Africa, the use of condoms is a highly charged issue. For example, there is a widespread belief that persons "who die childless cannot be accepted in the spirit world by the ancestors" and are evil (Scott and Mercer, 1994:86). To use condoms would repudiate this and other long-entrenched religious beliefs. It would also challenge the growth of an individual's tribe. These are significant personal costs, which, along with other costs, inhibit the use of condoms. Consequently, other than some increased use by prostitutes, increases in condom use in Africa will be most limited (Larson, 1989:727). Thus, for example, Barnett and Blaikie (1992:45) reported that, although a few people in trading centers in the Rakai district of Uganda said they used condoms, the use in the district was virtually zero. Richard Green (1994:1) reported that, despite the millions spent promoting and distributing condoms in Uganda, in 1993 only about 3 percent of men used them regularly.

Rationalization, Faith in Science, and Rational Norms of Preventive Behavior

In the final analysis, to avoid contracting an infectious disease, a person must avoid the agent. Avoidance is best accomplished if the individual knows how the agent behaves (is transmitted). Since this is generally known only through scientific study, most effective preventive behavior depends on scientific explanation. In this sense preventive behavior conforms to rational norms of behavior.

In the United States and the West in general, the acceptance of the scientific interpretation of an infectious disease is almost second nature, and since people want to avoid disease, they modify their behavior in light of that interpretation. Exceptions to the scientific interpretation of HIV-AIDS exist in the United States, as later chapters show. Nevertheless, this interpretation stands in contrast to interpretations in Africa.

As noted earlier, interpretations of infectious diseases in the West have been dominated by germ theory since the turn of the century. The influence of germ theory does not come from the theory alone but from a general cultural belief in rationality, which is the central feature of the rationalization process that Max Weber (1964) wrote about three quarters of a century ago (Ritzer, 1988:120–130; Westby, 1991:404–440). Although many believe the term *rationality* is value laden and otherwise fraught with ambiguous psychological qualities—and Weber's conception also involves certain ambiguities (Ritzer, 1988:122–125)—the central idea in the Weberian framework is that the primary basis for behavior is technical knowledge or empirical evidence that certain actions are more effective and efficient in achieving certain ends than other actions. This is true for action in legal, political, medical, childrearing, economic, and other areas. (Even clerics attempt to systematize religious beliefs and make them consistent.)

For example, rather than trusting to chance and luck in making business decisions, the businessperson depends on cost accounting and calculations of market forces. Rather than trusting to political convictions in an election, politicians use polling and other data to learn the sectors of the population where they might best garner votes, and they mobilize their efforts and resources accordingly. Or rather than depending on superstition, divine guidance, and rainmakers in making decisions about cultivating and harvesting crops, farmers depend on fertilizers, crop rotation, and the weather forecasts of meteorologists. In the rationalization process, the scientific vision penetrates into many aspects of life (Ritzer, 1988:125–130). A generalized norm of rationality is institutionalized in society, and its influence as a guide for behavior grows relative to guides based on emotion, traditional myths, superstition, and religious beliefs. Rational norms become the legitimate way to seek rewarding outcomes and avoid negative outcomes; to many people, just behaving in accordance with rational norms (doing things right) is rewarding in itself.

It was against the background of this cultural process, which had been under way in the West for many generations, that germ theory emerged. Rationalization provided a cultural umbrella for germ theory (and medical science in general) and provided for its social legitimation. Just as the rationalization process changed behavior in business, agriculture, law, and other areas, germ theory influenced behavior in medicine and disease prevention. Throughout most of history beliefs about the causes of disease have been anchored in morality, mysticism, religion, and supernaturalism. People who got a disease were assumed to be cursed by the gods for violating cultural taboos or religious tenets or were being punished by evil human agents (sorcerers or witches), an enemy, or someone retaliating for broken contracts and promises (Ackerknecht, 1982). In time, beliefs in natural causes increased, but before germ theory, these beliefs lacked empirical proof. Treatments included purgatives and emetics (sometimes together!), bloodletting, foul-tasting medicines and herbs, and blistering, among other measures that, on balance, probably did more harm than good (Haggard, 1929). Treatments based on natural causes were as outrageous as those based on supernaturalism and witchcraft. Germ theory changed this. Rather than avoiding the wrath of God or the curse of sorcerers and witches, or being guided by belief in traditional nostroms and the doctrines of quacks and sectarians, people followed the advice of medical science, which guided them in how to avoid contact with infectious microbes. People did not adopt more rational prevention habits because they wanted to avoid disease more. They changed because the norms for avoiding disease changed.

As Weber noted, rationalization was a product of the West. It did not, and still does not, characterize most of the world, including sub-Saharan Africa, where "efficiency and rational thought processes don't have much to do" with day-to-day life (Lamb, 1987:226–236; see also Okri, 1991:144). Invisible spirits are widely believed to be the cause of the social and natural orders, and superstition is widespread and central in social life. Such beliefs are not limited to backwater rural areas; their validity is recognized by urban elites and government officials as well. For example, in 1968, because of heavy rains that destroyed people's fields, the government of Tanzania put five "rainmakers" in jail (Cockcroft, 1990:95).

Many Africans, particularly the elites, do trust scientific interpretations of disease and seek scientifically trained doctors when sick. But among the masses interpretations of disease are infused with beliefs about witchcraft, sorcery, and supernatural spirits (Patterson and Hartwig, 1978; Shoumatoff, 1988:28; Ranger, 1992; Green, 1994), though faith in the healing powers (mostly mystical) of various plants (e.g., herbs) and animal parts (e.g., blood) is strong, as it is in most nonliterate societies (Ackerknecht, 1971, 1982; Murdock, 1980). John Mbiti (1969:153) stated, "By far the commonest cause [of death] is thought to be magic, sorcery and witchcraft. This is found in every African society, though with varying degrees of emphasis." Many explanations of HIV-AIDS are no different and include supernatural forces, witchcraft, sorcery, sin, morality, or "moral misdemeanor" (Caldwell et al., 1989:225; Barnett and Blaikie, 1992:42). In South Africa some tribal doctors are said to believe AIDS is caused by "wizards" (Thurow, 1986).

Africans fear HIV-AIDS, but much of their behavior to avoid the disease is based on myth rather than science. Men in Uganda believe they will avoid the disease "if they pay women for sexual intercourse [and hence] propitiate one of the lesser gods, [which] if not properly placated, are well-known for activating the infection" (Barnett and Blaikie, 1992:43). Men also believe that marriage and pregnancy may protect against AIDS (Barnett and Blaikie, 1992:45). They may refuse to use condoms because this would "waste" or "belittle" sperm (Barnett and Blaikie, 1992:160). Many men are indifferent to the risk, have machismo attitudes, and may simply deny that they themselves are at risk, and some question whether AIDS is even caused by sex (Barnett and Blaikie, 1992:44, 61, 83, 165).

And when people do believe HIV-AIDS is contracted through sex, their reasoning may be based on spiritualism, which may actually increase, rather than decrease, the risk of infection. Groups in Zimbabwe interpret AIDS in a number of ways, but a survey found that about 25 percent believed AIDS is contracted through sex (Scott and Mercer, 1994). However, they believe that it, like other STDs, is due to *runyoka,* a curse that faithful marital partners put on their partners if they engage in taboo sex outside marriage. Since fear of a hex may reduce extramarital sex with taboo partners, *runyoka* may prevent the transmission of HIV due to philandering, but it does not deter a faithful partner from having sex with a philandering infected partner who is seropositive for HIV. The disease is perceived as due to moral failing rather than to sexual intercourse itself, so that being faithful to a philandering (and infected) partner is thought to guarantee immunity to infection (Scott and Mercer, 1994:86–87).

And even when beliefs about HIV transmission are accurate, myth and superstition may nevertheless lead people to engage in sexual behavior they know may cause infection, as in the cleansing ritual. Shortly after a man dies, a custom common in several African groups obligates the widow to have sex with a designated person, usually a brother of her husband, who, in turn, is obligated to have sex with her (Gregersen 1983:193–194; Barnett and Blaikie, 1992:156). This purges or cleanses the widow of her husband's spirit. If the deceased had more than one wife, the brother is obligated to cleanse them all. The hold of myth may be so strong that the ritual is performed even when a person knows that the designated partner(s) is (are) infected and that the risk of infection is high. A Zambian man who cleansed his deceased brother's two wives, both of whom he knew had AIDS, declared, "What could I do? I was bound by tradition" (Tierney, 1990a:A-1). Rationality told the man he ran the risk of getting AIDS, but disease and death weighed less than the reward of being ritually pure.[23]

Supernatural beliefs about HIV-AIDS also exist in the United States and the West but are fundamentally different from African beliefs. In rationalized societies such as the United States, the common interpretation of disease accords with the scientific interpretation that disease is due to natural causes. Supernatural interpretations are the exception. In contrast, the magico-spiritual interpretation of disease is widespread and ingrained in the culture of African groups, and the interpretation of AIDS is a specific manifestation of this general view. Thus, even though some Americans believe that God has a hand in HIV-AIDS, this has not deterred people, particularly gays and IDUs, from modifying their behavior to avoid contracting HIV. Unlike so many Africans who try to avoid infection by pleasing (and hence being rewarded by) the spirits or avoiding magical agents, the behavior of Americans is controlled more by the rewards that come from avoiding physical contact with HIV.

Conclusion

The trends in AIDS in the United States and sub-Saharan Africa are understandable from the social behavior perspective. All people wish to avoid disease. Therefore, as people have learned how HIV is transmitted, they have modified their behavior to avoid contracting the virus. But more than knowledge—even knowledge emanating from science—is needed. Although this is frequently sufficient in the United States, Americans who are marginal to society and do not enjoy the usual rewards of life have less reason to try avoiding HIV and other diseases. The same is true for the masses of poverty-stricken Africans. In addition, the value placed on reproduction and the beliefs in gods, spirits, and hexes may encourage high-risk behavior. It is thus not quite correct to say that "the rapid recent growth of the disease [in Africa] probably reflects the normal development of an epidemic" (Anderson and May, 1992:59). The statement has the tone of too much natural history, which ignores the effects of cultural norms and social institutions. It implies that there is something inevitable about the way the epidemic has grown in Africa (and that it will follow a similar course elsewhere as the epidemic matures). The epidemic in Africa has been and will continue to be normal only in the sense that it is sustained by behavior that is normal and rewarded in accordance with the beliefs and values of African culture.

NOTES

1. This view of humans as pleasure-seeking creatures is an old one but was not explicitly incorporated in sociological theory until relatively recently (Parsons and Shils, 1951; Homans, 1961).

2. That the U.S. Public Health Service (1986b) has not raised its estimate of HIV infections from the 1–1.5 million it estimated in 1986 indicates that the agency with the most information believes the increase in HIV-AIDS has slowed.

3. However, 76 percent of the respondents who tested positive were males, which is not much lower than the 87 percent that the CDC (1993a:9) reported for AIDS cases of those people thirteen years and older for 1992. Consequently, the proportion of respondents who were gay may not be greatly different from the proportion of the total population of eighteen- to fifty-nine-year-olds who are gay, though IDUs would appear to be underrepresented.

4. Just how devastating saturation effects may have been is suggested by a study of a New York City cohort of almost nine thousand eighteen- to thirty-four-year-old male homosexuals between 1978 and 1988. More than 10 percent died during that period, and the overall annual mortality was twenty-four times greater in 1988 than in 1978. Of those for whom a cause of death was identified, 75 percent of the deaths were attributed to AIDS, and for another 7 percent AIDS was listed on the death certificate but was not considered the primary cause of death (Koblin et al., 1992:649). Since the subjects were recruited from clinics, bathhouses, gay organizations, and largely gay residential areas to participate in a study of hepatitis B viral infection, the cohort may not have been representative of gays in New York City (not to mention the entire country). However, some estimate that 50 percent of the gay populations in San Francisco and New York City were infected with HIV in the mid- to late 1980s (Fineberg, 1988; Montgomery and Joseph, 1989; Eckholm, 1990c).

5. Some theorists argue that the effort to maximize outcomes is also rational (Heath, 1976). Another view of rationality is presented later in the chapter.

6. Reference here is not to the formal segregation of large numbers of infected persons but to the informal avoidance of sick persons and their dwellings. Formal quar-

antines of large numbers of people seem never to have controlled epidemics (Musto, 1986).

7. Johnston and Hopkins (1990:81) argued that the changes are deceiving because they were limited mostly to urban areas with cohesive gay subcultures (e.g., San Francisco, New York City, Los Angeles) and did not occur in places such as Mississippi. However, it is precisely in the places with vibrant gay subcultures that the HIV-AIDS rate among homosexuals is so high. In a nationwide survey of the sexual practices of eighteen- to fifty-nine-year-olds, Laumann et al. (1994:305) reported that on the basis of responses to a question about sexual identity, 9 percent of men in the twelve largest cities identified themselves as homosexual or bisexual in comparison to only 4 percent for the next eighty-eight largest cities and 1 percent for rural areas. And a high proportion of infected rural gays may have actually been infected while living in urban areas and returned home to die or to be cared for by kin (Verghese et al., 1989; Verghese, 1994).

8. Some projection models have incorporated estimates of behavioral changes (microsimulation models). However, because the estimates are far off, the projections, such as those by Johnston and Hopkins (1990:129–146, 183–210), are far off. Johnston and Hopkins (1990:83–85) used the the very flawed study of Masters et al. (1988) to derive estimates of changes (or the lack thereof) in the sexual behavior of heterosexuals. (For a criticism of the study by Williams Masters et al., see Zilbergeld and Evans, 1990; see also Fumento, 1990:259–263.)

9. How widespread safe-sex clubs are is not known, but they definitely exist in cities with lively gay subcultures, such as Los Angeles, New York City, and San Francisco (Krieger, 1992; Navarro, 1993c).

10. A focus group is a small number of individuals who are interviewed intensively to gain insight into the dynamics of attitudes and behavior, even though the group is not a representative sample of the population.

11. Unless otherwise indicated, all references to the *New York Times* are to the national edition.

12. For example, CDC (1992a:11) statistics indicated that 2.8 percent of 1981–1991 male cases were due to nondrug-related heterosexual contacts. However, the New York City Health Department (which employs a more intensive interview and reinterview program) found that through September 30, 1991, only 0.66 percent of adult male cases appear to have been infected through heterosexual intercourse (Kolata, 1991).

13. Furthermore, if the trends were for rates, in which the number of cases is divided by the population, the epidemic significance of the heterosexual trend would recede still more. The exact numbers of non-IDU heterosexuals, gays, and IDUs in the total population are unknown, but since the first group is much larger than the other two (from which most HIV-AIDS cases come), differences in rates would be much greater than that shown in Figure 4.4.

14. For example, wives who had engaged in polygamous behavior in the previous year "commonly had only one outside sexual experience" (Blumstein and Schwartz, 1983:277). Since the respondents in this study were volunteers from New York City, San Francisco, and Seattle, the results may not be typical of the general population, though they are consistent with surveys of representative samples as previously reviewed.

15. The Mormons are the only significant population in the United States for whom polygamy (polygyny) was ever explicitly sanctioned, and as a condition for Utah being admitted to the Union, they changed their social policy.

16. For the most part, features of African society that are so supportive of premarital and extramarital relations (see Chapter 2) do not exist in the United States. The contrast in normative sexual patterns is exemplified by the fact that alleged past sexual peccadilloes may derail an American politician's presidential candidacy and endanger his presidency, whereas many African political leaders are known for having plural wives, mistresses, and other sexual partners outside their formal marriage.

17. All the evidence is not positive, however (Kegeles et al., 1988; Darrow, 1991; Lewin, 1992). For example, a survey in 1991 found that men who perceived their risk of contracting HIV as higher than other men had sex only slightly less frequently than other men (Klepinger et al., 1993:79), and a survey of college women showed that the number of sexual partners and anal intercourse (which was rare) had not declined (DeBuono et al., 1990).

18. Nevertheless, HIV-AIDS does present special problems. The behavior through which a person contracts HIV obviously gives physical pleasure, and people infected with HIV do not experience ill effects until months or years after they are infected. Consequently, fear of infection probably does not deter risky behavior as much as for other diseases.

19. Because of the way data are reported by NCHS, figures in Table 4.5 exclude persons born in pattern II countries, most of whom are classified as black. This exclusion has no apparent effect on the percentages or trends in Table 4.5. The CDC (1994a:9) reported figures for 1993 in which heterosexuals born in pattern II countries were not listed as a separate category. Percentages for African Americans who are heterosexual remain almost the same (52 percent) as for 1992 in Table 4.5, though they increase slightly (again 52 percent) for heterosexuals who do not have sex with IDUs.

20. Trends from 1981 to 1989 showed that the rate was at least ten times higher for African Americans in every year from 1981 to 1989 and that the difference was greater in 1989 than in 1981 (Rolfs and Nakashima, 1990; Moran et al., 1989). STDs may be especially high for African Americans who use drugs. One study of African-American adolescent drug (crack) users reported that 41 percent had a history of STD (Fullilove et al., 1990). Laumann et al.'s 1992 survey also found that a substantially higher percentage of blacks report ever having had STD (Laumann et al., 1994:388), though the black-white difference is not as great as in the studies based on official statistics.

21. Even so, monogamy is still the normative ideal in the African-American population. For example, Michael Williams (1990:189) noted that, although "many types of romantic and temporal affairs [exist] between black men and their multiple partners, ... most women, if not the majority of men, still regard this as 'cheating.'" Findings of Laumann, et al. (1994:518–529) suggest that differences between black and white Americans in normative orientation toward sex may differ somewhat depending on gender.

22. Some anecdotal evidence and considerable political rhetoric suggest an apparently similar pattern of social rewards that encourages polygamous behavior among

African-Americans who are in the underclass. For example, in writing about life on a block in Harlem, *New York Times* reporter Felicia Lee writes that children "are valued here for the usual reasons, but also because ... babies [bring] a welfare check, a subsidized apartment ... or a way to keep a man." And "Many men see their offspring as emblems of masculinity" (Lee, 1994:A–14). While such behavior may indeed occur, anecdotes are not sufficient to conclude that the behavior is common; the behavior may be far less frequent than much political rhetoric suggests. I mention this pattern here only to observe that *to the extent that a pattern actually exists,* it is much different from the African pattern, despite the apparent surface resemblance. The American pattern would be part of a largely urban underclass welfare subculture built on socioeconomic forces, whereas the African pattern is rooted in a traditional tribal culture. For African Americans, the pattern might be partly influenced by African cultural heritage, as some believe, but it would be cut largely from the cloth of socioeconomic forces that are unique to industrial urban America and would affect members of the underclass regardless of race or ethnicity. So although social rewards associated with sex and reproduction in the African-American pattern would impede the adoption of preventive behavior, as in the African pattern, it would be anchored largely in social and cultural forces that are quite different from those in Africa.

23. Anthropologists have observed the importance of ritual purity or cultural (moral) purity in many nonliterate societies. This may be more important than physical cleanliness, even if it contributes to infectious diseases. For example, the Gopalpur in the villages of North India believe that leather is morally polluted, so they drink well water, which is often physically polluted, rather than water from taps and hand pumps because both employ washers made of leather (Khare, 1977:249).

PART TWO

SOCIETAL REACTIONS

The societal reactions to HIV-AIDS—to the way people with HIV-AIDS are defined and treated by others—constitute some of the most striking features of this disease. HIV-AIDS has been the most feared infectious disease since the emergence of germ theory and the most stigmatized disease in modern times. As with any disease, societal reactions to HIV-AIDS are not just a function of the medical definition and physical aspects of the disease. They are also a function of social conditions. In the next four chapters, I examine several different aspects of the societal reactions to HIV-AIDS in the United States as products of social conditions from four sociological perspectives: collective behavior, social construction, the sociology of science, and deviant behavior.

Although medical sociologists have been investigating societal reactions to disease since Talcott Parsons (1951a:428–479) highlighted their significance in his seminal writings on the sick role, they have given little attention to infectious diseases and epidemics. By contrast, historians have conducted a number of studies of societal reactions to epidemics of the past (Marks and Beatty, 1976; Mack, 1991; Ranger and Slack, 1992). The Black Death in Europe in 1347–1351 and the cholera epidemics in Europe and the United States during the nineteenth century have received the most attention. In the chapters that follow, reactions to these epidemics are compared to those to the AIDS epidemic. Such comparisons serve to show that the latter are specific expressions of general types of social behavior.

In historical studies the primary aim is to record a historical event (i.e., epidemic) in detail as accurately as possible. Unlike in sociological analysis, generalizing about the similarities and differences between epidemics, and about the causes of these similarities and differences, is a secondary aim, if it is an aim at all.[1] Nevertheless, historical studies provide good material for arriving at such sociological generalization. They reveal that two features are especially prominent in societal reactions to lethal epidemics: the fear of contagion and the social definition of disease.

Fear of Contagion

Because many infectious diseases may be transmitted in person-to-person contact, they have a social dimension that noninfectious diseases do not have: The sick may be feared, leading people to avoid contact with them. Noninfectious diseases are frequently feared, but no one fears getting them from *another person*. This is significant sociologically since those with infectious diseases and those with many noninfectious diseases are treated differently.

For example, in three nationwide polls in 1985 and 1986, respondents were asked the question, "Which two or three disease or medical problems are you most concerned about getting?" The most frequently mentioned condition was cancer (mentioned by about 60 percent of respondents), with heart disease next (in two of the polls, 31 percent mentioned this). HIV-AIDS was mentioned by only about 12 percent of the respondents (Singer et al., 1987:585). Nevertheless, people with HIV-AIDS are more apt to be avoided than persons with cancer and heart disease because, among other reasons, HIV-AIDS is contagious, whereas cancer and heart disease are not. (In 1985–1986 many thought HIV could be transmitted through casual contact.)

When an infectious disease affects only one individual or a few persons, the sociological significance of the fear of contagion is limited to its effect on those who are sick. If the disease is widespread and becomes an epidemic, the fear of contagion and its social effects are more widespread. Then, according to historical studies, a "traumatic shock on a societal level" (McGrew, 1965: vii) may occur, accompanied by extreme collective actions: massive migration; desertion, persecution, punitive quarantines, and ostracism of the sick; riots; and accusations that certain groups cause the disease (scapegoating) or that it is due to a government conspiracy (Zinsser, 1938; Langer, 1958; Marks and Beatty, 1976; Rosenkrantz, 1987:xiii; Ranger and Slack, 1992).

Such reactions do not appear in all epidemics, however. They occur only when four conditions are met: (1) the disease is highly lethal; (2) the disease appears suddenly; (3) the death rate increases rapidly, and many people believe the general population is in danger of contracting the disease; and (4) there is no apparent explanation for the disease. (These are similar to the four conditions for "the most radical responses" that accompany an epidemic as discussed by Paul Slack [1992:5–8].) Unless all these characteristics are present, an infectious disease is not apt to lead to collective fear of contagion and to extreme actions, even if it has devastating effects.

For example, in just a few months the Spanish influenza epidemic of 1918–1919 killed 20–40 million people worldwide (500,000 in the United States), yet there was little panic or extreme collective reactions (Marks and Beatty, 1976:271–277; Henig, 1992). Some consider this anomalous. In

America's Forgotten Epidemic, Alfred Crosby (1989:xiv, 322) observed that
the calm way people responded to this "demographic catastrophe" and then
forgot about it was an "odd fact" and "a mystery." Actually, Crosby told us
why: People had a ready explanation for this disease. The cause of Spanish
flu was known, and people believed they could take steps to reduce the risk
of infection. For example, officials in various American cities closed schools,
churches, theaters, saloons, and other places of public gathering; they had
city streets flushed nightly; and they urged people to wear gauze masks for
protection. In addition, a vaccine was available in major cities across the
country. Flushing streets, wearing masks, and being vaccinated were ineffective, of course, but few people knew this. They believed the measures protected them from the disease, and this "helped calm nerves" (Crosby, 1989:
74, 84, 100–102). People had an acceptable explanation for Spanish flu and
thus believed they could take steps to avoid it. (In Slack's [1992:5] terms the
disease was not a "novelty.")[2] This reduced the fear of contagion.

The AIDS epidemic meets the four listed conditions. Hence, societal reactions to this epidemic would be expected to have features in common with
societal reactions to certain previous epidemics.

Definitions of Disease

Medicine defines disease in terms of pathological neurophysiological processes that have natural (including emotional-mental and epidemiological)
causes. Many societies, however, do not define diseases by their biological
properties at all. Indeed, conditions that some societies recognize as signs of
disease other societies do not so recognize (Ackerknecht, 1971:21, 139–141;
Murdock et al., 1978:450). Some sociologists conclude, therefore, that
physical pathology exists only if a condition is culturally defined as a disease
and that disease has no meaning apart from cultural context.[3] Such extreme
relativism views the scientific medical conception as just another framework
for defining disease (Mishler, 1981a, 1988b); it is no more valid than radically different conceptions held in other societies.

Such a position is not tenable in this extreme form. For example, AIDS has
been variously defined as a gay disease, slim disease (in Africa), and a God-
inflicted disease. Such differences in definition do not change the underlying
biological reality. Regardless of how the physical state is defined, AIDS consists of a syndrome of physical pathologies deriving from an immune system
that has been impaired by HIV. But the point that people *respond* to their
definition of a disease rather than just to (and sometimes instead of) the
physical aspects of the disease is irrefutable. And that sick people have to
cope with the social definition as well as its physical aspects is also irrefut-

able. Most social definitions of disease fall in one of three categories: archaic, metaphorical, or medical scientific.

Archaic Conceptions

Through most of history people thought that disease was caused by spirits, witches, sorcery, and other magico-religious forces. This archaic conception is dominant in many nonliterate societies in the world today such as in Africa (Murdock et al., 1978; see also Ackerknecht, 1971:121–123; Murdock, 1980). Since in many instances archaic conceptions define disease as punishment for bad conduct and the breaking of cultural taboos (Hallowell, 1941; Ackerknecht, 1971:16; Murdock, 1980:26), disease is frequently viewed in moral terms. The sick person is considered responsible for being sick, and "blaming the victim" is typical. Action by witches, spirits, or sorcerers is the immediate cause, but the person who is ill is the ultimate cause.

Metaphorical Conceptions

Susan Sontag (1978) extended the archaic conception with the idea of "illness as metaphor." Sick people have frequently been (and continue to be) viewed as morally polluted. Their social worth may be questioned, and they are treated as deviants or despised outcasts, as lepers have been for many centuries.[4] Disease is a metaphor for morality.

Metaphorical interpretations of disease may reflect other aspects of society besides conceptions of morality. For example, hated marginal or outcast groups may be scapegoated and accused of causing a disease, in which case the disease is a metaphor for divisions in the social structure. But the general point is that as a social metaphor, a disease is interpreted in terms of a condition of society rather than of the biological organism.

The Medical Science Conception

According to medical science, disease is a biological phenomenon with natural internal and external causes over which the individual has little, if any, control. Since science aims for universal generalizations that do not vary by culture (e.g., the laws of thermodynamics are the same in all societies), definitions of disease vary less between societies where medical science provides the dominant conception of disease than in societies where archaic-metaphorical interpretations are common. The scientific conception is most apt to prevail in a rationalized society, but as anthropologist Richard Lieban (1977:21) stated, in scientific medicine "a recognized disease retains its identity wherever it occurs, regardless of the cultural context," so that the scientific taxonomy of disease serves as a "transcultural reference for diagnosis of disease." In the medical science conception, in contrast to the archaic and metaphorical conceptions, disease reflects biology more than culture (Ackerknecht, 1971:151).

Nevertheless, even in rationalized societies, societal reactions may reflect conditions of society more than they do the biological attributes of disease. Archaic-metaphorical conceptions may emerge and exert as strong, if not stronger, an effect on societal reactions to a disease than the scientific conception. Archaic-metaphorical conceptions have shaped the reactions to HIV-AIDS more than any disease since medicine was put on a sound scientific footing.

The dominant societal conception of a disease influences the way people react to it and those who suffer from it. However, reactions based on archaic-metaphorical conceptions have frequently accompanied infectious epidemics. Such reactions were not simply responses to a disease. They were also shaped by social conditions. Reactions based on archaic-metaphorical conceptions also appeared in the AIDS epidemic and were shaped by social conditions in much the same way.

NOTES

1. Some historians question whether valid generalizations are even possible. For example, in a study of the cholera epidemics in Russia from 1923 to 1932, Roderick McGrew (1965:12) contended that populations "did not react uniformly" in different places and that a particular epidemic must be treated "in terms of the particular environment in which it occurred." Other historians disagree. Slack (1992:5, 3) believes that, although historical studies show that societal reactions to epidemics "assumed a different shape in different social, cultural, and political contexts," studies also "show that the shocks of epidemics elicited very similar responses in very different historical and geographical contexts."

2. Another example of an apparent anomaly is leprosy. It has been highly stigmatized for centuries but has seldom led to collective panic reactions. This is probably because it does not usually appear suddenly and spread rapidly through a population and because it does not appear as a lethal epidemic. (It is not even mentioned in Geoffrey Marks and William Beatty's [1976] historical survey of epidemics, and only passing comments are devoted to leprosy in the compilation by Ranger and Slack [1992].)

3. For example, in *Disease and Civilization* Delaporte (1986:6) stated, " 'Disease' does not exist. It is therefore illusory to think that one can 'develop beliefs' about it or 'respond' to it. What does exist is not disease but practices."

4. Leprosy as a metaphor for social deviance continues today. One definition of leper in *Webster's New Collegiate Dictionary* (1977) is "a person shunned for moral or social reasons: outcast."

5. Fear of Contagion

A number of extraordinary reactions are associated with HIV-AIDS: The prevalence of HIV-AIDS has been wildly exaggerated; the fear of contracting HIV has far exceeded the reality of doing so; people with HIV-AIDS have been stigmatized, denied proper medical care, and brutalized along with members of high-risk groups; gay victims and their sympathizers, in turn, have disrupted scientific meetings and public hearings about HIV-AIDS; and some have even accused the government of genocide. To sociologists, these are forms of collective behavior.

Such extreme reactions to epidemics were common before the twentieth century. Therefore, in this chapter I describe collective behavior in past epidemics, especially the Black Death in Europe in 1347–1351 and the cholera epidemics in Europe and the United States in the nineteenth century, and I compare reactions to those epidemics to the AIDS epidemic. The purpose of the comparison is twofold: to show (1) that societal reactions to HIV-AIDS fit a general class of societal behavior and (2) that the social conditions under which societal reactions to the AIDS epidemic occurred typically lead to collective behavior and are not unlike the social conditions under which other socially turbulent epidemics occurred.

Collective Behavior

Collective behavior refers to emergent and extrainstitutional behavior rather than to institutionalized, routine, day-to-day behavior (Lofland, 1981:411). Dramatic expressions of such behavior—riots, widespread lawlessness, crowds, mobs—are called *elementary* forms of collective behavior (Lofland, 1981), in contrast to more orderly institutionalized forms, such as social and political movements (Zurcher and Snow, 1981). Since elementary forms are the focus here, references to collective behavior are to the elementary expressions.

Such behavior is precipitated by a new situation or by the perception of one. In all communities and societies most events are normally routine. Social definitions—the way people define the world around them—give everyday events their meaning. For example, in many small, simple societies of the past (and in many parts of the world today), much routine daily activity was defined in religious terms and viewed as expressions of God's will. In all communities everyday situations were defined in terms of beliefs, religious or otherwise, that people had in common.

Social definitions need not correspond to reality in any "objective" sense, but they do frame the way people perceive the real world and their reactions to it. Social definitions are analogous to a blueprint. For example, a common belief may be that people are poor because they refuse to work hard or because God wills their poverty. This belief guides the way many people perceive and treat the poor. People respond to the "social construction of reality" regardless of its validity (Berger and Luckmann, 1966). Such constructions make the world predictable and convey a sense of certainty.

Sometimes, however, events cannot be easily explained. For example, many infants are poor, but obviously this is not because they do not work hard. Then people may say these infants live in poverty because "God is testing them" or because "God works in mysterious ways." People may go to great lengths to stretch their definitions to fit the facts and thus make them seem normal. But sometimes an event is "to some extent defined as unordinary, extraordinary, and perhaps as unreal" (Lofland, 1981:413), and no social definition provides an understandable or acceptable interpretation for that event. Then the usual social construction of reality cannot adequately guide thought and action. The construction may be suspended, and people become uncertain about what is happening. This is "the beginning point of the possibility of collective behavior" (Lofland, 1981:413). If people believe the event is dangerous, strong emotional feelings, such as fear and panic, may be aroused and lead to extreme behavior that existing social norms cannot guide or restrain.

A homologous process occurs at the individual level. When individuals encounter strange situations, they may be uncertain and anxious, and they may lash out or act out of line with their habitual behavior. However, when a number of individuals encounter a strange or novel situation, crowds, mobs, riots, and other forms of collective action that are outside the norms of everyday communal life take place. "The idealized profile of collective behavior is ... unanimous [characterizing all members of the community] and maximum suspension of the attitude of everyday life [or the existing social norms] in a collectivity [is] combined with uniform and maximal emotional arousal and universally adopted extraordinary activities" (Lofland, 1981: 413–414). This, of course, is an ideal-typical formulation; it may never fit the expression of collective behavior exactly. It does, however, provide "a bench mark in terms of which we can gauge empirical cases we do see" (Lofland, 1981:413).

Collective Behavior and Epidemics

When a disease appears suddenly and its cause is unknown, it falls outside the usual interpretation of disease and the norms that guide how people normally react to those who are sick. Then if the disease is highly lethal and perceived to be contagious, and deaths increase rapidly, collective panic (fear of contagion) is common, and collective behavior of various forms may result.

In the idealized profile all members of the community would suspend their everyday construction of disease because it did not explain the epidemic. If the disease were perceived to be contagious, fear of contagion would ensue, which would lead all members of the population to act in extraordinary (extrainstitutionalized) ways. Rather than cooperating with others to solve community problems, people might desert families, flee the community, falsely accuse individuals and groups of causing and/or spreading the disease, and behave in other extreme ways.

This ideal-typical formulation may never fit reactions to an epidemic precisely. It is rare for *some* people not to find *some* way to explain the cause of an epidemic, *all* members of the population may not experience fear, and *everyone* will not flee the community, participate in riots, engage in mob actions, scapegoat individuals and groups for causing the epidemic, and so forth. Nevertheless, as with the generalized ideal-typical formulation of collective behavior, the preceding formulation "is useful as a domain-making approach exactly because it is so rare, and, as formulated, turns collective behavior [reactions to epidemics] into a variable, something that is ... a matter of degree in concrete instances" (Lofland, 1981:414). The pure case may never occur in the empirical world, but individual epidemics may be examined in terms of the generalized conception.

Reactions to different epidemics are never exactly the same and, as the next chapter reveals, one reason is that the social conditions under which different epidemics occur are never exactly the same. However, there are common elements in the reactions, and these elements are our focus here.

Records of epidemics in antiquity and the medieval period indicate that reactions to epidemics frequently fit the model amazingly well. According to Barbara Rosenkrantz (1987:xiii) and other historians, epidemics commonly led to widely disruptive actions. In a study of epidemics in ancient civilizations and the Middle Ages, Hans Zinsser (1938) described what he called the "secondary consequences" of epidemics, specifically panic, fear, and mass migrations. Widespread lawlessness sometimes occurred. For example, in the first recorded epidemic in the Western world, the Athenian epidemic of 430 B.C., Thucydides wrote about the breakdown of law and order. The epidemic "was responsible for ... introducing a greater degree of lawlessness at Athens. ... No fear of the gods or law of men restrained" the citizenry. The epidemic undermined the norms of everyday civilized behavior (Longrigg,

1992:25, 44). As Zinsser noted, and subsequent studies of individual epidemics affirmed, the reactions to disease were sometimes as socially disruptive as the disease itself, as reactions to the Black Death exemplify.

The Black Death

The plague bacillus that causes bubonic plague is transmitted to humans by fleas. The primary host for the bacillus is the black rat. Fleas then carry the agent from infected rats to humans, who are the secondary hosts. Persons who contracted the disease during the pandemic of 1347–1351 developed black swellings (buboes) the size of eggs in the armpits and groins, oozing blood and pus, followed by spreading boils, and the sick gave off a foul smell (Tuchman, 1978:92). Because of internal bleeding, the sufferers' skin was covered with black blotches—hence, the name Black Death, though it was also referred to as the Great Plague, Great Dying, Great Mortality, or, simply, Pestilence (Langer, 1973; Tuchman, 1978:101).

Interpretation of Disease and Fear of Contagion

How the black rat got to Europe is unknown, but it was probably brought on ships from the Black Sea area or North Africa to European Mediterranean ports. Regardless, plague spread across Europe as well as other parts of the world with devastating results. From 20 to 90–100 percent of populations in places from India to Iceland may have died (Tuchman, 1978:94). Historians and demographers today seem to agree that about one third of the world population perished (Tuchman, 1978:94; Cornell, 1982:200) and that it was one of the worst human disasters in history (Siraisi, 1982:9). According to one analysis, it ranks just below World War II, which is considered the greatest catastrophe in world history (Lerner, 1982:77).

Epidemics had wracked society for centuries, of course, and a variety of religious and other nonscientific interpretations existed to explain them. But the Black Death was too catastrophic for people to comprehend in terms of their existing beliefs (Langer, 1958:297; Cornell, 1982:65). For example, a common interpretation of sickness derived from the promise Christ gave his apostles that they would heal the sick, a promise that extended to the pope. The scope of the Black Death brought the validity of that promise into question since the pope, as one contemporary wrote, was "unable to stop this unhealthy air and heal the sick" (Wenzel, 1982:133). People were uncertain about the cause of the disease, and existing interpretations made no sense of what was happening. Italian poet Francesca Petrarca wrote, "Consult the historians; they are silent. Interrogate the physicians; they are dumbfounded. Ask the philosophers; they shrug their shoulders, they wrinkle their brows; finger to lip they command silence" (Marks and Beatty, 1976:82). Consequently, many adopted the view ("eschatological mentality") (Lerner, 1982) that the plague signified the end of the world (Tuchman, 1978:92–125). For example, Petrarca surmised that "the end of the world is at hand" (Marks and Beatty, 1976:82), as did another contemporary who wrote that he was recording "the extermination of mankind" (Tuchman, 1978:103). Rejection of everyday morality became widespread (Langer, 1973:109), and some contemporaries wrote of the general deterioration of moral beliefs in the population (Wenzel, 1982:132).

A number of interpretations of the Black Death emerged. Many people believed the disease was spread by miasmata (foul odors) and by air and water (de Venette, 1971:17). Some blamed the plague on earthquakes, which released foul fumes from the interior of the earth and hence were beyond the control of humans. Similarly, many physicians believed it was due to the movement of the stars, though the medical faculty of the University of Paris, after careful study, issued a report in which it acknowledged that the causes of the epidemic were "hidden from the most highly trained intellects" (Tuchman, 1978:102–103). But the dominant interpretation among the masses seems to have been that the epidemic was divine punishment. And because the disease and death were so widespread, they showed that God was unsparing in his punishment; all humankind was in danger. Interpretations emphasized forces over which people had no control, and this did little to alleviate the uncertainty. No one knew when he or she would be stricken or how to avoid being stricken.

Although most of the population seemed to believe that infected persons were stricken by God, many people still feared they could become infected through contact with the ill, and some believed that just being in the vicinity of the sick caused infection (Amundsen, 1977:403). (This belief was not altogether erroneous because the plague was contagious. Since it was spread by fleas, contact with a sick person or his or her dwelling or clothing could have led to the transmission of vectors bearing the bacillus. Also, if a sufferer was infected in the lungs [pneumonic plague], others could have become infected by breathing droplets of his or her breath, as when that person sneezed, coughed, or simply breathed.) Some believed that infection could occur simply by looking at someone with plague (Tuchman, 1978:102). According to one anonymous Flemish cleric in Avignon, it was "the most terrible of all the terrors" (Tuchman, 1978:102). Fear of contagion was rampant.

Reactions to Fear

As with any historical event, descriptions of collective reactions to the Black Death are incomplete. Nevertheless, enough is known to identify certain extreme reactions, including avoidance and desertion of sufferers, massive flight from communities, riots and lawlessness, self-flagellation, and scapegoating of groups, which became targets of violence (Risse, 1988).

Contempories from Florence and Sienna wrote about people deserting members of their families and other relatives (Boccaccio, 1971:10–11; del Grasso, 1971:13). In summarizing the historical record, historians Darrel Amundsen (1977) and Barbara Tuchman (1978:97) reported that desertion of family members was widespread and that many community officials left their posts and fled to rural areas.

Social order was imperiled. The writings of contemporary chroniclers of Florence (del Grasso, 1971:14) and Paris (de Venette, 1971:15) indicated that riots and lawlessness were rampant.[1] Tuchman (1978:100–101) wrote about "lawlessness and debauchery," and in a general review of the historical evidence on reactions to epidemics, including the Black Death, historian William Langer (1958:293–294) stated that during such periods murdering the sick and looting their homes were common. Self-flagellation was also widespread (Cartwright, 1972:46–47; Tuchman, 1978:114–115). "Organized groups of 200 to 300 and sometimes more (the chroniclers mention up to 1,000) marched from city to city, stripped to the waist, scourging themselves with leather whips tipped with iron spikes until they bled" (Tuchman, 1978:144). But scapegoating was the most well-known reaction.

For centuries there had been no scarcity of scapegoats for epidemics. The Spartans were accused by the Athenians of poisoning their wells during the Athenian epidemic, and lepers and Jews, in a perceived conspiracy to destroy Christianity, were accused of poisoning wells during epidemics in Europe, as in Bohemia in the twelfth century (Newall, 1973:118; Tuchman, 1978:109). During the Black Death, Jews were again accused of poisoning wells. Other groups also came under suspicion, such as nobles and cripples (Cartwright, 1972:46). People considered to be witches and human agents of Satan were identified as causes, and in Genoa such persons were persecuted for bringing the plague to that city (Langer, 1973:109–110). Even physicians were accused of spreading the disease, and some were stoned (Langer, 1973:110). But the Jews were the primary scapegoats, and a reign of terror was directed against them. They were lynched and burned by the thousands in communities across Europe (Ziegler, 1969:84–109; de Venette, 1971:16; Cartwright, 1972:46; Tuchman, 1978:109–111).

To conclude, the Black Death appeared suddenly, caused many deaths, and was believed to be contagious. Existing beliefs about disease could not explain it. These are the conditions under which fear of contagion and extreme reactions to an epidemic would be expected to occur, and they did on a wide scale.[2]

The Cholera Epidemics of the Early Nineteenth Century

For a person to contract cholera, the cholera bacillus must enter the alimentary tract, as when he or she drinks contaminated water or other fluids, eats contaminated fish, or consumes fruits and vegetables that have been washed in contaminated water or derived from plants that have been fertilized with excrement. Since the bacillus breeds in human excreta, it is primarily waterborne, and epidemics typically occur when the bacillus contaminates the community water supply. (Infection may also pass directly from person to person, as, for example, when one person touches her or his lips after having handled the unsterilized bedding or underclothes of an infected person and the bacillus migrates to the alimentary track.) Once infected, untreated sufferers typically develop a high fever, experience severe burning in the stomach, have convulsions and experience severe diarrhea, and become dehydrated. Swift death may result.

Cholera epidemics occurred in the late eighteenth century in India (McGrew, 1965:18–19; Marks and Beatty, 1976:192), and cholera may have appeared in Asia for centuries before then. Several epidemics raged through Russia, western Europe, England, and the United States in the early nineteenth century, around midcentury, and again in the latter part of the century, causing many deaths. There are several well-documented descriptions of societal reactions to these epidemics, for the United States in 1832, 1949, and 1966 (Rosenberg, 1959, 1962) and Europe then as well as other times (Briggs, 1961; Morris, 1976; Durey 1979; Delaporte, 1986; Evans, 1987, 1992; see also Marks and Beatty, 1976:191–212). The first ones occurred in Russia in 1823–1832 (McGrew, 1960, 1962, 1965) and the last one in Hamburg, Germany, in 1892 (Evans, 1987). All accounts agree that the epidemics caused panic and massive fear that were related to the failure of existing beliefs to explain what was happening.[3]

Interpretation of Disease and Fear of Contagion

In the nineteenth century infectious diseases were still the major causes of death, with tuberculosis the biggest killer.[4] Mortality rates were still high but had been declining since the mid-eighteenth century. Although statistics were not generally available at the time, people were aware that devastating epidemics had been declining. The Black Death was a distant memory, and the last plague epidemic occurred in 1665 in London. Many in the West believed that progress and civilization ("Western superiority") had eliminated most of the conditions that caused infectious epidemics. As for cholera, it was considered a disease of the uncivilized nations of the East and thus posed little threat to countries in the West (Delaporte 1986:1–14, 16–17, 97–106).

Although few medical ideas were valid (Delaporte, 1986:197), doctors held strongly to certain beliefs about the causes of disease. Theories stipulated such causes as topography, climate, body humors, and atmospheric phenomena (Delaporte, 1986:97–107, 115–137, 149–163). Two theories were especially prominent: miasma theory and contagionism or infectionism (Dowling, 1977:7).

Miasma theory stipulated that disease emanated from noxious smells and foul odors generated by decaying and rotting organic matter, with major sources being areas of poor drainage (e.g., swamps), human waste accumulation (e.g., cesspools), and garbage and dead animals in public areas (e.g., streets). Contagionism contended that disease was caused by person-to-person contact. The doctrine of predisposing causes, a corollary to both, held that certain individuals were particularly vulnerable to the influence of miasmata or contagion (or other factors) because of diet, overwork, intemperance and immorality, poor living conditions that were somehow translated into biological conditions (Delaporte, 1986:95), or simply "obscure internal states" (McGrew, 1965:44).

Miasma theory and infectionism left much unexplained (Delaporte, 1986: 177–189). Nevertheless, most physicians and government authorities were convinced these theories accounted for the causes of disease, which ostensibly had been largely eliminated with the progress of Western civilization. This was particularly true for a disease like cholera, which originated in the East. Even though outbreaks of cholera had occurred in European Russia in the 1820s (McGrew, 1965), populations to the West still felt protected from a disease that was associated with the conditions of "barbaric" society (Delaporte, 1986:97–113). In France "the Royal Academy of Medicine believed that France possessed all the advantages accruing to a highly civilized nation" and that "its inhabitants would be spared by the [cholera] epidemic" (Delaporte, 1986:15).

Confidence may have been strongest in France because medicine was more advanced there, but the belief existed elsewhere as well. In the United States, for example, prior to the outbreak of the first epidemic in 1832 "most Americans regarded the United States as a land of health, virtue, and rustic simplicity." Americans knew about cholera, but "they reassured themselves that this new pestilence attacked only the filthy, the hungry, the ignorant. There seemed few such in the United States" (Rosenberg, 1962:6, 7). In Russia "an optimistic tone pervaded the early cholera literature and persisted until 1830," and even the Asiatic peoples showed little fear of cholera as late as 1829 (McGrew, 1965:20, 46–47).

When the cholera epidemics appeared, the validity of the prevailing constructions of disease were undermined (e.g., miasma could not explain why cholera appeared in environments diverse in miasmata, and infectionism could not explain why cholera bypassed sanitary cordons and quarantined areas, such as vessels and ports of call). Confidence and security, especially among the middle class, were shaken. In describing the French epidemic of 1832, Delaporte (1986:49) wrote:

> What was surprising was that an affliction like cholera, which reminded people of the great medieval epidemics, should have appeared in an age of progress. Hence the devastation caused by the disease came as a shock, especially to members of the bourgeoisie, who with all the resources of civilization at their disposal never dreamed that they would have to contend with such a frightful calamity.

Alternative theories to miasma and infectionism were put forward. Some Americans claimed electricity and ozone were the causes (Rosenberg, 1962: 197); Europeans cited rain, fog, wind, electricity, and geological factors (Delaporte, 1986:87–89). In most countries doctors claimed that eating fish, vegetables, and fruit was hazardous (which was correct, though they did not know why) (Rosenberg, 1962:42); and in Russia vaguely defined environmental forces were invoked as causes (McGrew, 1965:5, 140). In general such explanations represented efforts, as in the epidemic of 1832 in New York City, "to fabricate a consistent conceptual apparatus with which to explain the inexplicable [and] provide security where there was only uncertainty" (Rosenberg, 1959:39). Cholera defied the dominant explanations, and doctors could not agree on its cause or mode of transmission (Briggs, 1961:91). Uncertainty abounded.

Widespread fear and panic ensued. (Bronislaw Malinowski [1954] was the first to write about the relationship between collective uncertainty and fear and panic, or anxiety, with specific reference to nonliterate society.) In contrast to Asa Briggs (1961:79), who observed that cholera "not only created panic: it posed puzzles," we may say that cholera created panic because it posed puzzles (uncertainty) by undermining the social construction of disease. Michael Durey's (1979:154) statement that "terror, panic, fear, alarm, fright, and dread were all words used to describe people's reactions" to the English epidemic of 1831–1832 no doubt held for the epidemics elsewhere as well.[5]

Reactions to Fear

Fear of contagion led many people to leave cities and towns for the country-side (Rosenberg, 1962:26–28, 37; McGrew, 1965:12, 72–73; Langer, 1973: 107–108; Durey, 1979:139–141; Delaporte, 1986:58). For example, seventy thousand of the two hundred thousand inhabitants of New York City are said to have fled the city during the epidemic of 1832. On July 3 the New York *Evening Post* reported that roads "were lined with well-filled stage coaches, livery coaches, private vehicles and equestrians, all panic struck, fleeing from the city" (Marks and Beatty, 1976:202). People deserted the sick, including relatives and family members (Durey, 1979:161, 183).

Fear of contagion sometimes turned into violence. For example, in 1832 in Chester, Pennsylvania, "several persons suspected of carrying the pestilence" were killed, as was "the man who had sheltered them," and militia fired on people traveling from cholera-infested areas (Rosenberg, 1962:37). In all countries brutal actions by authorities were recorded. In some places in tsarist Russia "police officials who enforced the sanitary [e.g., quarantine] regulations were notorious for their brutal methods," with quarantines amounting to "virtual house arrest" so that "even food and water were difficult to get" (McGrew, 1965:50). In St. Petersburg "no person was safe on the streets. The sick and the well, the inebriates and the infirm, were collared, dumped unceremoniously into the dreaded cholera carts, and hauled off willy-nilly to lazarettes, often with whole families trailing the wagons wailing and weeping" (McGrew, 1965:109–110). Elsewhere "the police, who were charged with bringing suspected cholera patients to the hospital, ... [seized] anyone who looked suspicious. Those who were taken, cholera and non-cholera cases alike, were hustled into the hospitals, stripped of their clothes, dosed with calomel and opium, thrust into hot baths, and, when they resisted, were beaten into submission" (McGrew, 1965:69).

Scapegoats were found. Foreigners were blamed. The Russians accused the Poles of spreading the disease, the Poles accused the Russians, Europeans further west accused both the Poles and Russians (McGrew, 1965:101–102), and Americans accused immigrants, especially the Irish (Rosenberg, 1962:62). But the major scapegoats were the poor. The nature of the disease caused it to be concentrated among those who lived in dirty hovels and slums, where drinking water was most apt to be contaminated. Consequently, the wealthy and well-to-do accused the poor or masses of causing the disease and spreading it to the rest of the population. Beggars, vagrants, and itinerant workers were chased from the streets and even expelled from communities in England (Morris, 1976:117–125). The stricken poor were quickly quarantined in hospitals, and after death their bodies were commonly disposed of in mass secular burials, which denied the relatives the traditional religious wake (Delaporte, 1986:49; Evans, 1987:367).[6] Although many of the well-to-do fled their communities, many others were indifferent and felt protected because the poor were kept segregated from the rest of the community.

The poor, in turn, had their scapegoats. Sometimes they initially denied that cholera was widespread (McGrew, 1965:110; Morris, 1976:94–101; Delaporte, 1986:47), but as the epidemics spread and deaths mounted, they were also gripped by fear of contagion. They even feared their own sick relatives, whom they isolated and treated as pariahs (Durey, 1979:154, 161).

Beyond the simple fear of contagion, many of the poor thought cholera was a genocidal plot. They suspected the wealthy and the government of conspiring to kill them off (McGrew, 1965:116; Delaporte, 1986:49, 65). Some thought their water supplies were being poisoned (Briggs, 1961:85, 91; McGrew, 1965:116; Langer, 1973:110; Morris, 1976:108–109; Delaporte, 1986:48–50; Evans, 1987:244, 367). In St. Petersburg people distrusted government officials, and "the cry of poison was raised again and again" (McGrew, 1965:100, 106). Doctors were accused of conspiring with the wealthy and the government to control the population of the poor (Delaporte, 1986:51–52, 55–57). The peasants in Hungary thought the remedies that doctors were giving were "poisons designed to get rid of them" (Marks and Beatty, 1976:194). In France hospitals were considered death houses and "death traps" (Delaporte, 1986:37); in Tamrov, Russia, a hospital was a "place of horror" where "people [were] cut up and cooked!" (McGrew, 1965:69). Sometimes doctors were accused of "body snatching" (Morris, 1976:108–117) and killing patients to have bodies for dissection and study (Briggs, 1961:91; Morris, 1976:183–184; Durey, 1979:184; Evans, 1987:367). The poor often responded with mob action and riots, and physicians along with city authorities were frequently attacked (Rosenberg, 1962:33; Morris, 1976:108–117; Durey, 1979:157–159; Evans, 1987:244). Sometimes they were beaten to death (McGrew, 1965:111).[7] In short, collective behavior was widespread.

Even though cholera is much different from plague and wide sociocultural differences separated feudal Europe of the fourteenth-century and the developing industrial European societies (and tsarist Russia) of the nineteenth century, societal reactions to the two epidemics were similar. Beliefs about the causes of the diseases were found wanting, fear of contagion emerged, and extreme and violent reactions followed. Flights from cities, desertion of the ill, scapegoating, riotous and violent behavior, and accusations of poisoning and conspiracy occurred.

There were differences, of course. The Black Death was far more devastating than all the cholera epidemics combined, and by all accounts it generated more fear and terror. The primary scapegoats for the Black Death, the Jews, were apparently no more afflicted by the disease than the rest of the population, whereas the primary scapegoats in the cholera epidemics, the poor, were. Also, the Jews were accused of conspiring to kill the Christians, whereas no comparable charges were leveled at the poor, though they believed that the wealthy and official authorities were conspiring against them. The point is, however, that reactions to both epidemics were similar and collective behavior was widespread. Certain reactions to the AIDS epidemic were similar.

The HIV-AIDS Epidemic in the
United States

As a blood-borne disease, HIV-AIDS is much harder to contract than plague or cholera. Also, in comparison to the periods when the other epidemics occurred, HIV-AIDS appeared during an age when ethnic and religious hatred was not as intense and the class structure was not as oppressive. Most significantly, scientific medicine was far advanced. Since World War II the popular media had constantly brought messages of medical progress, from new drugs, to laser and microsurgery, to artificial implants and transplants. Life expectancy had increased from 43.3 years in 1900 to 73.7 years in 1980. Medicine was not without its critics (Carlson, 1975; Illich, 1976), but most people were awed by what medicine could do.[8] And progress against infectious disease had been particularly great.[9]

Society's View of Infectious Diseases

Penicillin, which cures many bacterial infections, came into wide use in the 1940s. After World War II antibiotics and vaccines were developed for many infectious diseases, including diphtheria, measles, typhoid, poliomyelitis, and tuberculosis, and some infectious agents (e.g., smallpox) were eradicated worldwide. The polio epidemics of the 1950s were the last major epidemics of infectious disease. Except for mild diseases such as influenza, infectious epidemics were considered to be past history. By the 1970s "the fear of epidemic [was] almost gone" (Dowling, 1977:241). Even syphilis and other venereal diseases, which had been scourges in the West for centuries, could be cured with antibiotics so that society had even lost its fear of them.

Some medical experts were confident that infectious diseases would be eradicated. For example, in 1961 Cockburn (p. 1058) wrote in *Science* that "we could look forward with confidence to a considerable degree of freedom from infectious disease at a time not too far in the future" and that, indeed, within one hundred years "all the major infectious diseases will have disappeared." In 1968 Surgeon General William Stewart told Congress it was time to "close the books on infectious diseases," declare the battle against infectious disease over, and shift resources to other diseases (Garrett, 1992:825). (Congress complied.) By the early 1970s the conquest of infectious diseases appeared so complete that microbiologists Macfarlane Burnet and David White (1972:263) wrote in their widely acclaimed text on infectious disease that, although there "may be some wholly unexpected emergence of a new and dangerous disease" in the years ahead, "the most likely forecast about the future of infectious disease is that it will be very dull," and any outbreak of new diseases "will presumably be safely contained." (For one scientist who was not so secure, see Dubos, 1965:374–375.)

The public felt as secure as the medical scientists were confident.[10] People knew that "for a generation scientists had rapidly identified new infectious agents and devised tests for their presence, vaccinations against them, and drugs to treat their victims" (Fox, 1986:17). By the 1980s less than 5 percent of U.S. expenditures for disease went for infectious disease (Fox, 1986:9). Writing in 1977, Harry Dowling (p. 241) stated that, "dimly aware of the many diagnostic tools available to doctors and hearing that 'miracle' drugs had now been placed in their hands, people expected doctors to cure just about everything," especially infectious diseases. Therefore, "a person died of infection only if very young, very old, weakened by alcoholism or physical injury, or *extremely* unlucky" (Crosby, 1989:xi). Accordingly, the public believed the appearance of any new microbe would pose no particular problem. Scientists would quickly identify the germ and develop a vaccine or medicine, and the danger would pass.[11] Eliminating the danger of infectious diseases with drugs was simply routine (Fox, 1986:9). Therefore, in 1983 on the eve of the AIDS epidemic, McNeill (p. 28), author of the outstanding *Plagues and Peoples,* stated, "One of the things that separate us from our ancestors and make contemporary experience profoundly different from that of other ages is the disappearance of epidemic disease as a serious factor in human life." Infectious diseases had been almost defined away as any kind of threat at all.

Then AIDS appeared. Medicine did not just lack a cure or vaccine for this disease. In the early stage of the epidemic medicine did not know what the cause of the disease was. Nevertheless, since it was overwhelmingly concentrated among gays and IDUs, most people did not feel threatened. Consequently, in the early years the media gave AIDS limited coverage or suggested that AIDS was a "gay disease" (Albert, 1986; Baker, 1986; Check, 1987). As with the poor during the cholera epidemics, gays were confined to their physical and social space (many still lived in the closet and displayed their sexual orientation only in the gay subcultures, which were invisible to most straights). And as with many of the better-off during the cholera epidemics, most nongays were indifferent to the problem (Bayer, 1985:587; Weitz, 1991:17–18; see also Altman, 1986:184; Shilts, 1987).

Security and apathy were soon shattered. In the early 1980s it became known that persons with no history of homosexuality or drug injection had AIDS. Reports of these cases signified that, whatever the cause of AIDS or its mode of transmission, the general population was at risk and that there was nothing medicine could do. Fear and panic resulted. "The AIDS epidemic ... aroused the return of irrational fear because it exposed the impotence of modern medicine just when we had begun to believe that infectious disease had been vanquished for good" (Grmek, 1989:41). The irrational fear was fear of contagion. And with no rational—that is, scientific—explanation for the disease, estimates of the number of infected persons were advanced that were not based on rational thought and scientific fact.

Doomsday Estimates and Projections

Erroneous projections based on the automatic pilot analogy were compounded by the use of two other deficient methodologies. One was the iceberg analogy for estimating the number of persons who were infected with HIV (Fumento, 1990:302–303). This analogy assumed that there were many unreported carriers of HIV (as many as fifty to one hundred) for each known AIDS case. The other method was to use erroneous estimates of the presumed percentage of U.S. males who are homosexual. Many of these estimates were based on the statistic reported by Kinsey et al. (1948) that up to 10 percent of adult American males are homosexual (Appendix; Fumento, 1990:205–210). One English writer even claimed that "*at least* ten percent of the overall population" are gay men (Watney, 1988:83). When this or an approximate number is multiplied by the presumed prevalence of HIV in the gay population (some have estimated that upward of 50 percent of the gay populations in San Francisco and New York City are infected [Fineberg, 1988; Montgomery and Joseph, 1989; Eckholm, 1990c]), the percentage of the population infected with HIV is frighteningly high. For example, in a special report, "The AIDS Epidemic" for the *New England Journal of Medicine* in February 1985, Sheldon Landesman et al. (1985:522) maintained that if the Kinsey estimate were correct (Landesman et al. did not question its validity), "the implications of the presence of [HIV] in a community are staggering." When this figure is then used in conjunction with the iceberg analogy, the resulting number staggers even more. And when this number is used in the automatic pilot analogy, the number of persons who are estimated to be infected with HIV simply boggles the mind. And *then* with assumptions about the domino analogy and risks of secondary and tertiary transmissions, sex between heterosexuals is a very risky matter. In fact, it is a death threat.

Therefore, statements began to appear warning about the heterosexual transmission of the AIDS virus. For example, in *The AIDS Cover-up: The*

Real and Alarming Facts about AIDS, former Christian minister Gene Antonio (1986:147; emphasis added) warned that "prolonged intimate sexual contact of *any* kind is potentially lethal." Such warnings were not limited to persons who had negative moral attitudes about sex. They also came from the mainstream—from the media, government officials, and scientists.[12]

In 1983 the Canadian magazine *Macleans* stated (erroneously) that U.S. public health officials believed that "AIDS could claim 100,000 victims" in three years and 1.6 million in five years (Fumento, 1990:264). The cover of the July 1985 *Life* stated, "Now No One Is Safe from AIDS." The August 2, 1985, issue of *Newsweek* warned that, although AIDS had once been dismissed as the gay plague, it was now "the No. 1 public-health menace" and quoted a CDC official as stating that AIDS was potentially "much worse than anything mankind has seen before" (Clark et al., 1985:20). Some warned that the heterosexual spread of HIV-AIDS would become as widespread as in Africa. The November 24, 1986, cover of *Newsweek* stated, "AIDS in Africa: The Future Is Now," and the February 1987 cover of *The Atlantic Monthly* stated, "Heterosexuals and AIDS: The Second Stage of the Epidemic." The *Newsweek* issue had a section, "The AIDS Epidemic," in which an article by Morganthau et al. (1986:30) entitled, "Future Shock," warned readers that "by 1991 an estimated 5 million Americans may be carrying the AIDS virus."[13] And as noted in the last chapter, in January 1987 *U.S. News & World Report* declared that HIV-AIDS was now "a plague of the mainstream" and had found "fertile growth among heterosexuals" (McAuliffe et al., 1987:20). The magazine then warned in June of that year that *everyone* was at risk and that as many as 10 million persons would likely be infected by 1991 (Kramer, 1987:13).

Representatives of government agencies and commissions made even more alarming statements. Theresa Crenshaw, sex therapist and member of the president's AIDS commission, was reported to have suggested in testimony before a House of Representatives committee on February 18, 1987, that the world was "facing the threat of extinction during our lifetime" (Fumento, 1990:301). Later that year Crenshaw wrote, "The AIDS epidemic is the greatest threat to society, as we know it, ever faced by civilization— more serious than the plagues of past centuries" (Fumento, 1990:324). And on January 30, 1987, under the headline "AIDS May Dwarf the Plague" (meaning the Black Death), the *New York Times* (p. A-42) reported that the leading health officer in the United States, Secretary of Health and Human Services Otis R. Bowen, had stated, "If we cannot make progress, we face the dreadful prospect of a worldwide death toll in the tens of millions in a decade from now" that would make the Black Death seem "pale by comparison." And to drive the danger of heterosexual transmission home, he warned that, because of the relatively long time after infection before AIDS appears, "when a person has sex, they're not just having it with that partner, they're having it with everybody that partner had it with for the past ten years."

As alarming as these statements were, they were affirmed by some medical professionals and scientists. On the February 18, 1987, Oprah Winfrey show, a physician from Infectious Disease and AIDS Services, Cook County Hospital, endorsed Winfrey's statement that "one in five heterosexuals could be dead from AIDS at the end of the next three years" (Fumento, 1990:4, 181). An orthopedic surgeon wrote in January 1988 that by the end of 1991 there would be 13–27 million carriers in the United States (Fumento, 1990:203). As noted in Chapter 4, in the same year another medical doctor, who acknowledged the research assistance of two "experts in the field of virology and infectious diseases" who were "sources of information about AIDS and of scientific data obtainable only from [technical] journals and meetings," wrote that 250,000 persons would die from AIDS in 1991 (Kurland, 1988:v, 55). (As of mid-1994 only 35,308 persons were reported to have died from AIDS in 1991 [CDC, 1994b:14].) Some of the most well-known sex researchers wrote that "the AIDS virus is now [1988] running rampant in the heterosexual community" (Masters et al., 1988:7) and that medical scientists and the CDC were ignoring some ways in which HIV might be transmitted. And in an April 19, 1987, statement in the *New York Times Magazine,* Gould (p. 33) wrote that the AIDS epidemic "may rank with nuclear weaponry as the greatest danger of our era. ... AIDS has begun its march through our own heterosexual community." Persons afflicted will be "our neighbors, our lovers, our children and ourselves." HIV-AIDS was "potentially, the greatest natural tragedy in human history."

Such statements, and their accompanying apocalyptic projections of infection and death, seem to have reached their peak around the end of 1986 (Fumento, 1990:235; for an analysis of the British media, see Wellings, 1988:98). They were certainly enough to scare, especially given the sources.[14] Some were not dissimilar to statements by people who believed the Black Death signaled the end of the world in the fourteenth century. These statements also generally went unchallenged. No one knew what the situation really was, so extreme statements were what much of the public read and heard.

The Public's Fear of Getting HIV-AIDS

Several polls indicated that the level of fear was indeed high. In 1985 and 1986 three national polls found that more than 75 percent of respondents believed HIV-AIDS would spread beyond homosexuals and IDUs and was "now a threat to the general public" (Singer et al., 1987:586), and Gallup polls for *Newsweek* revealed that the percentage of respondents who thought it "very likely that AIDS would become an epidemic for the public at large" increased from 27 percent in August 1985 to 36 percent in November 1986 (Morganthau et al., 1986:33).

Many people felt personally threatened. In five polls in 1985 and 1986, from 10 percent to 42 percent said they were "afraid [they] might get AIDS" (Singer et al., 1987:586). A 1987 Gallup poll found that 20 percent of a national sample were "very concerned" that AIDS would strike them personally and that another 22 percent were "a little concerned" (Lipset and Wattenberg, 1988:36); the finding of a *U.S. News*/CNN poll by the Roper Organization was similar (Corey et al. 1987:56). A 1987 survey of 2,303 adults conducted by the NCHS found that 5 percent believed their personal chances of contracting AIDS were "high" or "medium" (Dawson et al., 1987). A Michigan survey of emergency medical service professionals found that 57 percent believed their chances of becoming infected were "somewhat high" or "very high" (Smyser et al., 1990:499). Fear increased over time. The percentage who were "very worried" or concerned that they or someone they knew would get AIDS was 7 percent in August 1983, 14 percent in August 1985, and 19 percent in November 1986 (Morganthau et al., 1986:32).

In light of the actual risks, to say that such fears were unrealistic grossly understates the matter. The 1988–1991 NCHS seroprevalence survey indicated the number of Americans with HIV was probably no more than 1 million (it could have been considerably less), which would give percentages for nineteen- to fifty-nine-year-olds of 0.57 percent for men and about 0.15 percent for women.[15] Although men were far more apt to be infected than women (in the 1980s men were about ten times as likely to get the disease), women were just as fearful as men. A Gallup poll showed that in 1987 about the same percentage (19 percent and 21 percent) were "very concerned" about contracting AIDS and 22 percent and 23 percent were "somewhat concerned" (*New York Times*, November 19, 1987:I-6). And a 1987 survey by the NCHS showed a difference of only 5 percent to 4 percent between males and females. Clearly, then, by the mid-1980s the general population no longer indifferently considered HIV-AIDS a gay disease (as well as one in which IDUs were at high risk). It was now seen as a disease that "ordinary" heterosexuals were apt to get.

Casual Contact and Fear of Contagion

Although most warnings about people contracting HIV focused on sexual intercourse or drug injection, cases of babies with AIDS were reported in two articles in the May 6, 1983, issue of the *Journal of the American Medical Association* (Oleske et al., 1983; Rubinstein et al., 1983). The articles also reported that the babies had had close household contact with persons from high-risk groups (e.g., IDUs). Although the primary mode of infection for newborns is through placental transfer or during delivery, this was not known at the time (it was not known for certain that HIV-AIDS was a blood-borne disease, and the virus was not identified until 1984).

Neither article claimed that AIDS was transmitted through casual contact, but one stated that "sexual contact, drug abuse or exposure to blood products is not necessary for disease transmission" (Oleske et al., 1983:2345). And in *JAMA*'s editorial, Dr. Anthony Fauci (1983:2875) of the National Institutes of Health wrote, "The finding of AIDS in infants and children who are household contacts of patients with AIDS or persons with risks for AIDS has enormous implications with regard to ultimate transmissibility of this syndrome" because it reveals "the possibility that routine close contact, as within a family household, can spread the disease." Although Fauci only pointed to the *possibility* of AIDS being spread through casual contact, this is not how his remarks were interpreted by the press, and the media response fanned public hysteria (Fettner and Check, 1984:157–158).[16] In commenting on this episode, Grmek (1989:39) stated, "Amplified by the print and broadcast media, physicians' fears fed a wave of collective hysteria that seized some Americans, especially in the middle classes." (Compare Grmek's quote with the quote from Delaporte about the shock cholera caused the French bourgeoisie.)

For example, in July 1987 the Roper Organization conducted a nationwide survey of a representative sample of 1,997 persons that revealed widespread ignorance about the way HIV is transmitted. Thirty-six percent said they would not shake hands with someone who had AIDS, 44 percent would not work alongside such a person, and 48 percent would not send their children to a school where a child had AIDS. A substantial majority (71 percent and 74 percent) would not kiss someone on the cheek who had AIDS or eat in a restaurant if they knew a kitchen worker had AIDS (Stipp and Kerr, 1989:100). Similar results were obtained in a survey conducted by the NCHS in 1987 in which respondents were asked more directly about the chances of getting HIV from such casual contacts (Dawson et al., 1987). A 1987 *U.S. News*/CNN poll found that 67 percent thought restaurant workers should be tested (Corey et al., 1987:57). A large proportion of the population was simply ignorant about the way HIV is transmitted. In the eyes of many people, AIDS was "an omnipresent, insidious threat" to the general population (Weitz, 1991:23), and transmission was not limited to sexual contact. Even many health care providers feared infection through casual contagion (Wertz et al., 1987; Wormser and Joline, 1988; Smyser et al., 1990). Business firms concerned about the health of their workers fired employees who had AIDS (Roth, 1985; Wallis, 1985). Fear of casual contagion was so serious that the *New England Journal of Medicine* began its editorial of February 6, 1986, with the statement, "The epidemic of Acquired Immunodeficiency Syndrome (AIDS) is an epidemic of fear." It urged doctors to take a more active role "to counter the public's fear of casual contagion" (Sande, 1986:380, 382).

Never mind that not one verified case of infection from casual contact had been reported (and still has not) and that almost all medical persons with scientific authority, including those at the CDC, were convinced by 1986 that the chances of casual transmission were extremely remote (Curran et al., 1985, 1988; Friedland et al., 1986; Sande, 1986; Friedland and Klein, 1987; Lifson, 1988). Warnings about the danger of casual contact still went out. On March 18, 1986, in an article in the *New York Times*, Harvard law professor Alan Dershowitz (p. A-27) quoted Harvard professor and expert on infectious disease William Hazeltine as stating in an address to a university audience on some scientific facts about AIDS that "anyone who tells you categorically that AIDS is not contracted by saliva is not telling you the truth" and that there "are sure to be cases of proved transmission through casual contact." Dershowitz quoted another university scientist as having said, the "fact is that the dire predictions of those who have cried doom ever since AIDS appeared haven't been far off the mark."

One of the most prominent medical hysterics was Dr. Lorraine Day, chief of orthopedic surgery at San Francisco Hospital. In the late 1980s Dr. Day went around the country addressing groups of physicians and appearing on national television (e.g., on ABC's "20/20") expressing her views. She (1991) put her views in writing in a book (available in paperback) in which she claimed the government (the CDC) was not telling the full story about HIV. Dr. Day claimed that a person might contract HIV from shaking hands, kissing, and breathing airborne viral particles.

Religious and political conservatives were especially insistent that HIV could be transmitted through casual contact (Fumento, 1990:181–187). Antonio (1986:147) wrote that homosexuality was a major source of AIDS (as well as other diseases) and that HIV "exuded from almost every bodily orifice, pore and secretion, probably including sweat," and he warned against using public toilets and eating in restaurants with gay waiters, among other things. Presidential candidate and televangelist Pat Robertson insisted to the editors of New Hampshire's *Concord Monitor* on December 19, 1987, that infected people could spread the disease by "breathing various things in the atmosphere."[17] But fears were not limited to extremists; they were widespread in the population, as the results of surveys showed.

Therefore, as with the Black Death and the cholera epidemics in the nineteenth century, there was much ignorance about the cause of HIV-AIDS and its mode of transmission, and fear of casual contagion was high. (Actually, since AIDS is far more difficult than plague and cholera to transmit, the belief that it could be passed through casual contact actually reflected greater ignorance than beliefs about the Black Death and cholera.) Of course, unlike during the cholera epidemics and the Black Death, people were not dropping dead before others' very eyes. Thus, even though panic during the AIDS epidemic paled in comparison to the other epidemics in light of the obviously far more limited threat, the fear of contracting HIV was as extreme as the fear that accompanied the other epidemics.

Avoidance and Mistreatment of People with HIV-AIDS and Members of High-risk Groups

A number of surveys in the mid-1980s revealed that people believed children with AIDS should be prohibited from attending school with other children.[18] Parents boycotted schools in New York City, Florida, and other places to protest HIV-infected children attending school. The most well-known example is the case of Ryan White, a hemophiliac child in Kokomo, Indiana, whose parents had to go to court in 1985 to overcome the opposition of other parents and school officials to their son attending school. (For an analysis of the New York boycott and subsequent court case, see Nelkin and Hilgartner, 1986.)

Numerous other examples of avoidance and mistreatment of AIDS patients or persons from high-risk groups were reported (Nelkin and Hilgartner, 1986:118). For example, a Florida minister barred two hemophiliac children with AIDS from attending church (Ansberry, 1987:A-1). People even deserted relatives. On August 12, 1985, *Newsweek* reported that "horror stories abound of families who ... leave their sons to lonely deaths" (Seligmann and Reese, 1985:24). A gay forced his infected lover to leave their apartment (Seligmann and Greenberg, 1985:26). Reports appeared that landlords were evicting gay tenants and that health care workers were refusing to have contact with persons who had AIDS (Wallis, 1985:45; Trager, 1988:174). Even funeral homes denied proper services to persons who had died from AIDS (Wallis, 1985:45; Hancock and Carim, 1986:94). Some reactions were probably stimulated by a moral interpretation of AIDS, but for many people fear of contagion was paramount, as was obvious in efforts to exclude "innocent" children from attending school and church. In the September 12, 1985, issue, *Time* referred to hemophiliac children as "The New Untouchables." After the court ordered that three hemophiliac children of the Ray family in Arcadia, Florida, could attend school, the family's home was destroyed by arson on August 28, 1987.

These examples and other anecdotes do not reveal how general extreme reactions were, of course. However, in light of the survey data just reported, the avoidance of people who had AIDS and support for programs to isolate (e.g., quarantine) them were probably as widespread as the anecdotes suggest. Fear of casual contagion was widespread and certainly not limited to isolated instances. Many people were still ignorant of the modes of transmission, although they had been known since 1986, or simply responded to fear rather than facts. This is particularly clear in the following example.

On November 12, 1987, the *Wall Street Journal* reported that a Texas man with AIDS, which he believed he had contracted in a homosexual encounter years earlier, was brutally beaten by three men. The man screamed, "What are you doing?" "Killing AIDS," one replied. Fear of contagion was so great that one of the men added, "When we're done with you, we're going to kill your wife and kids, just in case they've got it" (Ansberry, 1987:A-1). (Recall that persons with cholera were killed during the cholera epidemic of 1832.) The man subsequently moved to Williamson, West Virginia, his hometown. After he swam in the local pool Myers (1987) reports mothers fled with their children, and the pool was closed. Townspeople then circulated a petition to ban his younger sister and her boyfriend from school because of a belief that *they* were infected with HIV.[19]

As with the fear of contagion itself, reactions to fear during the AIDS epidemic in the 1980s were not unlike certain reactions during the plague in the fourteenth century and the cholera epidemics in the nineteenth century. People with HIV-AIDS were deserted and mistreated and, like the poor in the cholera epidemics, were prominent targets of hostility and violence. Although hostility to homosexuals had declined with gay liberation, gays had long been the object of hostility in the United States. This intensified during the epidemic, with an increase in open hostility and physical attacks being reported (Fumento, 1990:212). *Time* magazine reported that in New York City alone, attacks against male homosexuals increased from 176 in 1984 to 517 in 1987 and that authorities attributed much of the increase to AIDS (Zuckerman, 1988).

Scapegoating

Some contend that gays have been used as scapegoats for AIDS. Altman (1986:74) argued, for example, that since HIV does not distinguish between the blood of male homosexuals and that of heterosexuals, to say that male homosexuality is a causal factor in AIDS is to make male homosexuals scapegoats for the disease just as the Jews were scapegoats for the Black Death. "The idea that the nation's blood supply was contaminated [by male homosexuals] became a twentieth-century version of [Jews] poisoning wells [during the Black Death]."

In fact, male homosexuals were not scapegoats and not comparable to Jews during the Black Death. Scapegoats are individuals and groups accused of causing a social event that they could not have caused. Altman's analogy is faulty because Jews did not poison wells (and would not have caused the plague if they had), whereas gays were contributing disproportionately to HIV in the donor blood supply. HIV does not distinguish between the sexual orientation of individuals, and all gays do not have HIV, but to dehomosexualize the disease simply ignores that in the United States anal sex between gays is the major way HIV is spread. Consequently, to say that a disproportionate percentage of the spread of AIDS is attributed to homosexuals is a statement of fact.[20] For gays to be targets of collective hostility similar to other groups in past epidemics does not make them, by that fact alone, scapegoats. Scapegoats were found, however.

In the early 1980s Haitian immigrants were believed to be a source of AIDS in the United States, and, as noted in Chapter 2, many believed that Africans are the origin of HIV. Since the scapegoating of these two groups as well as prostitutes is more closely related to social structure and social attitudes than to fear of contagion, this scapegoating is examined in the next two chapters. The belief that health care providers were spreaders of HIV was more directly related to fear of contagion.

Physician-to-patient infection is rare, if it even exists. In only one case is there evidence that a provider (a dentist) may have infected patients, and it would be incorrect to say that physicians and other health care providers were *major* scapegoats for AIDS. Nevertheless, they did not escape the scapegoating process altogether. Indeed, accusations against physicians and health care providers came from persons in high places. A U.S. senator and a U.S. representative each introduced legislation that would have required, among other things, that health care workers be tested for HIV and that infected workers be prohibited from performing invasive procedures. Some people believed health care workers were a major source of HIV-AIDS. Indeed, the representative, William Dannemeyer of California, wondered, "Have we been lied to about the way we can get AIDS?" (Berke, 1991:IV-14), suggesting that medical scientists had lied about how much physicians and other health care workers had been involved in the spread of HIV. To informed persons such a charge was (and is) irrational in the extreme. The risk of being infected by a health care provider is so remote—in the words of the former Surgeon General C. Everett Koop—"as to be unmeasurable" (Hilts, 1991:A-11). Nevertheless, scapegoating occurred and implied that the medical profession was somehow involved in a conspiracy.[21] Other charges of conspiracy and genocide were more explicit.

Charges of Conspiracy and Genocide

Charges of conspiracy came from two primary directions: from people who believed HIV-AIDS was a gay plot, on the one hand, and from gays and members of other high-risk groups who believed the government was engaged in a genocidal plot, on the other.

One version of the gay-plot theory held that gay leaders had intentionally allowed HIV to spread in order to further the "political agenda" of gays—for example, to evoke public sympathy (Rueda and Schwartz, 1987:7–8). Representative Dannemeyer suggested that gays might have deliberately contaminated the nation's blood supply to pressure the federal government to spend more money on AIDS treatment and research (Weitz, 1991:22). Antonio (1986:xii, 77–81) wrote that the federal government, in an effort to protect gay leaders, deliberately underestimated the number of infected persons and the ease with which HIV could be contracted (e.g., eating in restaurants where gays worked, using public toilet seats). Thus, he claimed, male homosexuals had deliberately introduced HIV into the nation's blood supply as a form of "blood terrorism." A number of other charges along the same lines were made (Fumento, 1990:181–187), particularly by conservative religious and political leaders (Weitz, 1991:21–22). Some found such charges by these leaders to be simply bizarre.

But these claims were no more bizarre than charges made by members of high-risk groups. One of the first charges was made in 1985, when political activist Dick Gregory argued that AIDS was due to germ warfare. He noted that AIDS had not appeared in ancient Greece when male homosexuality was common, and he wondered why such a large percentage of the victims were in the United States. He also hinted that Haitian refugees were being used as guinea pigs (Davidson, 1985).

Probably the most well-known, and certainly most explicit, statement about AIDS being a conspiracy against gays appeared in the book *Reports from the Holocaust* by playright Kramer. "AIDS is our holocaust and Reagan is our Hitler. New York City is our Auschwitz" (Kramer, 1989: 173). Kramer accused persons on the political Right, including President Ronald Reagan, of *intentionally* killing male homosexuals by opposing government expenditures to find a cure for AIDS. They *knew* that more gays (and African Americans and Hispanics in the United States) would die as a result. "I believe it is a conscious act," Kramer (1989:173–174) wrote. Government officials and others who failed to inform the public about the dangers of the disease and resisted or failed to mount efforts to find a cure for AIDS were engaging in genocide. They were "equal to murderers." (See also Wojnarowicz, 1991:107.) Similarly, Simon Watney (1987:74, 85–86) suggested that European governments' indifference to the epidemic among gays was "the active legacy of [the] eugenic theory" of the Nazis.

To some African Americans, HIV-AIDS was a form of racial genocide. In *U.S. News & World Report* Matthew Cooper and Greg Ferguson (1990) wrote that Louis Farrakhan, leader of the Nation of Islam, charged that the high rate of HIV-AIDS in Africa was caused by whites trying to steal Africa's natural resources, a view he did not deny on April 19, 1994, on ABC's "20/ 20," in which he also said HIV was created in a government laboratory outside Washington, D.C., thus implying that it was a government conspiracy against African Americans also.

Belief in racial genocide was not limited to extremists. Surveys showed that a significant minority of African Americans believed HIV-AIDS was a genocidal racial plot. A 1990 survey of church members found that 35 percent believed this; another survey found that 10 percent of respondents believed the AIDS virus was "deliberately created in a laboratory in order to infect black people," and another 20 percent thought this might be the case (*New York Times,* May 12, 1992:A-14). A Gallup poll in March 1992 revealed that somewhere between 7 and 16 percent of African-American respondents believed HIV-AIDS among African Americans was a racist conspiracy (Morganthau et al., 1992:22). To the editors of the *New York Times* this was a "bizarre" response that reflected "paranoia" among African Americans.

Sociologically, however, these beliefs, along with the beliefs that gays and the government are involved in conspiracies of another sort, are understandable forms of collective behavior. Collective fear causes extreme (bizarre and irrational) reactions. The records of other epidemics reveal that it is not uncommon for groups with high death rates from a mysterious disease to adopt irrational and paranoid views and to charge the government and other groups with conspiring to kill them off. The reactions of some gays and African Americans significantly resembled the paranoia of the poor in the cholera epidemics more than 150 years earlier. Actually, societal reactions to HIV-AIDS added a twist to the conspiratorial reactions. To some people, including the U.S. representative, the very group that had been most devastated by HIV-AIDS was using the disease to further its own goals!

Conclusion

In comparison to the Black Death and cholera epidemics, the AIDS epidemic in the United States occurred in an advanced industrialized society where science and scientific thought were institutionalized to a high degree and the sociocultural environment was vastly different from that existing in preindustrial or early industrial societies. But as with the earlier epidemics, AIDS appeared suddenly, had a rapid increase in deaths, was perceived to be contagious, and had an unknown cause, at least in the early years of the epidemic. Consequently, societal reactions were similar to the reactions during the Black Death and cholera epidemics.

Overall, of course, the reactions to AIDS were not as extreme as to the earlier epidemics. There were no mass flights from communities, lynchings and burnings, or self-flagellation crazes. Anarchy did not occur, and there was no forceful isolation of masses of people in hospitals and murderous attacks on doctors. But common elements in the reactions are clear. People avoided, ostracized, neglected, mistreated, or brutally beat people who had HIV-AIDS as well as members of high-risk groups, specifically gays. Some demanded that infected persons be quarantined. Demonstrations and moblike actions bordering on riots by high-risk groups took place. Scapegoats were found. Similarly, some members of high-risk groups believed that HIV-AIDS was a genocidal plot against them, while others held conspiratorial beliefs about gays, doctors, and medical scientists, which some found to be bizarre, irrational, and paranoid. The similarities are too great to dismiss. McGrew's statement about the cholera epidemics in Russia in the 1820s is illuminating in this regard.

McGrew (1965:12, 10) emphasized that the reactions varied in Russia depending on "the particular environment in which [cholera] occurred." Nevertheless, widespread fear and the failure of existing social norms to restrain violence and rumor-based fastasies, which are hallmarks of collective behavior, were common threads in the cholera epidemics at different places in Russia. "The cholera [epidemics] created a nameless dread, a paralyzing fear, which neither public proclamation nor learned articles could dissipate, and fear in turn dissolved normal reticence, eroded behavioral standards and ethical norms, and left men stripped of their dignity as men." Even though expressions of collective behavior in the AIDS epidemic were mild in comparison to expressions in the Russian cholera epidemics of 1823–1832, the hostile reactions to persons with HIV-AIDS and members of high-risk groups occurred despite public proclamations and scientific pronouncements that casual contagion was not possible. Even though such reactions, along with some of the counterreactions of high-risk groups, may not have been so extreme as to strip people of their dignity as humans, they were far enough outside the range of rational and civil norms so as to bring people's standing as members of a rational and civil society into question. Whenever epidemics occur under certain social conditions, people react in extreme ways, even though the extent to which they do depends on the exact nature of those specific conditions.

NOTES

1. Some historians question whether the socially disruptive effects of epidemics, especially the Black Death, were as severe as many have claimed (Amundsen, 1977; Siraisi, 1982). Social disruption was continually high because the populations were under the continual stress of moral confusion, political conflict, and a miserable material existence (Langer, 1958:297; Siraisi, 1982:17; Collins and Makowsky, 1989: 20). Nevertheless, even if the Black Death did not evoke entirely new social forces, it did intensify those already operating (Langer, 1958:294 and references cited therein).

The social order was already fragile; epidemics made it more so (Lyons and Petrucelli, 1987:351).

2. Unlike in Europe, the Black Death did not lead to fear of contagion and social disruption in the Islamic societies of the Middle East (Dols, 1977; Conrad, 1992). Religion played a different role there; it maintained certainty in the face of disaster. Medical explanations were altogether subordinate to religious explanations so that the social construction of plague was tightly integrated with religious beliefs. Religious doctrine stated that disease was caused by God and therefore that a person should *not* flee from plague, which (along with other diseases) was not contagious. It was visited on the individual as punishment for nonbelief or, in the case of Muslims, as martyrdom (Dols, 1977:109). Therefore, religion provided certainty and even interpreted infection as a reward (martyrdom), which prevented fear of contagion and hence collective reactions based on such fear.

3. Medical authorities did not know the cause of the disease or its mode of transmission for most of the century, though some physicians, such as John Snow of London in 1854, did show that cholera was a waterborne disease. However, Snow's insights and beliefs were not widely accepted until the bacillus was identified by Robert Koch in 1884.

4. Despite a high death toll, tuberculosis never led to the collective panic associated with other infectious diseases. Significantly, tuberculosis does not spread rapidly through a population, causing many deaths in a short period. It is not included in Marks and Beatty's (1976) review in *Epidemics* or in the essays compiled by Ranger and Slack (1992). Rather than evoking fear in nineteenth-century Europe, the physical symptoms of consumption (sunken chest, pale color, fragility) were sometimes considered expressions of creativity and genius, and for women these symptoms set the standard for beauty (Dubos and Dubos, 1987). (For a different view, see Trachenberg, 1994.) No one has been able to explain the fascination nineteenth-century industrial society had for this disease.

5. The connection between suspension of the prevailing social construction of disease and fear is especially explicit in Delaporte's (1986:xii, 1–57) analysis of the French epidemic of 1832.

6. One regulation stated, "Those who died of this disease should be buried as soon as possible, wrapped in cotton or linen cloth saturated with pitch, or coal tar, and be carried to the grave by the fewest possible number of persons" (Morris, 1976:104).

7. On one occasion in Paris "six persons were murdered and naked corpses dragged through the streets under" the belief of secret poisoning (Garrison, 1929: 774–775).

8. Progress was so great that medicine seemed to search for conditions, such as drug addiction, to define as illness (Conrad and Schneider, 1980). In 1989 members of the American Society of Plastic and Reconstructive Surgeons even defined small breasts as "deformities" and "a disease" (Weitz, 1991:35).

9. Most of the historical decline in infectious diseases was due to factors other than medical treatment, but many physicians and almost all laypersons did not know this.

10. "People no longer have to bar their doors to friends or flee their cities in droves at the approach of a dread disease" (Dowling, 1977:241).

11. "The most obvious way to control microorganisms that are not affected by the known antibiotics or chemical remedies is to devise new ones. ... Each effective rem-

edy further increases the total number of infections over which man has control" (Dowling, 1977:243).

12. Fumento (1990:235–248, 301–325) reviewed in detail the alarmists' projections and misrepresentations of the prevalence of AIDS.

13. The article also excerpted a hypothetical speech that the president might make on November 21, 1991, in which he would state, "We can no longer doubt that the continued spread of the AIDS virus represents a clear and present danger to millions of our fellow citizens, particularly the young. ... It is estimated that 5 million Americans are now infected with the AIDS virus, and it is medically certain they are infectious to others. Their dilemma—and ours—is that many of these people do not know they are spreading the epidemic" (Morganthau et al., 1986:30).

14. Extreme statements were still appearing in the 1990s, including statements in scientific and technical publications (Johnston and Hopkins, 1990; Anderson and May, 1992). On December 9, 1993, *New York Times* columnist Anna Quindlen warned her readers about the domino effect: "One day you ... will find yourself in the shadow of the plague [HIV-AIDS]. ... One day soon it will grip someone you know and love. Here is the real domino theory: Gay man to gay man, bisexual man to straight woman, addict mother to newborn baby, they all fall down and someday it will come to you." She then stated that the World Health Organization (WHO) reported that 14 million were now infected and predicted 30–40 million as the millennium approached. WHO reported these figures for the entire world, but since Quindlen's focus was a *New York Times* reporter's death from AIDS, her remarks suggested the figures were for the United States, particularly since the domino effect referred to a pattern of spread that, if typical anywhere at all, would be typical of the United States (and the West) rather than Africa and other parts of the world where transmission occurs mostly in sex between heterosexuals and the domino effect that Quindlen wrote about hardly exists.

15. Percentage calculations are based on cases reported by the NCHS (Altman, 1993) and population figures from the U.S. Bureau of the Census (1992:23).

16. Even the American Medical Association's news release was headlined, "Evidence Suggests Household Contact May Transmit AIDS" (Fettner and Check, 1984: 158). Dr. Fauci contended a short time after his editorial that he had been badly misinterpreted (Fettner and Check, 1984:158), and a review of his editorial would substantiate the claim.

17. "Robertson Disputes Doctors on AIDS," *Washington Post* (December 20, 1987:A-12).

18. In a *Wall Street Journal*/NBC nationwide poll in January 1987, 24 percent of the respondents thought that "children who have been diagnosed as having AIDS should [not] be allowed to attend school with other children." The *Journal* noted instances in which parents had opposed a child with AIDS attending kindergarten (*Wall Street Journal,* October 7, 1987:31). The *American Pharmacy* (NS28, 1988: 50) reported that in a 1987 survey by the American Medical Association, only 57 percent of nonphysician respondents believed that children with AIDS should be allowed to attend regular school classes; 80 percent of responding physicians believed this.

19. Many other examples of mistreatment were reported. An AIDS sufferer in Baltimore received a death threat, and the investigating police officer refused to enter the

man's office and wore rubber gloves to handle the evidence (Conrad, 1986:52). The *Wall Street Journal* and *Time* reported a number of episodes: denial of services ranging from pedicures to health care, a teacher transferred outside the classroom so he would have no contact with children, a mother who tried to prevent her former gay husband from having contact with their child because he might infect the child with HIV (denied in a court decision) (Ricklefs, 1987; Wallis, 1985:45). Mistreatment of infected prison inmates was reported. In a prison in Alabama, according to *New York Times* reporter Bruce Lambert (1990), inmates with AIDS had to scrub telephones with alcohol after using them, and one inmate reported that he had to scrub the shower stall as well as toilet seat with pure bleach after using them and then the floor behind him as he returned to his cell.

20. Altman's (1986:175–176) position that male homosexuals are scapegoats was based on the following reasoning. "AIDS is American and homosexual only in the sense that the first group in which the disease was discovered was American homosexuals. ... AIDS [in the United States] is intrinsically no more gay or American than Legionnaires' disease is an illness of ex-soldiers or than rubella (German measles) is inherently German." Fumento (1990:199) was correct when he noted that "the comparison is hardly fair: Germans do not account for 73 percent of all rubella victims, as did homosexuals of AIDS victims, at the time of Altman's writing; nor have the tens of thousands of American homosexuals who contract AIDS just happened to be in the wrong hotel at the wrong time," as were the Legionnaires.

21. In a discussion with a member of the nursing profession in December 1992, I was told that the government and medicine were not telling us everything they knew about AIDS

6. *Moralizing and Scapegoating*

In the archaic-metaphorical conception of disease (hereafter referred to as the metaphorical conception), disease is defined in social and cultural terms, as when the sick are viewed as deviants and people believe disease is caused by religious forces or actions of human agents (sorcerers) that would have been avoided were it not for the sufferers' social or moral failings. This has been the dominant conception throughout most of history, and it prevails in many nonliterate societies today. In the scientific conception of disease, which dominates in the United States and other rationalized societies, disease is defined in terms of deviation from normal neurophysiological states and is caused by natural forces that the individual has little, if any, power to ward off by his or her own action. Even without a technical, scientific understanding, most people believe diseases are due to natural causes.

At the same time, people may still view disease in terms of metaphor. Some diseases are viewed as dirty, and people with a particular disease are sometimes stigmatized and avoided. This may be true even though the danger of contagion is minor (e.g., leprosy) or nonexistent (e.g., cancer) (Sontag, 1978). The idea of disease as a social metaphor is the focus of the social construction perspective. This perspective stipulates that people respond to disease in terms of their definition of it, regardless of the scientific validity of the definition, which may derive from social and cultural conditions and not just biological conditions. A considerable literature has developed around this idea (Mishler, 1981a, 1981b).

In this chapter I examine some of the major aspects of the metaphorical construction of HIV-AIDS. My objective is to show that HIV-AIDS as a social metaphor is produced by underlying social conditions and is part of a social process. In pursing this goal, I compare the metaphorical construction of the AIDS epidemic and the constructions of the Black Death and cholera epidemics. First, however, I need to review two related but analytically distinct issues: (1) the general relation of metaphorical constructions to fear of contagion and (2) the difference between metaphorical constructions and collective behavior.

Disease as Metaphor, Fear of
Contagion, and Collective Behavior

The relationship between metaphorical constructions of diseases and fear of contagion is ambiguous, and any generalization is fraught with risk. We can say, however, that metaphorical constructions are never solely responses to epidemics and to fear of contagion. The same epidemic may evoke entirely different metaphorical responses in different societies. For example, the response of Islamic societies to the Black Death was much different from the response of European Christian societies. There also appears to be little evidence of massive panic in response to disease in nonliterate societies. Significantly, the foremost medical and anthropological expert on medicine in nonliterate societies, Edwin Ackerknecht (1971:24), noted that the magico-religious character of "primitive medicine" gives it a great deal of certainty, which reduces fear of contagion. But where such fear does exist, certain metaphors may be intensified; accusations that human agents (sorcerers, witches), in particular, may be especially intense. But these and other metaphorical responses are never simply responses to fear; they are also part of cultural tradition. A society that vehemently accuses sorcerers of causing a sudden outbreak of disease traditionally believes that sorcerers cause disease.

Collective behavior in epidemics differs from social metaphors of disease in the following way: Collective behavior may be precipitated by fear of contagion, but such behavior is also shaped by the social context in which it occurs and is infused with social meaning. For example, sorcery (and by extension, scapegoating) in response to an infectious epidemic may be intensified when social tensions are high (Hartwig, 1978:37). And the search for sorcerers, or for witches or scapegoats, almost always focuses on groups that have been traditionally viewed with suspicion or considered enemies of society. Sorcery and scapegoating in an epidemic may be metaphors for intergroup hatred. Therefore, the same response to an epidemic may be a form of extraordinary or extreme behavior when viewed from the collective behavior perspective but a metaphorical response when viewed from the social construction perspective. The difference is analytic, not concrete. A concrete expression of extreme actions may contain elements of collective behavior and social metaphor.

The difference may be seen another way. Collective behavior occurs because the everyday interpretation of disease is suspended (hence evoking fear of contagion) and the disease has little social meaning. People may attack or persecute witches and scapegoats. But such suspension also gives rise to new metaphors or intensifies existing metaphors that make the epidemic understandable in social and cultural terms. If people believe disease is caused by human agents, scapegoating and other forms of accusation give an epidemic social meaning. As collective behavior, societal reactions in epidemics are responses to fear. As metaphors, they symbolize social conditions and give the disease meaning. This is true for AIDS as well as other epidemics in history.

The Black Death and Religion

Since the Black Death occurred during a period in which scientific knowledge of diseases was virtually nonexistent, societal responses were controlled largely by metaphorical conceptions.

Moralizing, Blaming the Victim, and Religion

Prior to the development of scientific medicine, religion was a dominant force in the social construction of disease. Even though physicians had begun to separate medical interpretations of disease from religious interpretations by the time of the Black Death, religious interpretations still played a major role. However, the Black Death was so catastrophic that the usual religious interpretations were strained and found inadequate. Other interpretations emerged to fill the void but were themselves forged mostly out of religious beliefs. It was thought that individuals and humankind in general were being punished for sinful conduct. Other beliefs did exist, as, for example, physicians' belief that the disease was caused by astrological forces. But any opinions physicians had about natural causes had no chance with most people, for whom there could be but only one explanation: the wrath of God (Tuchman, 1978:103). This shaped the reactions to the disease.

Blaming the victim is inherent in the moral interpretation of disease. People believe the sick are the cause of their own disease. Therefore, avoidance (even desertion) of them during the Black Death, as was described in the previous chapter, prevented the blamer from being morally contaminated and in any case could be defended in the name of God. The underlying reality of the plague was rats, fleas, a lack of sanitation, and close contact. The social construction was, of course, altogether different. People believed the cause was moral and religious, and they responded to that belief. They blamed the victim.

Self-Flagellation. Blaming of the victim led logically to punishment of the self and self-flagellation. Even though this was a form of collective behavior, it also symbolized sinful conduct and the atonement for that conduct. Since the disease was divine punishment for sin, a metaphor based on religious beliefs, the flagellants believed that by punishing themselves, they could divert the punishment of God from themselves and humankind in general (Tuchman, 1978:114).

Psychologically, self-flagellation may be considered a form of collective masochism. When the cause of disease and death is unknown, it may generate widespread uncertainty, fear, and anxiety. People may turn to religious and moral beliefs in a search for certainty and confidence in the future. (For the classic statement on the relationships among uncertainty, fear-anxiety, and religion, see Malinowski, 1954.) Sociologically, however, self-flagellation symbolized evil, and this construction gave the epidemic social meaning.

Symbolization is always adapted to the wider culture. Self-flagellation, a part of the cultural tradition for many years before the Black Death, was meant to induce God to forgive people of their sins (Langer, 1958:295; Tuchman, 1978:114). Although an extreme form of collective behavior, the specific expression of self-flagellation was guided by a social construction built on traditional cultural beliefs. Within this cultural context, self-flagellation made the epidemic meaningful. It symbolized the Black Death as punishment from God.

Scapegoating, Religion, and the Social Structure

Which individuals and groups are selected as scapegoats is usually a function of the social structure. In this connection McNeill (1976:107) stated that there is a "universal human penchant for attributing the origin of an unfamiliar nasty disease to foreigners." More generally, members of any group (foreign or not) against whom the dominant population harbors suspicion or hostility and considers to be outcasts are apt candidates. The Jews were social pariahs who had long lived on the fringe of society. Their historical isolation was predicated on the idea that "contact with them brought the Christian faith into disrepute" (Tuchman, 1978:112), so Christians who had contact with them were also brought into disrepute. Social barriers had been established to prevent such contact—marriage between Jews and Christians was forbidden, Jews could not be servants for Christians or sell certain goods and products, and Jews were barred from certain guilds (Tuchman, 1978:112). Jews were thus convenient scapegoats for the Black Death. Scapegoating was a metaphor for social division, and the brutal treatment of Jews symbolized and reinforced the division. As with the moral interpretation, scapegoating was a social symbol.

The Cholera Epidemics and the Class Structure in the Early Nineteenth Century

During the course of the nineteenth century, evidence that cholera was related to environmental conditions accumulated. The cholera bacillus was isolated by Robert Koch in 1884. The effect of increases in scientific knowledge on the societal reactions to cholera epidemics over the course of the century is described in the next chapter. Here reactions to the earlier epidemic are examined.

Cholera as a Metaphor for Class Conflict: Fear of Violence and Conspiracy

By the nineteenth century, although religion was still a pervasive feature of society, a heightened sense of class identity and consciousness had emerged in the industrial societies of Europe and America, and the class structure was perhaps the dominant feature of society, as Karl Marx and his followers contended. The working and living conditions of the working class were brutal, and the oppressive practices of the wealthy (capitalist) class were severe. The privileged and wealthy feared the violence and riotous behavior of the poor, the "dangerous" classes, and erected physical and social barriers to keep them segregated. The poor masses of the working class, for their part, resented and distrusted the capitalists and wealthier classes. This was the social context in which the cholera epidemics occurred.

Policies to isolate people with cholera and restrict the movement of people, as reviewed in the last chapter, were especially severe for the poor, as were the brutal way the sick and suspects were treated. The poor experienced these actions as directed against *them,* not against cholera, and they viewed cholera itself as a genocidal plot. Some thought the wealthy were using it to control the population of the lower class. (There was probably some real basis for this belief because since the seventeenth century, physicians had commonly considered an increase in population to be a cause of disease [Grmek, 1989:105].) "The poor all over Europe could not understand how a disease that [primarily] attacked the lower classes could be anything but intentional." Many concluded, therefore, that "the ruling class had chosen to use [cholera] as a weapon in the class war" (Delaporte, 1986:50).

For the wealthy, hospitalization (and other isolation measures) "isolated [the sick] and kept them at a reassuring distance from the healthy," but this was "actually of benefit mainly to the wealthy." Isolation protected the rich from being contaminated by the poor, or so the rich believed, but it also protected them from the violent behavior of the poor. For the wealthy, then, "fear of disease alternated with fear of riot," so that actions were "directed not only against a disease but also against a class—the dangerous class—whose hostility might at any moment be unleashed" (Delaporte, 1986:61). And mob action and riots by the poor did sometimes occur (Rosenberg, 1962:33; Morris, 1976:108–117; Durey, 1979:157–159; Delaporte, 1986: 65–67, 69–72; Evans, 1987:244). Since the poor believed the wealthy and powerful were using cholera as a weapon in the class war, the former's acts of violence were expressions of class hatred, not simply reactions to cholera itself.

Interpretations of cholera reflected a variety of other social tensions (Durey, 1979, 188–189), but class tensions were dominant. Interpretations rose out of fear of contagion, of course, but they also rose out of the class structure and symbolized class hatred and fear and, for the poor, class oppression and a lack of social justice (Morris, 1976:95–126; Evans, 1987: 367–368). "The rich feared lethal contamination" by the poor, and the "poor feared that the rich were poisoning them" (Delaporte, 1986:157–159). Cholera was more than a biological disease. It was a social metaphor for class conflict. The class structure and class hatred were to cholera what religion and religious hatred had been to the Black Death.[1]

Moralizing, Blaming the Victim, and the Class Structure

Moralizing about disease and blaming the victim were still common in the early nineteenth century. However, a belief that disease had natural causes had begun to take hold, at least among physicians, most of whom subscribed to the idea of miasma or infectionism. Neither could account for cholera, leaving physicians squabbling about the nature of the disease and its cause (Briggs, 1961:91–92; Rosenberg, 1959:39; Morris, 1976:129, 161–162; Delaporte, 1986:116–130; Evans, 1987:235–236). Thus, as with the Black Death, a cultural vacuum existed that allowed for the introduction of moralistic interpretations (Morris, 1976:161). By all accounts, the dominant interpretation in Europe and the United States was that cholera was God's punishment for vice, sin, and moral flaws (Briggs, 1961; Rosenberg, 1962; Morris, 1976; Durey, 1979; Delaporte, 1986:107–113).[2] The dominant reaction was to moralize and blame the victim.

As early as 1832, a few people recognized that cholera was associated with filth and the environment (Rosenberg, 1962:58–60), but to most people it symbolized sin. The disease was caused by moral failing and was punishment from God. Many members of the medical profession (probably most of them) believed this (Evans, 1987:355), though as predisposing, rather than as primary, causes. (Even so, in *The Treatise on Epidemic Cholera* in 1832, Dr. Amariah Brigham wrote that boards of health should be given "the power to *change the habits of the sensual, the vicious, the intem-perate*" [Musto, 1986:106].) Cholera was a metaphor for immorality.

Moral metaphor was intertwined with the metaphor of class conflict (Morris, 1976:95–126). Since cholera took such a heavy toll among the poor, the combination of metaphors came easily. The poor (the dangerous class) were sick because of their immoral habits. "In America, as in Europe, cholera was specifically associated in 1832 with 'the most miserable and degraded of our population—white, black, and coloured'—and it was said to 'arise entirely from their habits of life'" (Briggs, 1961:88; see also Delaporte, 1986:63).[3] The higher classes did not believe that the poor lived "in accordance with bourgeois ethical principles" (Delaporte, 1986:112). Moreover, they also believed that the lower class lived as "primitives" and "savages" and thus were not civilized (Delaporte, 1986:105). Many realized, of course, that the poor lived in filthy environments, but these same people also believed that this circumstance simply "mirrored accurately [the poor's] inner [moral] decay" (Rosenberg, 1968:133). Cholera was "God's justice" for such decay (Rosenberg, 1962:40–52). This decay could even infect the air. For example, on July 23, 1832, the *Evening Post* of New York City wrote of the "vilest brutes" who lived in a local red-light district, "Be the air pure from Heaven, their breath would contaminate it, and infect it with disease" (Rosenberg, 1962:34). The poor were the cause of their own suffering.

The class-related moral interpretation of cholera influenced other reactions by the propertied and "respectable" classes. Although some fled cities and towns out of fear and panic (Rosenberg, 1962:26–28, 37; Durey, 1979: 139–141), many did not. They felt secure in the fact that their habits were temperate and their conduct moral (Rosenberg, 1962:29–30; Morris, 1976: 144; Durey, 1979:150–151). That medicine had no acceptable explanation reinforced the moral interpretation. Indeed, Morris (1976:164) stated that "the confusion and failure [of medicine] provided [people] with more proof of the power of God, and was a reason for the widespread acceptance of religious comfort and explanation."[4] Just as the suffering of the poor was due to their immoral habits, the lack of suffering among the higher classes was due to their higher moral standards.

Scapegoating and the Class Structure

The moral construction of cholera also scapegoated the poor. Since immoral habits caused cholera and the habits of the poor were immoral, it followed that poor people *caused* the disease and its spread through the population. It is not clear what people thought the causal mechanism of such contagion was. Many believed that mere proximity to the poor was sufficient. To some extent cholera is contagious, but many viewed contagion in moral terms, as though physical proximity to persons of poor morals put a person in jeopardy of contracting the disease (Rosenberg, 1962:133). Hence, contact with the poor was to be avoided for fear of moral contamination. Keeping a distance from the poor was a matter of *social*, not just physical, distance.

It is clear that moralizing, blaming the victim, scapegoating, and charges of conspiracy were not simply irrational flailings and forms of collective response to fear of contagion and death. They were reactions guided by the social metaphors of class conflict and the immorality of the poor (Durey, 1979: 188–189).

HIV-AIDS and Deviance

More than victims of any disease in modern times, people with HIV-AIDS have been viewed with disgust and hatred and treated as social pariahs. One reason for this is that HIV may be sexually transmitted, and persons with STDs have long been stigmatized in the United States (Brandt, 1987). However, the dominant factor is that HIV-AIDS is concentrated among deviant groups that are already stigmatized, especially male homosexuals. The association of HIV-AIDS with deviance is especially important in moralizing and blaming the victim, which are the most prominent metaphorical reactions to HIV-AIDS, as they were to cholera.[5]

Unlike in the nineteenth century, when belief in natural causes of disease had strong competition from religious and other mythical reasoning, AIDS appeared when belief in the natural cause of disease was thoroughly institutionalized in the culture. However, since no firm estimate of the number of infections could be given, no one knew how fast the epidemic was growing, particularly among heterosexuals. Such uncertainties brought forth conjectures that were horrifying, if true. By 1987 it was clear that the time between HIV infection and the onset of AIDS was longer than experts had originally thought, and this compounded the uncertainty. The New York City health commissioner, Stephen C. Joseph, stated that "the hardest thing for the public, for all of us, is that we desperately want certainty" about the disease, but there was no certainty, even about the number of infections (Lambert, 1987). And like the Black Death and cholera, no one knew what the cause of AIDS was, at least during the early years of the epidemic. Recall that the AIDS epidemic began in 1981, but the virus was not known until the spring of 1984, and the mode by which HIV was transmitted was not clarified for some time thereafter. And it took several more years before such knowledge was diffused in the population. Therefore, uncertainty abounded, and a situation not unlike that of the earlier epidemics existed: Uncertainty created a cultural vacuum, permitting moralistic and other metaphorical explanations to move into the void.

Moralizing, Blaming the Victim, and Deviance

During the early years of the epidemic, there was little fear of contagion in the general population, with many viewing AIDS as a gay disease. However, in the absence of a scientific explanation, moralistic interpretations were introduced (Hancock and Carim, 1986:40–41). Some religious groups admonished that AIDS was "God's revenge" or a "message from God," and that there would be "no epidemic in the West if the laws of Moses had been followed" (Plummer, 1988:32). Jerry Falwell, president of Moral Majority, was one of the first to claim, at a news conference in July 1983, that AIDS was divine punishment—God was "spanking" gays for their sins (Bayer, 1985:588–589; Hancock and Carim, 1986:40).[6] In 1984 an election advertisement in Australia referred to "the satanic spread of the AIDS homosexual 'wrath of God' disease" (Altman, 1986:185). Probably the most well-known example of AIDS as moral retribution appeared on May 24, 1983, in the *New York Post* by syndicated columnist and subsequent presidential candidate Patrick Buchanan (1983). Buchanan, who believed that, according to Christian doctrine, homosexuals were "leading a life of sin" (Buchanan, 1991:9), wrote the *Post* column under the headline "AIDS Disease: It's Nature Fighting Back." He exhorted, "The poor homosexuals—they have declared war on Nature and now Nature is exacting an awful retribution."

Moralizing did not stop even when AIDS was affirmed to be a bloodborne disease caused by a virus and explained entirely by natural causes. The American Council of Christian Churches declared in 1989 that HIV-AIDS was God's judgment against male homosexuals (Weitz, 1991:22). *Time* reported on a Vatican meeting about HIV-AIDS in November 1989 in which Pope John Paul II claimed that the connection between homosexuality and HIV-AIDS was due to an "abuse of sexuality" and that the AIDS crisis was due to an "immunodeficiency" in values. Since the biological cause of AIDS is a deficiency of the immune system, the moral versus scientific interpretation of the disease is clear. In case there was any doubt, at the same meeting Father Rocco Buttiglione of Liechtenstein's International Academy of Philosophy suggested that the AIDS epidemic could indeed be "divine punishment" (*Time*, November 27, 1989:58).

Such statements, as strange as they may seem, resemble the statements church officials had made about the Jews during the Black Death (Tuchman, 1978:110) and the clergy's exhortations in the nineteenth century that cholera was God's justice for moral failing. The idea that AIDS among gays was a "spanking" from God is not unlike the belief held by much of the clergy during the early cholera epidemics that cholera was a "rod in the hand of God" (Kraut, 1994:31–94). More generally, compare the above positions on AIDS and those held by the clergy and others during the cholera epidemic of 1832, which Charles Rosenberg (1962:45) summarized as follows: "The pestilence was an inevitable result of man's failure to observe the laws of nature. Man has free will, and when he fails to observe those laws, brings inescapable punishment upon himself." Similarly, people with AIDS, especially gays, chose their "lifestyle," and punishment from God was the inevitable result of that choice.

As noted, moral metaphors of cholera by the well-to-do were also metaphors of class conflict and symbolized fear of lower-class violence and revolt. By the same token, moral attacks on people with HIV-AIDS were moral metaphors and a repudiation of groups (especially gays) that many viewed as morally deviant. In this connection, some wrote and spoke of "innocent victims." For example, Robin Maranz Henig (1983:36) referred to hemophiliacs and others as "innocent bystanders" caught in the path of HIV-AIDS, a theme repeated by many journalists (Wellings, 1988:86–88).[7] President George Bush stressed that "innocent babies" could be infected (Weitz, 1991:28). To refer to such people as innocent is to imply that persons who contract HIV in male-to-male anal intercourse or in the exchange of needles in drug use must be guilty (Brandt, 1987.201). Buchanan and religious leaders were explicit.

Since HIV-AIDS was so highly concentrated in deviant groups, especially gays, moral reasoning was easy to come by. Gays (IDUs) *chose* to be gay (and drug injectors) of their own free will. A Supreme Court decision in June 1986 reinforced the moral interpretation. In *Bowers* v. *Hardwick* the Court upheld Georgia's sodomy statute, which makes homosexual acts a crime. In conveying the majority opinion, Chief Justice Warren Burger wrote, "To hold that the act of homosexual sodomy is somehow protected as a fundamental right would be to cast aside millennia of moral teaching" (Bayer, 1989:7). The decision said nothing about HIV-AIDS, but it did ratify a statute that made illegal certain acts, common among gays, that increased the risk of HIV-AIDS and that many viewed as immoral, a view with which the Supreme Court judges seemed to agree. By implication, therefore, the legal interpretation of homosexual sodomy supported the moral interpretation of HIV-AIDS. But note the process went in the other direction as well. The moral interpretation ("millennia of moral teaching") influenced the justices' legal interpretation concerning male homosexuals, the group at greatest risk of contracting HIV. In addition, as we see in Chapter 7, some physicians' views of people with HIV-AIDS were also influenced by the morals of society.

If a moral view of HIV-AIDS exists among religious leaders as well as judges and physicians, its acceptance by much of the general population would be expected. In fact, a Gallup poll in October 1987 found that 51 percent agreed it was the person's "own fault if [he or she] gets AIDS" (Lipset and Wattenberg, 1988:39). More significantly, 43 percent agreed that AIDS represented "divine punishment" (*New York Times,* October 11, 1987: I-18), which meant that tens of millions of Americans believed this. Even a middle-class mother who was infected with HIV through a blood transfusion and who considered herself a sacrificial innocent stated in an interview with Rose Weitz (1991:70), "AIDS is a punishment from God. I just feel like he's telling the gay population to knock it off. And if they continue to do so, and infect each other knowingly, then they deserve what they get."

As with cholera, to many people HIV-AIDS was the result of moral failing and a form of God's justice. Impressions of journalists are in accord with this view. For example, in the January 1987 issue of the *Atlantic Monthly* (in what was actually an alarmist article about the heterosexual spread of AIDS), a journalist stated, "To travel around this country talking to people about AIDS is to learn quickly that most Americans still regard the emergence of the disease, which struck gays first, as an act of God" (Leishman, 1987:39). For many people, then, HIV-AIDS was a metaphor for evil, and this gave it social meaning and an interpretation that they could understand. People who had HIV-AIDS did not just (or even) have a physical disease. They were sinners, and God was punishing them for their sins. As with cholera, HIV-AIDS was gauged in terms of moral standards. Gays (and IDUs) fell below the norms. Straights (and especially those of zealous religious convictions) rose above them.

Such thinking is strange, bigoted, and irrational to persons who do not think this way, but to many this was exactly what HIV-AIDS meant (and still means to some). This belief was obviously contradictory. If HIV-AIDS were God's punishment for homosexuality, why was the punishment so extreme for gays only in the United States? Why did the punishment begin in the early 1980s? More fundamentally, why were lesbians not being punished? It is a sociological truism that lack of logic is no barrier to moral reasoning. Inconsistencies are simply ignored if they cannot be explained away; to believers God works in mysterious ways. Besides, He had condemned and punished male homosexuals before (e.g., in Sodom and Gomorrah more than two thousand years ago), and so it makes perfect sense that He would do so to gays in the late twentieth century. In the early years of the epidemic, scientists did not agree on an acceptable interpretation to counter moral interpretations, which made the latter all the more persuasive, just as disagreement among doctors had made religious interpretation of cholera persuasive 150 years before (Morris, 1976:164).

Mistreatment, Stigma, and Deviance

In a 1987 nationwide Gallup survey reported in the *New York Times* (November 22, 1987:I-18), 17 percent of respondents said landlords should have the right to evict people with HIV-AIDS, and 71 percent thought victims should not be isolated from the rest of society (implying that 29 percent thought they should be quarantined). In a study of people with HIV-AIDS, Weitz (1991:124) reported that most persons who disclosed their illness "were either fired immediately, demoted, or forced to quit by co-workers or employers who made their situations intolerable." A Harvard-educated lawyer who was forced out of a job at a top Texas law firm said that to have AIDS was "like wearing the scarlet letter." He said that when coworkers find out, "there is a shading, a variation in how they treat men. There is less familiarity. A lot less" (Wallis, 1985:45). Such reactions, along with the increase in physical attacks on male homosexuals (Zuckerman, 1988), may have been based to some extent on fear of contagion. But not all were: In a 1988 Gallup poll 11 percent believed it was possible to get AIDS just from working alongside someone with AIDS, whereas in a 1987 poll 25 percent said they would actually work beside a person with AIDS (Lipset and Wattenberg, 1988:29, 37). It was necessary for coworkers to maintain *social* distance and not be too familiar with workers who had AIDS. People feared *social* contamination and not just physical infection. The responses of psychology students at Stockton State College (New Jersey) to a questionnaire exemplifies the point (their responses may well be representative of the general population). Only 50 percent said they would be "willing to work in the same office with someone dying of AIDS" (in comparison to 89 percent for cancer), and only 62 percent would "buy a house next to someone dying from AIDS" (versus 89 percent for cancer) (Lester, 1988).

As noted in the last chapter, religious and political conservatives in particular expressed alarm about casual contagion. To Fumento (1990:183), among others, this was "certainly a mystery." The scientific community had dismissed casual contact as impossible. Furthermore, the conservative moralizers themselves had little to fear from being infected through casual contact since they had little contact with gays and drug users. (They no noubt deliberately avoided contact with them.) So why raise the alarm? They did so for the same reason that moralizers feared contact with victims of the cholera epidemics, most of whom were poor: to reinforce the *social* distance between themselves (the general population) and members of high-risk groups (and especially male homosexuals), not just the physical distance. When viewed this way, the moralists' concern about casual contact during the AIDS epidemic is no more mysterious than the moralists' concern about keeping a distance from the poor during the cholera epidemics.

This is not to say that all of the moralists advocated mistreatment. The pope and other church officials at the Vatican meeting admonished that people with HIV-AIDS should not be discriminated against and should be treated with compassion (*Time,* November 17, 1989:58). Priests and other religious leaders may be up to treating "sinners" with compassion, but this is not the case for most ordinary members of society whose moralistic zeal the leaders inspire. (Here is another parallel with the Black Death. In 1348 the pope issued a statement urging that the persecution of Jews be stopped [Tuchman, 1978:113], with no apparent effect.)

Scapegoats, Foreigners, and Deviance

As with most epidemics, the primary scapegoats for HIV-AIDS were either foreigners or outcast groups. They included Haitian immigrants and prostitutes. (The Africa as origin hypothesis scapegoated Africans and is examined in the next chapter.)

Haitians. In the early 1980s, Haitian immigrants were accused of spreading AIDS. Early statistics showed that a disproportionate number of Haitian immigrants did have AIDS. The reasoning advanced for this, however, reflected social attitudes about the Haitians. As noted in Chapter 2, one theory, based on sheer conjecture, was that Haitians had contracted the virus from the ingestion of animal blood in voodoo ceremonies (Moore and Le Baron, 1986). A more common belief among scientists (Gallo, 1988:56) was that Haiti was a "bridge" between Africa and the United States. Haitians visited Africa as workers, contracted HIV, returned to Haiti, and either by having sex with gay American tourists or by immigrating were responsible for HIV in the United States. However, the HIV strains in Haiti resemble the American strains more than the African strains (Grmek, 1989:154), and it is equally plausible, and probably more likely, that HIV was introduced to Haiti by gay tourists from the United States (Shoumatoff, 1988:163; Grmek, 1989:154, 174). This was not the first time in American history that Haitians had been blamed for bringing an infectious disease to the United States. They had been blamed for the yellow fever epidemic in Philadelphia in 1793 (Kraut, 1994).

Haitians continued to be classified as a high-risk group even after it had become apparent they were not the source of HIV. Thus, the scapegoating followed a typical pattern (McNeill, 1976:107)—namely, society attributing a new disease to foreigners and Americans attributing a new disease to immigrant pariahs (Kraut, 1994). Haitians were subsequently declassified as a high-risk group, but we must wonder: If the same kind of evidence had been found for Canadians or the English, would these groups have been labeled the way the Haitians were?

Prostitutes. Prostitutes probably have a higher rate of HIV-AIDS than the rest of the American population, though existing evidence is very limited in this regard and indicates no increase over time. Studies in the United States and Europe show that for nondrug-using prostitutes, HIV infection is not particularly high (Root-Bernstein, 1993:39–43) and not nearly as high as many earlier believed (Lambert, 1988). In addition, the customers of prostitutes may have a rate no higher than 1 percent (Wallace, 1989). Prostitutes are thus not a significant threat for transmitting HIV in the United States (Root-Bernstein, 1993:39–43; Fumento, 1990:97–106).

Nevertheless, as with other STDs (Brandt, 1987), prostitutes have been considered major sources of infection and singled out as scapegoats. Television talk shows and the print media have charged that prostitutes are a major source of heterosexual transmission (Fumento, 1990:98). For example, in June 1987 Mark Kleiman (1987:22), a teacher of public policy at Harvard's Kennedy School of Government, wrote in the *Wall Street Journal,* without citing any evidence at all, that "between 1,000 and 10,000 men will become infected with the AIDS virus by having sex with female prostitutes."

Scapegoating seems to have reached its height during the period of extreme fear of heterosexual transmission. Rumors were rampant that prostitutes were deliberately giving HIV to their customers, and on the popular television program "Geraldo," prostitutes with HIV were called "AIDS assassins" (Fumento, 1990:97). Prostitution and HIV-AIDS were a topic in *Newsweek* on June 25, 1990, and a picture of an apparently infected prostitute from Oakland, California, was shown. The *New York Times* reported (July 15, 1990:I-8) that an Oakland police officer, who knew the woman, saw the picture and arrested her for "attempted murder."

As noted in the previous chapter, health care providers were also made scapegoats. However, in this instance their scapegoating derived from their close contact with patients and the American tendency to distrust officialdom and social institutions, including physicians and the medical establishment, not from any status as social pariahs (Musto, 1986:114).

The Racial and Moral Context of Charges of Genocide and Conspiracy

To understand charges by African Americans that AIDS was a racial conspiracy and genocidal plot, we must understand the social-racial context in which such charges were made. To label these charges bizarre, irrational, or paranoid, as some have done, implies that those making the charges suffer from some form of psychological malady. In fact, the charges reflect a *social* malady instead—namely, historical racism against African Americans and their oppression in American society. The charges resemble those of the poor during the cholera epidemics, which were responses to class oppression.

To many African Americans, the validity of the belief that AIDS was racial genocide was driven home by something that came to light in the late 1980s: It was revealed that the U.S. Public Health Service had conducted an experiment, known as the Tuskegee syphilis study, earlier in the century in which African-American men in rural Alabama who had syphilis went untreated so the experimenters could see what the effects of the disease would be. Under the circumstances, why would it be bizarre and paranoid to believe the same thing was happening with respect to HIV-AIDS? Thus, an African-American journalist stated, "If some African-Americans feel that a secret white American cabal is trying to kill us off, there might be some reasons" (Cary, 1992: 23).[8] Racial genocide would be consistent with the way many African Americans had been treated in the past.[9]

As noted in the last chapter, gays and conservatives (religious and political) made charges and countercharges about a conspiracy. Conservatives charged that gays were intentionally spreading HIV, and gays charged that political conservatives were trying to kill them. Even though some may view such charges as irrational or bizarre fantasies, they were guided and given meaning by existing social and cultural conditions. The gay liberation movement had enjoyed considerable success, but a high proportion of the American public still believed (and continues to believe) that sex between persons of the same sex is immoral. Moral conflict between gays and religious and conservative political leaders (e.g., Jerry Falwell, Pat Robertson, Anita Bryant, Pope John Paul II and other officials of the Roman Catholic church, Senator Jesse Helms, Patrick Buchanan) was (and is) especially intense (Greenberg, 1988:466–468). Gays felt others were trying to oppress them, whereas the "oppressors" believed gays were degenerate and had no legitimate place in society. In this context charges and countercharges of conspiracy are not bizarre at all. They are simply extensions of moral conflict, just as the charges during the Black Death and cholera epidemics were extensions of religious and class conflict.

To charge that gay leaders were allowing HIV-AIDS to spread in order to advance their (immoral) political agenda or to pressure the federal government to spend more money on HIV-AIDS research made plenty of sense to the moral opponents of gays. Gays were immoral lowlifes, and such persons, after all, would go to any means to achieve their aims (the "gay agenda"). By the same token, gay accusations of genocide made plenty of sense to some gays. After all, their opponents hated them, considered them immoral degenerates whose "life style" polluted the culture, wanted their rights suppressed, and otherwise simply wanted them to disappear. Although many who disliked gays did not go beyond exhorting them to change their sexual orientation, for gays to believe a conspiracy of gay genocide was underfoot was not at all bizarre in light of the contemptible and hateful epithets hurled at them as well as the types of brutality they had historically experienced from the police and others. As David Black (1986:40) wrote, gays wondered, "How could a disease pick out just gays?" They answered, "There had to be medical homophobia." The poor had asked a similar question and arrived at a similar answer for why cholera took such a heavy toll among them.

Charges and countercharges by gays and their moral opponents were not just reactions to HIV-AIDS as a disease; they were expressions of moral conflict. They were social constructions of HIV-AIDS that, in the context of this conflict, gave the AIDS epidemic social meaning to some gays and their moral opponents no less than the charges and countercharges by many of the poor and wealthy had made the cholera epidemics meaningful to them. In a moral war enemies will make outrageous charges about each other, just as they do in class war or any other (political, military) war. There is nothing bizarre about this. Given the social conditions, it is altogether normal.

Conclusion

Despite great differences in the nature of the diseases and social and cultural conditions under which they occurred, parallels among the interpretations and social meaning of the bubonic plague, cholera, and AIDS epidemics are clear. Social constructions included moralizing, scapegoating, and charges conspiracy. As metaphors, they gave each epidemic a social meaning. People responded to these constructions rather than just (or even) to the biological attributes of the disease. In some instances such reactions were responses to unrealistic fear, whereas in other instances they probably reinforced fear. But regardless, in the absence of an explanation in terms of prevailing conceptions of disease, they gave meaning to the epidemics.

The previous chapter examined societal reactions as collective behavior, as extreme and extraordinary responses to fear of contagion. The analysis in this chapter complements that analysis. The extraordinary responses were patterned on existing conditions of society. This was especially clear in scapegoating and charges of conspiracy. These were patterned on preexisting divisions and conflicts (religious, class, sexual orientation) in the social structure, out of which metaphorical constructions were fashioned. At the same time, the metaphors widened the divisions and intensified the conflicts; the epidemics led to more extreme forms of collective behavior than would have otherwise occurred. Thus, in general terms, to quote again from McGrew's (1965:11) observation of the cholera epidemics in Russia in the

1820s: "An epidemic sharpens behavior patterns, but those patterns, instead of being aberrations [bizarre and without a factual basis], betray deeply rooted and continuing social imbalances [in society]." The AIDS epidemic did this in the United States in the 1980s.

Reactions to the AIDS epidemic are especially illuminating because they occurred in an age when the medical science conception of disease was widely accepted throughout society. Almost everyone believed diseases were due to natural causes, and that infectious diseases were due to infectious agents. However, metaphorical reactions guided by moral beliefs and symbolizing fractures in the social fabric were simply more powerful than the medical science conception in the minds of many people. Such reactions overrode the force of scientific interpretation in a way not seen since the articulation of germ theory. Even in an age of science, the view that the causes of disease are natural forces may not be sufficiently strong to eliminate the influence of cultural myths, social prejudices, and moral reasoning, thus validating a major tenet of the social construction of disease. However, as the growth of rationalization makes clear, science is also a powerful social force. It may weaken and dissipate reactions that are guided by metaphorical constructions of disease, as the analysis in the next chapter shows.

NOTES

1. It was not just the upper classes that the poor feared; it was also the government, which protected the interests of the upper classes. McGrew (1965:116) contended that the reactions of the poor in the Russian epidemics were to the oppression of autocratic government rather than to the wealthy and propertied as such.

2. This may have been less so in Russia. McGrew (1965:12) observed that, although in some places cholera was attributed to God's will, this was not true everywhere; the particular response varied with local conditions.

3. The quote by Briggs is from Adams (1947:82).

4. "To put the matter ... sociologically, religion thrived in conditions of social instability and physical danger [as during the cholera epidemic of 1831–1832 in England], as men needed to reassert their values and seek security in the promises and community of faith. Church attendance improved as the epidemic approached" (Morris, 1976:144).

5. A number of authors have written about reactions to AIDS as metaphor, though in somewhat different ways (Altman, 1986; Conrad, 1986; Treichler, 1987; Alcorn, 1988; Brandt, 1988a; Sontag, 1988; Padgug, 1989; Patton, 1990a; Weitz, 1991).

6. To say that AIDS is a spanking by God is not just archaic thinking; it is also a horrible insult to the people who have this awful disease and to all caring people. It is also an insensitive confusion of metaphors. If Falwell felt the need to use a religious metaphor, "kiss of death" would have been more apt than spanking.

7. In a review of media coverage in Great Britain, Kay Wellings (1988:87) observed that "on the whole, the deaths of those who have contracted the disease as a

result of what some may see as 'illicit' or 'morally unacceptable' practices (by being gay, by being bisexual, by being a prostitute or by being an intravenous drug user) have been evaluated far more negatively by the media than those of people who have become infected as a result of accidental or iatrogenic infection."

8. A panel discussion of the Tuskegee study was held in February 1993 at Meharry Medical College, a predominantly African-American medical school in Nashville, and was covered by a reporter from the *Tennessean* (Ippolito, 1993). One participant (a Fisk professor) observed that the belief that HIV-AIDS was a plot to kill African Americans was circulating on college campuses, including Meharry. He stated, "When you hear young medical students, when you hear future doctors, when you hear the concerns they have, then you know it's a serious concern." To him, the connection between this belief and the Tuskegee study was clear: "If racism is the residue of slavery, certainly mistrust and fear of genocide [from HIV-AIDS] must be the residue of the Tuskegee study" (Ippolito, 1993).

9. The history of the Hispanic social experience in the United States has been different; Hispanics were never legally enslaved and have not been oppressed the way African Americans have. Significantly, despite the high prevalence of AIDS among Hispanics, charges of conspiracy and genocide seem not to have been made by members of this group.

7. Science, Societal Reactions, and Social Control

The overall reactions of the scientific community to HIV-AIDS are well known. Once AIDS and the groups at high risk for the disease had been identified, a great deal of scientific research activity began in which the cause of AIDS was investigated, HIV identified, and the development of drugs for the prevention and treatment of HIV-AIDS pursued. While such activity involves technical aspects of virology, immunology, and other biomedical sciences, there are also social aspects to this activity that may be examined from the sociology of science perspective. I am concerned with two general approaches to the sociology of science perspective.

In one approach, science is viewed as being socially embedded. In this approach, the influence of social factors on scientific belief and research is the focus. In the other approach, the consequences of science for the beliefs and behavior of nonscientists is the focus, and science is viewed as an institution of social control. In the first part of the chapter I examine science and HIV-AIDS in terms of the first approach. In a much longer section, I examine medicine in terms of the second approach, that is, the effect of the reactions of science in controlling societal reactions.

The Social Embeddedness of Science and HIV-AIDS

Some social factors that influence scientific thought and activity are internal to science; others are external. Both types of influence may be seen in scientists' beliefs and research with respect to HIV-AIDS.

Internal Influence

The internal influence of science has been described by Thomas Kuhn (1971) in his well-known statement. Through logical reasoning and empirical discovery, scientists develop ideas about the nature of various aspects of the real world. As ideas accumulate about a particular phenomenon, a scientific consensus emerges about it and its underlying causes. This becomes the dominant interpretation and shapes the way scientists view the phenomenon in question. The interpretation provides the framework within which scientific research on the phenomenon is conducted, and ideas that do not conform to the interpretation or research findings that cannot be explained in terms of it are rejected or ignored. Scientific activity is thus more than the simple pursuit of truth. It is also social behavior, being guided by the beliefs and opinions of scientific peers in which the acceptance of an idea or a datum as empirical fact depends on whether the idea or datum is consistent with or can be explained by the dominant interpretation. A scientist with a discovery or an idea that is subsequently accepted may actually be discredited when the discovery or idea is first made or presented. A new interpretation emerges only when the accumulation of evidence becomes so great that ideas and facts that are inconsistent with the dominant interpretation cannot be ignored or rejected any longer.

With respect to HIV-AIDS, as knowledge accumulated in the 1980s, a dominant interpretation emerged. Research discoveries led scientists increasingly to agree that the explanation of AIDS was a special case of germ theory and that AIDS is a syndrome of infectious diseases due to impairment of the immune system. Most scientists came to believe that HIV is sufficient and necessary to cause the immunosuppression that leads to AIDS. In addition, HIV is classified as a special kind of virus (a retrovirus) that is blood-borne and not transmissible through casual contact, and the primary modes of transmission in the United States are anal sex between homosexuals and needle sharing by drug injectors. Gradually, ideas contrary to these were rejected, a consensus was formed, and the dominant interpretation of HIV-AIDS emerged. This interpretation now shapes the perceptions and beliefs most scientists have with respect to HIV-AIDS.

It is conceivable, however, that the dominant interpretation represents premature scientific consensus. Michigan State physiologist Robert Root-Bernstein (1993), among others, believes this is in fact the case. Root-Bernstein questions the idea that HIV is necessary and sufficient to cause AIDS, and he believes that some of the ideas that are inconsistent with the dominant interpretation are valid. Nevertheless, some scientists who have proposed that factors other than HIV cause AIDS or challenged the orthodox view in other ways have been ostracized and discredited by the scientific community: They have lost positions on research boards and editorial boards of scientific journals; editors of scientific journals have denied them opportunities to express their views in their journals; and committees that control how funds for research agencies are allocated have denied them funds to conduct research on their ideas (Root-Bernstein, 1993:339, 349). There are few scientists who do not realize the consequences for their careers if they challenge the validity of the view held by most scientists.

The point here is not to question (or affirm) the validity of the dominant interpretation of HIV-AIDS.[1] Neither is it to assert that scientists' perceptions and beliefs about HIV-AIDS are controlled by the dominant interpretation simply for social reasons, namely, fear of ostracism and discreditation by scientific peers. Rather, it is to note that if the interpretation is in fact premature, social factors are in part responsible. Furthermore, the interpretation is the result of a social process. Of course, most of the beliefs that most scientists have about AIDS derive from research on the disease, but the research efforts have been (and are) controlled by more than the pursuit of the truth. They are also controlled by what other scientists find acceptable. The dominant interpretation of AIDS emerged the way any communal belief or norm emerges. There was a social process in which the beliefs of scientists converged, the beliefs and research of individual scientists were shaped by the dominant view of the scientific community, and scientists who expressed dissenting views were rejected by their peers. In this sense, scientific beliefs about HIV-AIDS have come to be controlled by social developments internal to science. They have also been influenced by social factors external to science.

External Influence

External influence refers to the role that social beliefs, values, and attitudes in the surrounding society have on scientific activity. The most famous case of external influence occurred during the Inquisition when Galileo was forced to recant his Copernican view of the universe. This does not mean that Galileo actually changed his beliefs, but it is certainly probable that fear of retribution for heresy influenced what many scientists believed about the natural world. Even today, religious views influence some scientists' beliefs about evolution. The more subtle influence of religion may be seen, as in Merton's (1970) tracing of the emergence of modern science in England to religious values associated with the puritan ethic. Social attitudes and beliefs may have influenced scientists' belief about the origin of HIV, and they have definitely influenced the view that at least some physicians have held about the cause of AIDS.

African Is Origin Hypothesis. As noted in Chapter 2, the mere fact that heterosexual transmission of HIV is more prevalent in Africa has led many to believe that the disease is more advanced in Africa and indeed that Africa is the historical origin of HIV. Scientists have presented several variations on this hypothesis, but as physician and AIDS researcher Samuel Duh wrote (1991:61–62), all hypotheses follow the same line of reasoning:

> There is a close similarity between [SIV] and [HIV]; SIV is isolated in African green monkeys, and the green monkeys have close contact with humans in Central and East Africa. ... The speculation is that green monkeys bit humans and transmitted SIV. Alternatively, humans ate green monkeys with SIV infection and thus contracted the virus. SIV underwent mutation to become HIV and somehow maintained a silent infectious state. During the immediate postindependence years (the early 1960s), many of the countries in Central and East Africa acquired expert knowledge; the experts who came included Haitians. The Haitian experts (mostly men) had sex with African women who were infected with HIV. They returned to Haiti and spread the virus in heterosexual and bisexual populations. Homosexuals from San Francisco went to Haiti on vacation, had sex with bisexuals, and contracted the virus. They brought it to San Francisco. Meanwhile, some of the European experts also had sex with infected African women and similarly introduced the virus to the homosexual populations in Europe. The virus spread from homosexual IV drug users to heterosexual IV drug users, and then it finally spread to the rest of the population.

Duh (1991:62) reported that this story "has been the 'official' scenario of the origin of HIV-AIDS infections" and that he has heard it from officials from the CDC and state public health departments as well as from infectious disease specialists and experts. "The story is told so matter-of-factly that there seems to be no doubt about it." Clearly, however, in light of the evidence reviewed in Chapter 2 (see also Duh, 1991:60–65), there are several reasons to doubt the story. If this is so, why have so many scientists and experts clung to the story ("hypothesis")? Gallo's reasoning suggests an answer.

In December 1987 Gallo presented a hypothesis that the first known human retrovirus, HTLV-1, originated in Africa. He hypothesized that HTLV-1 infected many species of Old World primates, including human beings (who may have actually been infected by monkeys) and reached the Americas via the slave trade (Gallo, 1987:95–96). Gallo knew his argument was flawed by the fact that the virus had appeared among people in areas that slave traders out of Africa had never visited (specifically, among the Ainu on an island in the northernmost part of Japan); and there were other questions as well (see Grmek, 1989:189–191). For example, green monkeys and chimpanzees, whose viruses are most closely related to HTLV (Gallo, 1987:95), are most apt to be found in Central and East Africa, but the African slave trade to the Americas was out of *West* Africa. Nevertheless, Gallo

(1987:96) contended, "for the time being, it remains a plausible explanation of the global pattern of the spread [of HTLV]." What is plausible about this? And what is plausible about the hypothesis that Africa is the origin of HIV? There is certainly no compelling evidence that makes either one plausible.

The strained reasoning of Gallo and the easy, almost nonreflective manner with which scientists accepted the hypothesis about the African origin of HIV suggest that it derived, not from science at all, but from a social tendency with deep historical and cultural roots: social prejudice against foreigners, the general tendency to attribute strange diseases to them, and the specifically Western tendency to believe new and strange diseases have their origin in Africa, which has been a cultural force in the West for centuries (Grmek, 1989:101). (Thucydides wrote that the disease of the Athenian epidemic originated in Ethiopia [Marks and Beatty, 1976:20].) Thus, Grmek (1989:124, 28) stated that, despite the evidence from serological analysis that HIV was present in the United States in the 1960s, "some specialists still have difficulties believing this story, because it challenges the scenario whereby AIDS is presented as having been imported into the United States [from Africa]." He mockingly asked, "[Did not] long-standing experience teach us that the dark continent was the cradle of strange microbes?" Age-old myths and social attitudes are hard to overcome and may influence the perceptions of scientists and their assessment of the facts about a new and mysterious infectious disease.[2]

Social Attitudes and Physicians' Views of AIDS. Although physicians are not scientists in the strict sense, they have been trained in the physical and life sciences and to view disease as caused by natural forces. However, in some instances physicians' views about HIV-AIDS depart widely from science and reflect the moral beliefs and social prejudices of the wider society.

For example, in the February 1984 issue of the *Southern Medical Journal*, Dr. James L. Fletcher (p. 150) of the Medical College of Georgia wrote an editorial that echoed Patrick Buchanan's moralistic diatribe. He suggested that AIDS among homosexuals was divine punishment—"a fulfillment of St. Paul's pronouncement: 'the due penalty of [the homosexuals'] error.'" Dr. Fletcher announced that "our society's approval of homosexuality is an error and that the unsubtle words of wisdom of the Bible are frighteningly correct."

At the time, the viral cause of AIDS was not known. However, the relationship between homosexuality and AIDS was known, which prompted Fletcher (1984:150, emphasis added) to question, correctly, "Could it be that a causal relationship exists between [homosexuals'] behavior and *their* disease?" However, rather than wondering what the natural cause might be, as his medical education had trained him to do, he suggested the cause was a *supernatural* force! The title of the editorial, "Homosexuality: Kick and

Kickback," captured exactly what he meant: Homosexuals had insulted ("kicked") God, and He was punishing them for this ("kicking back").

How common this view was among physicians in 1984 no one knows. But that a faculty member of a medical school would publicly express this view to his professional peers and that a major medical journal would publish it as an editorial strongly suggest that an archaic conception of disease overruled a medical science conception of AIDS in the minds of more than a few physicians.[3] This speaks volumes for the power cultural (moral) beliefs may have in the medical interpretation of disease.

Science, Metaphor, and Social Control

Medical science is nevertheless a powerful force. Recall that germ theory increased preventive behavior, as did knowledge about HIV. The effects of medical science in reducing collective hysteria, scapegoating, and moralizing about HIV-AIDS and the mistreatment of persons with HIV-AIDS were also significant. These effects are examined in the remainder of this chapter. To begin, however, a few general points about medicine as social control and how this compares with metaphorical (including archaic) conceptions are instructive.

From the standpoint of social control, the roles of medical science in rationalized societies and of archaic medicine in nonliterate societies are similar. This may be seen by comparing the roles of shamans and physicians. Shamans interpret many illnesses as due to immoral thought or behavior and as punishment from God or magical human agents. They have the power to mediate with these magico-religious forces, and they speak with moral authority. Consequently, they are agents of social control, and according to some anthropologists, this is their primary function. After their rituals are performed, the moral code of the community is reinforced for the patients as well as for others who may be present. Consequently, Ackerknecht (1971: 168) stated that shamans provide "at little expense the services that in our society are rendered by courts, policemen, newspapers, teachers, priests and soldiers." This is not to say, of course, that natives of nonliterate societies are aware of the role shamans play in social control. The consequences are, in Robert Merton's (1957) terms, unintended and unrecognized, or latent functions, rather than anticipated and recognized, or manifest functions.

The moral authority of modern physicians and medical scientists does not begin to approach that of shamans. Nevertheless, in a rationalized society medicine exerts much influence over the way society reacts to people with disease. It does this primarily through the institutionalization of medical knowledge. Such control is largely unanticipated and unrecognized. The intent of most medical scientists is to understand the biological and epidemiological features of a disease and arrive at an effective treatment or preventive, not to control the societal interpretation of a disease and the way persons who have it are treated.

Therefore, no less than metaphorical conceptions of disease, the medical science conception is a social construction that shapes reactions to disease. In pure form, this conception is based on physical reality, whereas metaphorical conceptions are based on social and cultural reality. The relativism of some social constructionists notwithstanding, the underlying reality of disease *is* biological and epidemiological. The social construction of disease may or may not be consistent with this. If people believe a disease is caused by supernatural spirits and is punishment for evil ways, the social construction is metaphorical and obviously deviates widely from reality as revealed by medical science. To the extent that the social construction is influenced by scientific knowledge and diseases are viewed as natural, rather than supernatural, phenomena, as they generally are in a rationalized society, this construction is more consistent with the underlying reality, and societal reactions will be more to diseases as biological states than to social and cultural forces.[4]

Consequently, as the social construction of a disease is controlled by the norms of science, the influence of metaphor declines, though it never disappears entirely. Since disease raises questions of death, dependency, physical and mental dysfunction, and, in many instances, contagion, societal reactions to disease will probably always be controlled to some extent by metaphor, even in highly rationalized societies. As Brandt (1988a:416) has stated, "Disease is simply too significant, too basic an aspect of human existence to presume that we could respond in fully rational or neutral ways." Nevertheless, as scientific knowledge about disease increases, social metaphors of disease lose force, and people are guided in their reactions more by rational and neutral norms of science than by fear and social metaphor.

There is, of course, no *one specific* reaction either in the scientific or the metaphorical conception. For example, the scientific conception leads people to avoid contact with persons who have influenza because of the fear of getting the infection, but there is normally no such avoidance of persons with diabetes, a far more serious disease. By the same token, metaphorical reactions are varied. Therefore, the scientific conception and metaphorical conceptions are cultural *frameworks* within which *specific* reactions to persons with different diseases may differ. The essential difference between the two conceptions is not that each leads to a uniform reaction that differs from the other but that one is based on empirical knowledge and scientific reasoning, whereas the other is based on cultural myths, social tensions, and moral reasoning.

The comparative influence of social metaphor and of science in controlling societal reactions to illness may be seen in changes in societal reactions to the cholera and the AIDS epidemics. In both instances societal reactions changed over time and were traceable to increases in scientific knowledge about the two diseases.

Changes in the Social Construction of Cholera and the Role of Science

Knowledge abut disease increased during the course of the nineteenth century. The relative importance of metaphor and science in controlling societal reactions to the cholera epidemics also changed.

The Early Epidemics

During the early epidemics, moral interpretations were far more powerful guides for societal reactions than scientific interpretations. In describing the epidemics of 1832 in England, Morris (1976:129) stated:

> In the face of terrible and inexplicable threat, individuals needed some guide which would enable them to carry on their lives with reasonable calm and order; governments needed some imperative which would gain the cooperation of their subjects in measures to combat the threat. Science could not provide this certainty. Science was unconvincing and could persuade no one of the value of public health measures. Therefore, religious and moral explanation and imperative [played the dominant role].

It was from the pulpit that people learned how to avoid cholera (or so they thought) (Rosenberg, 1962:5).

Epidemics at Midcentury

To some people, the early epidemics were lessons in public health (Briggs, 1961:84; Durey, 1979:204). Rosenberg (1962:147, 150) stated that by the time of the 1849 epidemic, more Americans were convinced that environmental reform was needed, and "a few ... suggested [that] cholera was a judgment demonstrating not that the poor were sinful, but [that they] were oppressed." Nevertheless, "most thoughtful persons were unable to discard an accustomed belief in the role of moral failing in the causation of disease"; they believed "it was the slum dweller who was responsible for the filth in

which he lived." Poverty was "a result—not a cause—of vice and imprudence," and vice and imprudence caused cholera. Thus, for example, rather
than authorities assuring that rental housing met sanitary conditions, they
urged landlords to be "more selective in their choice of tenants." Cholera
was still a judgment of God, and blaming the victim was the dominant reaction.

The situation in Europe was similar. In an account of the French epidemic
of 1832, Delaporte's (1986) general thesis is that physicians learned from
that epidemic, which led them to recognize that environmental factors
played an important role in disease, particularly cholera. The relationship
between sanitation and disease was also being brought to the public's attention in England, as in Edwin Chadwick's 1842 report to the British Parlia-
ment, "Report on the Sanitary Condition of Labouring Population of Great
Britain" (Flinn, 1965). English physicians began recommending measures of
environmental sanitation to prevent disease (Flinn, 1965:18–26). Medical
science still had little to offer, but a dent in European social attitudes had
been made (Briggs, 1961:84). So in the 1840s cholera was less apt to be
viewed as caused by class status and flawed character (Briggs, 1961:85).
Nevertheless, only a minority endorsed the sanitation movement, with most
of society paying the "sanitation idea" little heed (Briggs, 1961:85–86).
Even to believers in the idea, miasma was still the dominant notion. The role
of filth in disease was not understood, and sanitation measures were controversial. So, as in the United States, the prevailing interpretation of cholera in
Europe was still based on moral reasoning.

Epidemics in the Latter Part of the Century

By the time of the next epidemic in the United States, in 1866, "scientific
values and habits of thought had assumed a new prominence in the American mind" (Rosenberg, 1962:232). People were beginning to think about
disease differently. Statistics gathered by a generation of public health workers left little doubt that people "who lived in the worse conditions, in the
dirtiest, most crowded, and least ventilated houses" were most apt to be afflicted (Rosenberg, 1962:217). Although physicians still could not agree
about the causes of cholera (or disease in general), they increasingly accepted
secular theories, such as those of John Snow and Max von Pettenkofer,
which contended that cholera was a waterborne disease (Rosenberg, 1962:
194–200). Newspapers and magazines, in turn, urged readers to accept the
secular theories (Rosenberg, 1962:197). In general, then, the accumulation
of empirical evidence, the enhanced stature of science, and physicians' increasing agreement that cholera was due to natural causes helped change the
public's ideas about the disease.[5]

As the new thinking was incorporated in the political process and legal statutes, public reactions to cholera changed (Rosenberg, 1962:213). Sanitary reforms were introduced, and boards of public health could now use scientific evidence and the prestige of science to reinforce their reforms (Rosenberg, 1962:232). For example, the Metropolitan Board of Health in New York City imposed sanitation practices and showed that cholera could be prevented, "not with prayer and fasting," but with disinfection and other public health measures (Rosenberg, 1962:213). Cholera was increasingly seen as an issue of a filthy environment and less as a matter of "moral choice and spiritual salvation" (Rosenberg, 1962:228). The "gospel of public health" was gaining strength (Rosenberg, 1962:213–225), and societal reactions to cholera were being guided more by science.

The same changes occurred in Europe during the epidemics of the 1860s, 1870s, and 1890s (Briggs, 1961; Evans, 1992:171–173). Collective behavior was virtually absent during the last major epidemic in Hamburg, Germany, in 1892. "The absence of any rioting or public disturbance in Hamburg in 1892 contrasted sharply with the experience of cholera in other places and other times. ... [The] pattern of behavior—from terror released by the arrival of an epidemic, through the popular search for a scapegoat, ... to collective violence and revolt—was conspicuously lacking" (Evans, 1987: 367). Although this absence was due to several factors (Evans, 1987:366–372), preventive education based on Koch's isolation of *Vibrio cholerae,* the cholera bacillus, in 1884 was one reason:

> When the cholera epidemic hit Hamburg in 1892, ... Germany was a society on the threshold of [the] transition to mass medicalization. A last rotten bloom of the age of epidemics, [the epidemic] fell in a period when the educative influence of Koch and the bacteriologists—purveyed in Hamburg through leafletting, comprehensive disinfection, popular newspaper reports, and the like—was already having a substantial effect on public opinion. Thus political activists of all shades quickly accepted Koch's theory that cholera was caused by unfiltered water, poor housing, and inadequate sanitation. (Evans, 1987: 477–478)

As in the United States, scientific knowledge was incorporated into the political process and legal statutes (Evans, 1987:495–496). The Social Democrats, the party of the working class, endorsed the Koch-led medical explanation of cholera, giving it political sanction (Evans, 1987:370). By the time of the Hamburg epidemic in 1892, then, medical science was playing a more important role and religion a less important role in the social construction of cholera.[6] Rather than blaming the poor for cholera, people learned it was due to a bacillus, and they blamed society—"the state" and "the absence of constitutional democracy"—for cholera's concentration among the poor (Evans, 1987:478).

Moralizing and erroneous beliefs did not disappear, however. Indeed, in the United States in 1866 "cholera was still a sign of moral indiscretion" (Rosenberg, 1962:217), and many physicians continued to believe that moral failings were "predisposing causes" (Rosenberg, 1962:230). Also, some ministers viewed sanitary reform as "a necessary prerequisite for *moral* improvement" (Rosenberg, 1962:5, emphasis added). Some interpreted the laws of sanitation as God's laws, so that cholera was still punishment for neglecting the laws of God (Rosenberg, 1962:217). During the Hamburg epidemic of 1892, years after Koch had identified the *Vibrio cholerae,* some of the Hamburg clergy still preached that cholera was the Almighty's punishment for sin (Evans, 1987:358–362). It was not until "the twentieth century that social control [by public health] had become genuinely international" (Briggs, 1961:86). Religion and science existed together in uneasy contradiction in Europe as well as the United States.

Nevertheless, religious interpretation was losing the battle to "the strong and unified efforts of the authorities to educate the populace in simple ways of preventing infection, and the general acceptance of water-borne and person-to-person contagion as the major, and therefore in principle controllable, cause of the disease" (Evans, 1987:362). And outside the clergy itself, the moral interpretation of cholera was transformed from a spiritual morality into a secular morality, one in which individuals were simply careless and irresponsible rather than violators of God's will. According to Evans (1987: 363):

> In earlier epidemics, the advice had been to trust in God and obey the authorities; the explanation for cholera had been a moral decline of which irreligion was undoubtedly a part. But by the epidemic of 1892 the discourse on the moral origins of the disease had largely secularized itself. The working class was blamed because it was careless, and drunken, and irresponsible, but not— except by the church—because it was irreligious.

Thus, with each succeeding epidemic, as knowledge expanded, cholera was increasingly viewed as a specific disease caused by ingesting a specific (but until 1884 still unknown) type of poison. The social construction of cholera became more consistent with its natural causes, and science became the basis for the social construction of the disease. As scientific knowledge broadened and as consensus among medical scientists and physicians increased, scientific norms emerged and were incorporated in public health regulations and laws. Social attitudes changed, and the public began to react to cholera and its victims in ways that were consistent with scientific norms. The sick were less apt to be viewed as social deviants, and blaming the victim and scapegoating declined. Moral judgments did not disappear, but as evidence was gathered, "the hand of God was being withdrawn from the World," and "the role of the divine in causing cholera [became] a smaller one" (Rosenberg, 1962:220). The disease was increasingly viewed as a biological pathology, though one with environmental causes, and reactions became controlled by that view.[7] Cholera as a social metaphor was on the wane.

Expansion of Scientific Knowledge
and Changes in Societal Perception of HIV-AIDS

Although many have claimed that society and especially the federal government were slow to respond to the threat of HIV-AIDS, scientific achievement over a very short time was actually quite remarkable (Gallo, 1988). Starting in 1981 with no knowledge of HIV at all, medical science soon identified the groups in which AIDS was so prevalent, discovered HIV in 1984, and ascertained its modes of transmission shortly thereafter. A dominant scientific interpretation emerged. By comparison, a dominant interpretation of cholera in the nineteenth century took more than half a century to develop. Nevertheless, just as societal perceptions of cholera changed as a dominant scientific interpretation emerged, perceptions of HIV-AIDS changed as a dominant scientific interpretation of HIV-AIDS emerged. Media reports and efforts in public education were instrumental in this, just as they had been for cholera many generations earlier.

Science and the Media

Although there were many doctors of doom, there were also countervailing views in the scientific community. As early as 1983 in a speech to a conference of mayors, Margaret Heckler, secretary of the Department of Health and Human Services, reported that with the exception of individuals in certain groups, scientists had concluded that there appeared to be little risk of contracting AIDS, particularly through casual social contact (Bayer, 1989: 233); and in 1984, with Robert Gallo by her side, she announced that the viral cause of AIDS had been identified. In 1986 the Institute of Medicine of the National Academy of Sciences issued a report, *Confronting AIDS* (updated in 1988), and the surgeon general issued *Acquired Immune Deficiency Syndrome* (U.S. Public Health Service, 1986a). Both reviewed what was known scientifically about the transmission of HIV-AIDS and emphasized that it could not be transmitted through the air, insect bites, or casual contact with a person infected with HIV (such as shaking hands and living in the same household with such a person). The surgeon general repeated the message in 1988 in "Understanding AIDS," which was mailed to households in the country, and he also emphasized that transmission could not occur through casual contact or from the "saliva, sweat, tears, urine or bowel movement" of an infected person (U.S. Public Health Service, 1988:3).

Publications in the scientific and professional medical literature appeared in the middle to late 1980s in which the mode of HIV transmission was detailed (Friedland et al., 1986), international differences in the epidemiology of HIV-AIDS were described (Piot et al., 1988), and the possibility of transmission through casual contact was rejected (Sande, 1986; Lifson, 1988). As in other matters of medicial science, physicians and the media are the sources from which the public learns most of what it knows about a disease. As noted in Chapter 5, media coverage was not altogether balanced or undistorted (Albert, 1986; Check, 1987), and alarmist statements were still being reported in the late 1980s and early 1990s. Nevertheless, there was much accurate reporting. For example, on July 13, 1986, Harvey Fineberg (p. IV-29), dean of the Harvard School of Public Health, wrote in the *New York Times* that "we understand enough about the cause and spread of the AIDS virus to give people the knowledge they need to protect themselves."

By the end of the 1980s, the tone of media coverage had definitely changed. Four years after declaring that AIDS was "finding fertile ground among heterosexuals" and three years after declaring that "*everyone* is at risk," *U.S. News & World Report* carried an article on HIV-AIDS entitled, "Virus on the Run." Its contention that "scientists are making progress in the search for an inoculation against AIDS" (*U.S. News & World Report*, November 19, 1990:65–67) was naively optimistic, but it did reverse the alarmism of its everyone is at risk warning. In the August 12, 1990, issue *U.S. News* essentially admitted that its 1986 projection of up to 10 million carriers by 1991 had been an alarmist fantasy when Jeffrey Harris (1990:56) wrote that the number of persons under treatment for AIDS or HIV infection was between about one hundred thousand and two hundred thousand and that "the epidemic is slowing." In the July 2, 1990 issue *Time* observed that AIDS was not easily contracted ("No one gets it from the air, food or water"), that HIV-AIDS was still largely concentrated in the gay and IDU populations, and that the spread could be stalled through the use of condoms and the distribution of sterile needles to drug injectors (Thompson, 1990:42).

The record for retreating from a forecast of doom probably goes to former Secretary Otis R. Bowen. Just a few months after issuing his 1987 warning of a holocaust worse than the Black Death, he (1988:1) stated, "We do not expect any explosion into the heterosexual population." His retractions were noted in a *New York Times* (p. IV-24) editorial of February 28, 1988, in which the *Times* also observed that "most sexually active Americans are probably at little risk [of contracting AIDS and that] the urgent need is ... to deal instantly with transmission among drug addicts."

Several informative articles appeared in the the *New York Times* in the summer and fall of 1990. On August 28 Elizabeth Rosenthal (1990) explained why AIDS was concentrated among gays and cited the various risk factors in the disease; Erik Eckholm (1990a) followed on September 16 with a discussion of the mode of transmission and the relative vulnerability of the two sexes. A later article (December 16) by John Tierney (1990b) detailed the connection between drugs and HIV-AIDS. An excellent book by lawyer and journalist Fumento, *The Myth of Heterosexual AIDS*, appeared in 1990 and outlined in considerable detail the mode of transmission of AIDS, its international patterns, and why it was highly concentrated among gays and IDUs in the United States; he dispelled the myths that AIDS could be contracted through casual contact and that it was spreading rapidly among heterosexuals. (Curiously, this book did not receive as much attention as it deserved.)

Education of the Public

Despite much opposition, public education about AIDS did take place. Much of this education occurred incidently through the media. Beginning in the late 1980s, media accounts about whether hospitalized patients and health care providers should be tested for HIV necessarily involved a discussion of the mode of transmission. Thus, more accurate public perception was a positive, if unintended, consequence of the publicity. Discussions of whether health care workers were at risk looked at the danger of invasive surgery in which the surgeon could cut himself or herself and become infected from a patient with HIV or infect the patient if the surgeon were a carrier. These discussions highlighted the fact that HIV-AIDS is a blood-borne disease. Although much of the political action about testing health care providers (in July 1991 the Senate passed legislation requiring all health workers to be tested for HIV, but the legislation was later modified) was a response to and a prey on public fear, the discussion still contributed to the public being more informed about how HIV-AIDS was transmitted. The case of basketball star Magic Johnson undoubtedly had educational benefits. After he announced he had HIV in October 1991, the media were full of the account and of how HIV is transmitted. And even though Johnson apparently contracted the infection through heterosexual intercourse, in many, if not almost all, instances, the very low chance of getting the infection this way, especially for men, was pointed out. Johnson's appearance on television for interviews and talk shows could not help but shape perceptions and allay fears about contagion through casual contact.

TABLE 7.1   Adults Answering "Definitely Not Possible" or "Very Unlikely" to Questions About Contracting HIV from Different Sources

Questions	% in 1987 (2,230)	% in 1989 (40,609)	% in 1991 (42,726)
How likely is it to get HIV from			
Living near a hospital or home for AIDS patients?	74	83	N/A
Working near someone with AIDS?	53	71	80
Eating in a restaurant where the cook has AIDS?	36	49	55
Shaking hands with or touching an AIDS victim?	61	73	N/A
Sharing utensils and dishes with a victim?	27	47	50
Using public toilets?	40	60	64
Being coughed or sneezed on by an AIDS victim?	31	45	48
Attending school with a child who has AIDS?	58	76	80

SOURCE: Dawson et al. (1987); Hardy (1990); Aguilar and Hardy (1993).

Inaccurate perception of AIDS in the general population may have reached its peak in late 1986 and the first half of 1987, when the media really let loose with alarmist statements (Fumento, 1990:235). Recall that much ignorance about how HIV could be transmitted existed in 1987. Table 7.1 compares correct responses to questions about contracting HIV-AIDS in national surveys conducted by the NCHS in 1987, 1989, and 1991. An increase in knowledge over time is evident. On all eight questions relating to contagion through casual contact, accuracy of perception increased in every instance, sometimes substantially. For example, the percentage of respondents who believed that it was not likely or definitely not possible to contract AIDS by working near someone with AIDS increased from 53 to 80 percent. Media reporting undoubtedly contributed to the change, even if this was not the intent.

But some deliberate educational efforts had a positive effect. Ann Hardy (1990:632–633) found that many respondents in the 1989 NCHS survey had read brochures or pamphlets (such as the surgeon general's "Understanding AIDS"), which was related to knowledge about AIDS. Dorothy Wertz et al. (1987) reported substantial changes in the knowledge and attitude of health care workers after an educational program. Thus, although a high degree of ignorance and irrational fear still existed, erroneous beliefs and irrational attitudes were beginning to be dispelled and societal perception was changing.

Changes in Societal Reactions

On November 28, 1993, in the *New York Times Magazine,* Schmalz wrote an article, "Whatever Happened to AIDS?" In contrast to the 1980s, when

HIV-AIDS was constantly in the news, by the early 1990s it was "old news" and no longer appeared on the front page with regularity. His point was that the societal reactions to HIV-AIDS had changed.

An abundance of anecdotal evidence and some systematic evidence indicate that reactions had indeed changed. And there are strong indications that such changes were due to increases in scientific knowledge and correct perceptions with respect to HIV-AIDS and the way HIV is transmitted. In this way medicine became increasingly an institution of social control. (Note that my emphasis here on medicine as social control pertains to the research and knowledge-producing dimension of medicine, not its applied clinical dimension.) Foremost in this change was a decrease in fear of contagion.

Fear of Contagion

Several accounts indicate that fear of contagion declined toward the end of the 1980s and early 1990s, consistent with the results in Table 7.1. In comparison to 5 percent of adult (male and female) respondents in the 1987 NCHS poll who believed their personal chances of getting AIDS were "high" or "medium," in the 1991 survey only 2 percent felt their chances were "medium" (none felt their chances were "high") (Aguilar and Hardy, 1993:14). The case of dentist-to-patient infection in Stuart, Florida, a state in which children were prohibited from attending church and school in certain communities and where the home of two hemophiliac children was destroyed by arson in 1987, illustrates how fear declined in a very short time. In 1990 a deceased dentist acknowledged in a letter he left for his former patients that he had AIDS and urged that they be tested. Six of the approximately seventeen hundred patients the dentists had treated since being infected in 1987 had apparently tested positive for HIV by 1993.[8] After the first case, that of Kimberly Bergalis, was publicized, Stuart residents were reported to be unsettled, but there was no panic or anger. By the account of city and state officials, this was due to an increase in knowledge about AIDS. The editor and president of the *Stuart News* stated, "A few years back, I might have expected more outrage or anger, as if someone was to blame. Now the reaction is more sadness than outrage, for both the dentist and patient. I think people understand AIDS better then they once did." The deputy chief of the AIDS program for Florida was quoted as saying that persons calling and asking for information about the disease displayed little panic and hysteria and that he believed this reflected the fact that more people knew how HIV is transmitted. "I believe the reaction we're seeing reflects 1990, not 1985. Five years ago there would have been a lot more panic, more chaos. The level of knowledge about the disease now is pretty high" (Applebome, 1990:9; Altman, 1990; Barringer, 1991).

By the end of 1993, fear of causal contagion had virtually disappeared from the nation's consciousness. To illustrate, in December of that year television newscasts announced that the CDC (1993e) had reported that each of two adolescent boys with hemophilia had transmitted HIV to a brother, thus raising the specter of transmission through casual contact. It was explained that one of the boys shared a razor with his brother; another had frequent nosebleeds during sleep and shared a bed with a brother who had a skin disease and hence lesions on his body. Public health officials braced for an outpouring of public reactions, but they never came. The episode disappeared from the front pages and the newscasts as abruptly as it had appeared.

Fear of provider-to-patient transmission also declined. Bergalis's subsequent congressional testimony in October 1991 (when she aroused the moral issue—"I did not do anything wrong, yet I am being made to suffer") led some senators and representatives to call for mandatory testing of health care workers. However, more reasonable heads prevailed. The legislation that was eventually passed only made recommendations about testing, and the overall public reaction to the possibility of provider-to-patient transmission was one of calm rather than panic, as the following example illustrates.

Early in 1991 the CDC issued guidelines urging health care workers who were infected with HIV to stop performing invasive procedures or to inform their patients of the infection. In the first response to this recommendation, officers of a hospital in Dunkirk, New York, asked an HIV-infected physician to resign, which he did. The resignation was announced at a well-publicized news conference. However, it brought no panic from the community and former patients. A *New York Times* reporter quoted the president of the hospital as saying that, although the hospital had received more than one thousand phone calls in response to the resignation, "most people seem to be quite well informed and really want a little reassurance, and that's about it" (Wolff, 1991:10). Congressional testimony by former Surgeon General Koop, among others, undoubtedly quieted many irrational fears about patients being infected by health care providers.

Reactions to children with HIV-AIDS changed:

> As recently as two years ago, many children who tested positive for the AIDS virus ... spent their first months in hospital wards waiting for foster homes. But today [1990], foster-care experts say, that need is being filled. Greater knowledge of the disease has meant less fear of contagion. ... Around the nation, growing numbers of prospective foster parents are stepping forward. Some agencies even report waiting lists. (Navarro, 1990:A-17)

Anita Septimus, director of social services of the pediatric HIV-AIDS program at Albert Einstein College of Medicine, was quoted in the *Tennessean* (December 9, 1990:A-18) as saying it was now a "worthy cause" to care for children with AIDS. "Slowly but surely, every segment of the population has been forced to be confronted with AIDS, and there is more acceptance because there is more knowledge." On November 26, 1990, the Associated Press also reported in the *Tennessean* (p. A-14) that, although volunteer workers for HIV-AIDS patients in Ohio said they were still sometimes avoided by others, this response had declined. "Public fear toward people who work with AIDS patients has eased as general knowledge of the disease, which cannot be spread through casual contact, has grown since the early 1980s." In January 1993 the *New York Times* reported that in contrast to the Ray brothers in Arcadia, Florida, in 1987, who had been severely harassed by the community and prevented from attending school and whose house had been burned down, in 1992 another family was met with mostly acceptance in Lakeland, fifty miles from Arcadia (Smothers, 1993).[9]

In addition, the federal government began providing a "manager's kit" to employers, advising them how to inform employees about HIV-AIDS cases in the workplace. For example, one poster in the kit stated, "One million Americans have HIV. And not one of them got it from a coffee pot, a water fountain, a toilet, or any piece of office equipment touched by someone with HIV. So don't worry about getting HIV through casual contact at work" (Noble, 1992:IV-25). Some employers have offered employees or required them to attend educational sessions on the transmission of HIV (Navarro, 1992; Noble, 1992). These efforts plus the fact that more workers who have HIV-AIDS have become known and coworkers have grown accustomed to working with them have obviously reduced fear of casual contagion. Although employers continue to report, as of December 1992, that many workers still worry about contracting AIDS through casual contact with infected coworkers (Navarro, 1992), this type of workplace fear has been replaced with another type.

From Fear of Contagion to Financial Fear

With newer forms of treatment, the cost of medical care for persons with HIV-AIDS increased. Officials from Blue Cross and Blue Shield in New York reported that the average lifetime cost of treating a person with HIV-AIDS rose from about $60,000 in 1986 to $200,000 in 1992 (Navarro, 1992). Consequently, employer discrimination against persons with HIV-AIDS may have risen. Dismissals have been alleged, and civil rights lawyers contend that thousands of workers who receive health insurance benefits as part of their employment have had their benefits reduced once their employers learned they had HIV-AIDS (Barrett, 1992). Therefore, some civil rights groups contend that "employment-related discrimination against people

TABLE 7.2   Percentage of Respondents in Gallup Polls Who Agreed or Disagreed with Three Statements About AIDS

Statement	% in October 1987	% in May 1991
Agree: "I sometimes think that AIDS is a punishment for the decline in moral standards."	43	34
Agree: "In general, it's people's own fault if they get AIDS."	51	33
Disagree: "I would refuse to work alongside someone who had AIDS."	65	80

SOURCE: Lipset and Wattenberg (1988); *New York Times* (November 22, 1987:A-18, May 19, 1991:I-13.

with H.I.V. is based not on fear [of contagion] but on [fear of economic] cost" (Navarro, 1992:B-12; Noble, 1993).

Such discrimination is tragic, but sociologically it is fundamentally different from earlier reactions. Reactions stemming from economic fear are rational, whereas reactions based on fear of contagion through casual contact are not. Employers are simply responding to what employees with HIV-AIDS mean to the economic realities of the bottom line.

Moralizing, Prejudice, and Blaming the Victim

As noted in the previous chapter, moralizing about HIV-AIDS was widespread in the 1980s, and in a nationwide survey in October 1987, 43 percent of respondents agreed that HIV-AIDS was a form of divine punishment. Meanwhile, other surveys indicated that substantial changes in moralizing and prejudice had occurred in less than four years, from October 1987 to May 1991. Table 7.2 shows that, according to Gallup polls, the belief that AIDS is punishment (by God?) declined by 25 percent; a decline of greater magnitude in blaming the victim also occurred. In addition, more people were willing to work besides an infected coworker. (However, there is no way to know if this change reflected a decline in social prejudice and fear of moral contamination or a decline in fear of infection, but probably both were involved.) In just three months, from July to October 1987, Gallup polls showed that the percentage of Americans who rejected the idea that employers have a right to dismiss people solely because they have AIDS increased from 43 percent to 64 percent (*New York Times,* November 22, 1987:I-18).

In 1988 a conference of American corporations sponsored by Allstate Insurance Company produced a report—"AIDS: Corporate America Responds"—that urged humane corporate behavior toward persons with HIV-

AIDS (Chase, 1988:31). In October 1987 Congress declared an AIDS Awareness/Prevention Day. The World Health Organization designated December 1 as World AIDS Day. On that day in 1990 retailers in New York City and their employees, along with entertainers, contributed to a benefit in which the proceeds went to the New York AIDS Fund. The chairwoman of the event, Carolyne Roehm, said, "This goes beyond any charity I've ever been involved in" (Hochwender, 1990:B-7). In a segment of the 10:00 P.M. (EST) December 17, 1990, newscast, CNN sympathetically discussed the plight of Laguna Beach, California, in which a high proportion of the residents are gay and in which a very high death toll from AIDS had occurred. The devastating effect of AIDS on lovers and former lovers of infected gays was presented in a caring way. Similar episodes are commonly reported in the media today. That the federal government increased its funding for HIV-AIDS annually, from $6 million in 1982 to more than $2 billion in 1989 (Vanderveen, 1991:153) certainly sent a signal to the public that the disease is potentially preventable and/or curable. Whether this is *in fact* the case remains to be seen, but it signified that HIV-AIDS is not a form of divine punishment but a result of natural causes.

The change in the social standing of people with HIV-AIDS is exemplified by analyses such as that in 1989 of Joel Hay, a health economist of the Hoover Institution, which questioned whether the government was spending too much on HIV-AIDS in comparison to what it spent on other fatal diseases (Hay, 1989). (Many others have made this charge since.) This question implied that HIV-AIDS was being given a favored position relative to other fatal diseases.[10] Indeed, some states (California, Wisconsin) have passed laws prohibiting insurance companies from considering the results of tests for HIV when issuing health insurance policies. This means that the premiums of other policyholders must be increased to cover the higher medical cost of treating people with HIV-AIDS. The governor of New York, Mario Cuomo, proposed similar legislation for his state. The chair of the New York State Insurance Committee, who opposed the legislation, declared, "AIDS is the only politically protected disease" (Sack, 1990:A-17). Of course, such protection reflected the political power of the gay population as much as, if not more than, a change in the standing that people with HIV-AIDS had in the eyes of the public. Commonly in the United States, laws reflect the special interests of particular categories of people rather than the will of the general population, but it is inconceivable that people with HIV-AIDS would have been considered for such legislation in the early and middle 1980s by any state.

Nevertheless, cultural myths and social prejudice continued (and still continue). The Associated Press reported on August 22, 1990 (*Tennessean*:A-6) that the National Commission of AIDS had determined that fear and bigotry, even among dentists and physicians, were still widespread in many rural areas. (Significantly, this was attributed to a lack of knowledge, with the commission reporting that in "rural America, there is an epidemic of fear and bigotry, fanned by the absence of education and knowledge [about AIDS].") A nationwide survey also revealed considerable prejudice in the medical community toward persons with HIV-AIDS (Gerbert et al., 1991 [this study is reviewed in the next chapter]). Finally, the decrease in prejudice, moralizing, and discrimination may have occurred primarily for the *category* of persons with HIV-AIDS, as in organizational efforts to provide more funding for HIV-AIDS research and medical care and laws to protect the civil rights of persons with HIV-AIDS. The social acceptance of *individuals* on a face-to-face personal level may have changed very little (Weintraub, 1991).

Nevertheless, the moral and social atmosphere surrounding HIV-AIDS clearly changed as scientific knowledge about the disease and its mode of transmission increased and became known to the public. Although we do not know what President Bush meant when he declared Magic Johnson a "national hero" after Johnson announced he had HIV (presumably, Bush thought Johnson's public announcement was heroic), it is certain that no president would have dared make such a statement just a few years earlier. (Even with the change, however, it is most doubtful that President Bush would have made the statement if there were evidence that Johnson had gotten the virus through drug use or sex with another male.) Even though moralizing and blaming the victim in HIV-AIDS remain (and will probably always exist to some extent), there is also no doubt that these reactions declined as knowledge of the disease increased, and in some respects HIV-AIDS began to receive favored status.[11]

A final point on moralizing about HIV-AIDS: Recall that in 1892 members of the Hamburg clergy trumpeted the idea that cholera was a visitation from God for human sin almost ten years after the cholera bacillus had been identified as the natural cause of the disease. Similarly, years after HIV had been identified, some ministers were still proclaiming, over the airways as well as from the pulpit, to mostly white middle-class heterosexual listeners and viewers, that AIDS was punishment from God. For example, on ABC's "20/20" in 1994 (rebroadcast on August 28), the Reverend James Miller declared, "AIDS is unquestionably a message from God." Nevertheless, moralizing about HIV-AIDS had begun to take on a secular tone, just as moralizing about cholera had done a century earlier. Moral disapproval was voiced in terms of carelessness and irresponsibility as well as in terms of religious beliefs. An individual should have sex with fewer partners, select sexual partners carefully, use condoms, and if she or he injected drugs, do it hygienically. Responsibility was the message that the safe-sex commercials by the CDC brought in the late 1980s and 1990s. Many of those who believed at the start of the 1990s that HIV-AIDS among gays and IDUs was due to a decline in moral standards and who blamed the victim probably thought in terms of the irresponsibility of gays and IDUs, not in terms of divine punishment.

Scapegoating

Changes in scapegoating also occurred. Cultural, social, and medical factors that contributed to HIV-AIDS in Africa and Haiti were publicized in the late 1980s and early 1990s. Articles in scientific journals described international differences in transmission (Piot et al., 1988), and they simply provided no evidence that Africa was the source of HIV in the United States. Several informative articles appeared in the *New York Times* and elsewhere in which the differences between Africa and the United States were outlined with no reference to Africa as the origin (Wade, 1988; Rosenthal, 1990; Perlez, 1990; Eckholm and Tierney, 1990; Eckholm, 1990a, 1990b; Noble, 1990; Tierney, 1990; Fumento, 1990:107–128). Fumento (1990:37–38), among others, revealed that there was no evidence that a high prevalence of AIDS had existed in Africa for a considerable period before AIDS cases appeared in the United States. (Nevertheless, some scientists continue to believe that Africa is the origin of HIV in the United States.)

As for Haiti, where HIV was probably introduced by visiting American gays, the poverty, cultural customs, social conditions, and medical facilities and practices were similar to those in Africa (Fumento, 1990:125–178). It is not surprising, therefore, that a number of recent Haitian immigrants would be infected. However, once the causal linkages were known, Haitian status per se was no longer recognized as a risk factor. In 1985 Haitians were removed as an official high-risk group. The director of the CDC was quoted in the *New York Times* on April 10, 1985 ("Haitians Removed from AIDS Risk List," p. I-13) as saying they had been dropped because "the Haitians were the only risk group that were identified because of who they were rather than what they did." This was an admission that the Haitians had been scapegoats for HIV-AIDS.

Scapegoating of prostitutes was also undermined. The National Research Council reported that prostitutes were not a major source of AIDS spread. The *New York Times* (p. I-12) called attention to the report in its article on the arrest of the Oakland prostitute for attempted murder. It also quoted the director of the Health Department of Alameda County (California) as saying, "This kind of action, it seems to me, is scapegoating. Why do we go on this witch hunt and persecute this one individual when the action to remedy the situation can be taken on the part of the client taking personal responsibility for using a condom?" As with other STDs (Brandt, 1987), prostitutes will probably always be scapegoats for HIV-AIDS to some extent. Indeed, as of 1991 twenty-four states had laws permitting the testing of prostitutes for HIV.[12]

Physicians were late in becoming scapegoats and emerged primarily after the Bergalis case of provider-to-patient transmission was discovered. Since such scapegoating, however limited, was a response to actual knowledge about the way HIV is transmitted, it would seem to contradict the hypothesis that scapegoating declines as knowledge increases. The contradiction is only apparent. Had the Bergalis episode occurred in the mid-1980s, the demand for mandatory testing of health care providers (and especially surgeons) would probably have been too strong for legislators not to have enacted it into law.

Changes in the Law and the Courts

Knowledge about how HIV is transmitted has influenced court decisions concerning persons with HIV-AIDS. In June 1986 the U.S. Department of Justice ruled that employees may bar persons with AIDS from work; the decisions meant that federal protection of civil rights did not apply to persons who *might* be considered dangerous to others (Brandt, 1987:194). However, later court decisions were guided more by scientific evidence. For example, courts have ruled that discrimination and reactions based on fear and prejudice, as when children with HIV-AIDS are not allowed to attend school, are illegal. In one particularly important case, a federal court ruled that employers could not discriminate against or discharge employees simply because they were carriers of HIV. The ruling stated "that discrimination based solely on fear of contagion" is illegal (Hevesi, 1988:8).

In January 1992 a report based on a review of 372 of the more than 1,000 AIDS-related court cases stated that people were still going to court out of fear and prejudice and that judges "have tended ... to follow public fears more than scientific evidence" (Margolick, 1992:I-10). For science to have a pervasive effect on court decisions will take time. Nevertheless, the report itself will be an impetus to change. Indeed, one author of the report stated, "I hope the impact [of the report] will be to get judges to wake up to the idea that they have to follow public health advice" (Margolick, 1992:I-10).

Court decisions will be influenced further by the Americans with Disabilities Act, which Congress passed and the president signed in 1992 and which was phased in through 1994. The act prohibits discrimination against disabled workers, including persons with HIV-AIDS.

This brings us to public health regulation and law. In the case of cholera (and other diseases), scientific knowledge was incorporated in public health regulation, and law controlled the behavior of potential victims (by enforcing preventive measures) as well as the public reactions to sufferers. It is much easier to do this for infections other than HIV-AIDS because HIV is usually transmitted in intimate private acts and efforts to prevent infection may infringe on individual liberty (Bayer, 1989). This will always be a problem with HIV-AIDS (as it is with other venereal diseases). Nevertheless, certain public health regulations have been introduced and implemented. The best example is the closing of bathhouses. In general, however, short of harsh criminalization of gay sex, public health regulations designed to prevent the transmission of HIV will be virtually impossible to enforce. This and issues of individual liberty present greater barriers to implementing public health law than lack of knowledge. Unlike with many other infectious diseases, passing enforceable laws that prevent the transmission of HIV is virtually impossible. Closing the bathhouses may have reduced the frequency of anal sex between gay males, but it certainly did not prevent such sex altogether. This action just eliminated a major setting where such activity took place.

And whereas employer-related discrimination based on fear of contagion has declined, discrimination based on economic fear has increased. In a celebrated case a Texas employer who reduced the health insurance of an employee once he learned the employee had HIV-AIDS was sued in federal court. The court upheld the employer, and in October 1992 the Supreme Court refused to hear an appeal of the lower court decision, thus affirming the legality of the original finding.[13]

Conclusion

Despite much sharp criticism from some circles that American society and especially the federal government were indifferent and slow to respond to the threat of AIDS, especially in the early years of the AIDS epidemic, the reaction of the scientific community was quite vigorous. The accomplishments in the early 1980s have no equal in the history of biomedicine with respect to understanding a devastating disease. When one considers that the technology for identifying a retrovirus did not even exist until a few years before the epidemic began, the accomplishments are most remarkable. Sociologically, the effect of scientific activity and understanding, aided by the printed media and electronic communication, on the societal reactions to HIV-AIDS is also unequal in history. The socially embedded nature of science had an effect on the beliefs and research activity of scientists, of course, but the effect that scientific knowledge had on societal reactions to HIV-AIDS was dramatic. Fear of contagion through casual contact declined greatly, and even though beliefs about HIV-AIDS are still influenced by archaic and metaphorical conceptions of disease, such conceptions of HIV-AIDS have been greatly defused. The process was not unlike that which occurred with respect to cholera a century ago.

At the same time, there are obviously major differences between the cholera and AIDS epidemics. The biology of cholera and HIV-AIDS differs greatly, and the capabilities and social standing of medical science during the cholera epidemics were nowhere near what they were during the AIDS epidemic. Social and cultural conditions affecting the strength of moral reasoning and social prejudice against pariah groups also varied. And precise comparisons of the pace of change in the societal reactions to the two diseases cannot be made because the statistics that would permit such comparisons simply do not exist. Nevertheless, when the effects of medical science knowledge on societal reactions to HIV-AIDS epidemic are compared to historical accounts of those during the cholera epidemics, striking similarities are seen. As scientific knowledge increased, reactions changed. Interpretations became more rational and reactions calmer, though this change occurred much more rapidly for HIV-AIDS than for cholera (scientific progress was much faster for HIV-AIDS also). Science narrowed the window of opportunity for cultural myth, prejudice, and moral reasoning. For both diseases, biomedical science took much of the steam out of social metaphors, and fear of contagion virtually disappeared.

The later cholera epidemics and the HIV-AIDS epidemic both occurred in rationalized societies where science was widely accepted and institutionalized. This was especially so for the HIV-AIDS epidemic. In other types of society, such as nonliterate ones, science would not be expected to have this effect any more than it has affected preventive behavior.

But even in rationalized societies, medical knowledge and scientific reasoning do not always undermine archaic-metaphorical reasoning. When a disease is associated with what many consider to be immoral conduct, the social construction of that disease as due to natural causes must continually compete with a construction based on moral reasoning and ideas about sin and the wrath of God, even when the medical science conception of disease is broadly institutionalized in society. This is the case with HIV-AIDS. Medical knowledge has not eliminated reactions based on supernatural beliefs and moral reasoning by a long shot.

The reduction of stigmatizing and moralizing is not the aim of medical science, of course. The aim of those who produce scientific knowledge is to achieve scientific understanding of HIV-AIDS and to develop treatments and possible cures for the disease. Social control is unintended and is generally unrecognized by most people. Such control is more the result of medical science than of clinical treatment; it is due largely to the scientific arm of medicine and the diffusion of scientific knowledge in society. Indeed, clinical cures or vaccines are not necessary for changes in the social construction of disease to occur, as the change in the social construction of HIV-AIDS clearly shows. The role of medical science in maintaining social control may be considered as important as its role in providing cures for disease. Indeed, sociologically, this is medical science's most significant function.

NOTES

1. In fact, the validity of the dominant interpretation is assumed, as previous chapters revealed. However, if subsequent facts were to indicate that it needed to be modified, this would be of little, if any, consequence sociologically. This is because most of the scientific disputes about the dominant interpretation concern the physiological processes in the relationship between HIV and AIDS and whether there are biological cofactors (e.g., other viruses) with HIV to produce AIDS or whether HIV itself is a product of other biological factors (Root-Bernstein, 1993:327–349). Virtually no one questions that the dominant mode of transmission occurs through polygamous anal sex and needle sharing in the United States and polygamous sex between heterosexuals in Africa.

2. According to Duh (1991:63), Gallo announced at the Fourth International Conference on AIDS in Stockholm, Sweden, that HIV had not come from the green monkey after all. (More likely, it had come from an Asian monkey.)

3. The August 1984 issue of the *Southern Medical Journal* (pp. 1065–1067) published several letters criticizing Dr. Fletcher's editorial. Dr. Fletcher replied that the majority of letters he had received supported his position, and he reaffirmed the view that AIDS among male homosexuals is the result of a "moral choice." God punishes those who make this choice even if they are monogamous (presumably even with uninfected partners) since "homosexual monogamy repudiates the biblical norm of heterosexual monogamy."

4. This hypothesis is central to Sontag's (1978) thesis.

5. The importance of physician consensus for public opinion is reflected in a statement in the *London Times* in October 1869: "What is needed is first information and then faith on the part of the public, and doctors must agree among themselves, if that be possible, before the outside world can be expected to agree with them [about cholera]" (Briggs, 1961:92).

6. McNeill's (1976:122) description of the reactions to epidemics in northern Europe before the nineteenth century contrasts with reactions toward the end of that century: "In northern Europe the absence of well-defined public quarantine regulations and administrative routines—religious as well as medical—with which to deal with plagues and rumors of plague, gave scope for violent expression of popular hates and fears provoked by the disease. In particular, long-standing grievances of poor against rich often boiled to the surface." That boiling continued during the nineteenth century, though the extent to which it did so declined as medicine was put on a factual and scientific footing.

7. It would be an oversimplification to say that societal reactions to cholera were the same in all countries or that no other factors besides more knowledge were important in structuring these reactions. Political factors in Hamburg in 1892 (Evans, 1987) were not the same as those in New York City in 1866 (Rosenberg, 1962), and

such differences made for variations in societal reactions. Some countries were ahead of others in implementing public health programs. Thus, Britain was virtually untouched by the European cholera outbreaks of 1873, 1884, and 1892, apparently because public health programs were more advanced there (Briggs, 1961:86), which led to different reactions between England and countries on the Continent, where the mortality rates were higher.

8. No one knows with certainty how the transmissions occurred, but one of three modes seems probable: Blood from a cut on the dentist's hand entered the bloodstream of the patients, the dentist somehow contaminated his instruments with his own blood and failed to sterilize them, or he intentionally injected his patients with his blood, thus murdering them (Breo, 1993). However, that the infection rate from the dentist's patients was reported to be almost the same as for the two counties from which he got his patients may suggest the dentist was not the source of the infections at all. This was still a matter of conjecture and debate as of July 1994 (Altman, 1994).

9. Even so, reactions by a few people were so hostile that the family decided to move to another state.

10. A contrary argument is that HIV-AIDS should receive more funding because its economic effects on society are far more devastating than probably those of any other disease. Since HIV-AIDS is concentrated among young adults, losses of human capital and economic potential are great.

11. To appreciate this point, we need only observe the difference in the societal reaction to HIV-AIDS and other STDs. We can be sure that if Magic Johnson had publicly acknowledged that he had contracted syphilis (or some other STD), President Bush would not have declared him a national hero.

12. Such laws have been opposed by civil libertarians as well as persons who realize that female-to-male transmission is rare (*Wall Street Journal,* February 3, 1991: B-6).

13. However, the ruling applies only to employers who are their own insurers (that is, do not insure through an insurance company); it does not apply to insurance companies, which are regulated by individual states. Such actions may be ruled illegal under the Americans with Disabilities Act.

8. The Sick Role, Personal Responsibility, and Problems of Treatment and Prevention

Any society or group within society establishes norms of behavior to which its members are expected to conform. When people violate these norms, others express disapproval; deviants are ostracized, and if the violation is serious enough, they may be incarcerated or dealt some other form of physical punishment. Since 1951 and the writings of Talcott Parsons (1951a:428–429, 1951b), medical sociologists have been writing about disease as a form of deviance. This idea is particularly relevant to HIV-AIDS. The moral construction of HIV-AIDS is due largely to the fact that a very high proportion of people who have HIV-AIDS are social deviants, as foregoing chapters have shown. In this chapter I more extensively analyze the deviant aspects of HIV-AIDS. The way they differ from those of other medical conditions and how this creates special problems for the treatment and prevention of HIV-AIDS are the focus of my analysis.

Any discussion of disease as deviance must begin with Parsons's formulation. Although a number of criticisms have been made of this framework (Levine and Kozloff, 1978; Arluke et al., 1979; Cockerham, 1986:137–146; Wolinsky, 1988:105–111), it has stimulated much empirical and theoretical research on the relationships among sickness, society, and medical care. Sociologists agree that this formulation contributes significantly to understanding disease and medical treatment as social phenomena. (At least one sociologist believes it is the single most important idea in medical sociology [Wolinsky, 1988:105].) It is instructive, therefore, to see to what extent Parsons's formulation applies to HIV-AIDS, even though, as we see, the formulation is seriously deficient in this regard.

Parsons's Social Theory of Illness

According to Parsons, when people are sick they engage in a form of social behavior. The central tenets of the formulation are the conception of disease as social deviance, the sick role, and medicine as a form of social control.

Disease as Social Deviance

As viewed in medicine, disease is a deviation from biological norms. Parsons (1951b:436–437, 1975, 1979; Parsons and Fox, 1952) observed, however, that disease is also a deviation from social norms. But it is a special kind of deviation.

Parsons (1979:129–130) distinguished between "normative" and "situational" deviance. Normative deviance is motivated behavior and involves sin, immorality, or violation of law. The deviant is viewed as capable of conforming to social norms but chooses not to do so. He or she is responsible for the action. A normative deviant is typically met with negative reactions in the form of ostracism, incarceration, or other punishment. Situational deviance is due to the circumstances that just "happen to" people, as when they get sick (Parsons, 1951b:430, 440, 1979:129–130). Except for psychosomatic conditions, sickness is not motivated by or due to a lack of attitudinal commitment to obeying the norms of society; sickness is not a moral or legal issue. It is not the fault of the individual, and willpower will not make him or her well (Parsons, 1951b:440). Instead, sickness is deviance in terms of standards of "adequacy" of performance because the individual lacks the capacity to function normally (Parsons, 1979:126). In contrast to normative deviance, which is socially proscribed, sickness is *permitted* deviance.

An example is children who do not attend school because they are sick. The inability to attend school because of sickness is not motivated and immoral behavior (though truancy is), but it is still deviance because children are not performing their normal social role. The same is true for housewives or househusbands who do not perform housework or take care of children, soldiers who do not perform their assigned duties, and breadwinners who do not go to work, all because they are sick. Such persons are not behaving in ways normally expected of them.

Although this lack of action is not a violation of moral norms or law, it may still have socially disruptive consequences. Other people may need to adjust their own behavior and schedules and in some instances perform duties and roles usually performed by the person who is sick, as when soldiers assume the duties of a sick comrade (Schneider, 1953), or relinquish their own roles and perform those ordinally assumed by the person who is sick, as when a breadwinner stays home from work to do housework and take care of children. Therefore, sickness may endanger the functioning of families, business firms, military units, and, if widespread enough, society as a whole

(Parsons, 1951b:430). Consequently, social systems must keep the level of illness at a low level. The sick role and medical care do this.

The Sick Role

Sickness is not just a biological condition; it is also a social role, the sick role, which is defined by social norms and expectations. In return for permission to be exempt from the demands of normal social roles,[1] the individual is expected to try getting well. This includes seeking medical care and cooperating with professional providers. The individual is obligated to resume his or her normal social roles as soon as possible.[2] Therefore, the sick role is a temporary deviant role.

To be sick may also bring rewards, or "secondary gains" (Parsons 1951b: 437–438). People may enjoy being exempt from normal social responsibilities and receiving special attention and care. Parsons and Reneé Fox (1952) observed, for example, that children who are sick get additional attention from parents. Consequently, people may be motivated to adopt the sick role, in which case they are malingering and not sick. That problem is minimized by the social expectations that the individual should try to get well. Thus, the sick role, while a form of permissible deviance, is also a mechanism by which society controls, at least to some extent, the overall level of sickness behavior.

Medicine and Social Control

In the last chapter I examined medicine in terms of its control of societal reactions to HIV-AIDS. In Parsons's formulation, such control is simply assumed. Medicine as social control enters at a different point, namely, at the clinical, rather than research, arm of medicine. Since clinical physicians define what constitutes illness and treat people who are sick, they determine whether and for how long a person may occupy the sick role (Parsons, 1951b:436). As "gatekeepers" for the sick role and "legitimizing agents" for persons in that role (Parsons, 1951b:436), physicians screen out malingerers and reduce the level of sickness behavior in society. For example, by refusing to confirm a child's pretension of being sick or not legitimating complaints after a condition has been cured, they prevent the "contagion" of malingering among siblings (Parsons and Fox, 1952). In restoring people to normal biological functioning, physicians also restore people to normal social functioning. In bringing individuals back to within the range of biological norms, medical care returns them to the range of social norms, analogous to the rehabilitation of criminals. Therefore, since physicians both define who is a (legitimate) deviant and reduce deviance (sickness), they facilitate the smooth functioning of social units and are important agents of social control.[3]

Parsons's formulation provides significant insights into social aspects of sickness and the role of medical care as social control. It provides an understanding of sickness as a social process. At the same time, as several authors have noted, it has limited validity for certain forms of sickness. Its validity for HIV-AIDS is limited in several respects, deriving from the cultural bias in the formulation.

Cultural Bias of Parsons's Theory and HIV-AIDS

The cultural bias derives from the assumption that societal reaction is controlled and guided by the medical science conception of disease.[4] Even though this conception has become increasingly stronger for HIV-AIDS over time, archaic-metaphorical conceptions were widespread in the 1980s, and they remain problematic even today. Consequently, Parsons's formulation does not capture certain aspects of social deviance, the sick role, and social control as they pertain to HIV-AIDS.

Deviance

People with HIV-AIDS are not just (or even primarily) situational deviants. They are also normative deviants.[5] In fact, reactions to persons with HIV-AIDS are controlled to a large extent by an archaic conception. Recall that in 1987, 43 percent of survey respondents agreed that HIV-AIDS was divine punishment. Parsons recognized that his formulation assumes that the medical science conception is widely institutionalized in society, as in the rationalized societies in the West, and would not apply unless this were the case (Parsons, 1951a:456; 1951b:474). But he did not recognize that an archaic conception of a disease could flourish in a society that is as rationalized as the United States.

The limit of Parsons's conception is revealed in the way patients may experience guilt. They may feel guilty because they are physically unable to pull their weight in social and economic responsibilities, but sick people rarely experience *moral* guilt. They do not usually see themselves as normative deviants who deserve to be punished with sickness. In contrast, persons who had HIV-AIDS indicated in interviews with Weitz (1991:76) that they tended to see themselves as normative deviants and were "likely to feel guilt about the behaviors that led to their illness and, consequently, to believe that they deserve their illness." This is the principal tenet of the archaic conception of disease. One male homosexual told her, for example, "I reaped what I sowed. I sowed sin, I reaped death. I believe, biblically, I received AIDS as a result of my sexual sin practices" (Weitz, 1991:68, 69). Even though a society is arguably the most rationalized society in history, even persons who have HIV-AIDS may accept society's moral view of them and identify themselves as normative deviants. Parsons's conception simply does not recognize this possibility.

The Sick Role

Although many persons with HIV-AIDS are temporarily exempted from their normal social roles, for others this is not the case. Instead, they are *rejected* by spouses, lovers, family members, coworkers, and employers. Therefore, the sick role for persons who have HIV-AIDS is frequently not a temporary deviant role at all. In the eyes of many people, the moral status of persons with HIV-AIDS is permanently impaired.[6] Parsons's formulation does not allow for this status since it is not the usual way sick people are treated in a rationalized society.

Social Control

According to Parsons, sickness must be controlled to avoid its disruptive consequences for the functioning of social systems. Sickness from HIV-AIDS may disrupt the functioning of families, business firms (especially in industries where a large proportion of the employees are gays), systems of medical care (e.g., the additional burden of caring for persons with HIV-AIDS), and other social units. Medical care may alleviate these problems to some extent. But in the eyes of many people, perhaps most, this is not the most significant problem of social control and HIV-AIDS. The central problem is normative. HIV-AIDS is usually caused by immoral or illegal acts, and the problem of social control resembles that of ordinary deviance and crime as much as it resembles most forms of sickness. Consequently, the role of medical care in the social control of HIV-AIDS is different from almost all other forms of sickness. Medical care may enable people with HIV-AIDS to function better in their normal social roles, but it does not control (that is, reduce) the normative deviance that causes HIV-AIDS.

Nevertheless, the social construction of HIV-AIDS has changed. As the construction has become increasingly medicalized, it has more closely met the criteria associated with Parsons's formulation. The medicalization of HIV-AIDS is reflected in the statement we sometimes hear, "It doesn't make any difference how you get it [HIV]." But, of course, it does make a difference. Although persons who contract HIV in ways other than gay sex and drug use may experience less stigma (they are considered innocent bystanders), many people still view a person with HIV-AIDS as a member of a stigmatized deviant group rather than as someone who is simply infected with a virus.[7]

Personal Responsibility, Deviance, and HIV-AIDS

The idea that people have a moral reponsibility to preserve their health and avoid sickness is a growing idea in the United States (Knowles, 1976, 1977; Zola, 1978; Courtwright, 1980; Matarazzo, 1984; Califano, 1986). It has become a significant social movement and, according to some, has emerged as a political ideology (Crawford, 1977). It is based largely on the fact that behavior and lifestyle are major etiological factors in seven of the ten leading causes of death, as with cigarette smoking in heart disease and cancer (Matarazzo, 1984:15). Some view the association of behavior with disease in moral terms. For example, in 1977 prominent medical authority John Knowles (p. 80, emphasis added) stated, in an article entitled, "The Responsibility of the Individual," that a person has "the *moral* responsibility ... to maintain his own health by the observance of simple prudent *rules of behavior* relating to sleep, exercise, diet, alcohol, and smoking."

Some sociologists contend that this is not a new moral conception but represents the reemergence of the archaic conception of sickness. In a frequently cited article, Irving Zola (1978:84) stated, for example, that "the issue of morality and individual responsibility" as related to sickness "seems to be re-emerging" in American medicine. Weitz (1991:41–44, 48–49) observed that the attribution of disease to lifestyle factors connects sickness to sin and confers a moral status on sick people who have certain lifestyle attributes. The deviant and immoral status of HIV-AIDS is an extreme manifestation of this view.

In fact, however, this moral conception is not the reemergence of an old conception of sickness at all. It differs from the archaic conception in two important ways. First, the new morality is based in science, not on religion and beliefs about the supernatural. Smoking, eating habits (diet), excessive use of alcohol, and other behaviors are believed to be related to ill health because this is what scientific studies show. Although this leads to the idea of "personal responsibility for [one's own] health and illness" (Matarazzo, 1984:15), it is not the reemergence of an archaic conception. The relation between behavior and illness is empirical, not spiritual. Negative health behaviors are related to sickness as "behavior pathogens" (Matarazzo, 1984), not as behaviors that the spirits oppose.

Second, in the archaic conception the behavior that is assumed to have led to sickness is inherently bad. It is a form of sin because it is defined as such by religion. In contrast, the modern conception is a form of secular morality and follows a different logic based on economic interdependence in the cost of medical care. The behavior is not inherently bad (indeed, traditionally many behavior pathogens, such as smoking, have been socially accepted forms of behavior), but it may have negative economic consequences for others. Because health insurance is so widespread, the expense of an individual's medical care is not his or hers alone; it is shared with others. "The smoker who develops emphysema or lung cancer accumulates large medical bills, most of which are covered by private or government insurance. We all pay [with higher premiums or taxes]" (Courtwright, 1980:274). The community suffers.

In a sense, then, the new morality is an extension of traditional public health policy, which, since germ theory, has attempted to minimize the harmful effects a person's sickness has for others (e.g., by requiring that people with certain infectious diseases be isolated). This is justified under the harm to others doctrine. The evolving new morality is similar to this doctrine but with an important twist: "Indirect *monetary* effects are substituted for health effects" (Courtwright, 1980:274). "In the end, all such arguments [about adverse consequences of deviant health habits] come down to this: since your unhealthy acts hit the rest of us in our pocketbooks, we have a right to pressure you to change. The appeal is ultimately to [economic] utility; bad habits are penalized in the name of the greatest [economic] good for the greatest number" (Courtwright, 1980:274).[8] As Knowles (1976:62) put the matter, "One's man's freedom in health is another's shackle in taxes and insurance premiums." Consequently, if an individual does not follow healthy rules of behavior—that is, if she or he is a deviant, that person should have to pay. This is not an archaic conception. Sickness is not the price paid by people whose behavior has offended the spirits. Rather, people with certain habits should pay in dollars to compensate others whose medical costs are higher because of those habits. God's judgment and the spirits have nothing to do with this circumstance.

As suggested in the previous chapter, people with HIV-AIDS are increasingly being seen in terms of a secular morality that views them as having been careless and irresponsible. But to many people, the moral status of people with HIV-AIDS is closer to the archaic conception than to a secular moral conception. The relationship between certain types of behavior and HIV-AIDS is an empirical fact and explained by science, but many think an individual has HIV-AIDS because he or she is being punished for immoral conduct. Whereas smokers have lung cancer simply because smoking insulted their lungs, to many people gays and IDUs have HIV-AIDS because their behavior insulted God. The relationship between behavior and disease is spiritual, not just (or even primarily) secular and empirical. Gay sex and drug use that transmit HIV are viewed as immoral because of their inherent qualities, not because of the economic consequences they have for others. Gay activists, among others, protest, however, that HIV-AIDS is no different from any other behavior-linked disease, such as lung cancer. The problem is that many (probably most) people do not see the issue this way. They believe that people who get HIV-AIDS from gay sex or drug use are on a different moral level from those who get lung cancer from smoking or heart disease from having consumed too much animal fat and not gotten enough exercise.

The difference may be seen by noting the way sick people are often viewed in nonliterate societies, where the archaic conception is dominant. Among the Dobu, for example, "there is no tender feeling for the deformed and incurable. ... He is 'bad'" (Ackerknecht, 1971:45). This is exactly the way many Americans feel about people who have HIV-AIDS. They are bad. And, understandably, many of these people are apt to view themselves accordingly. For example, an HIV-infected male homosexual told Weitz (1991:68) that he was being punished by God "for not being a good person."

Thus, the moral and deviant status of people with HIV-AIDS is not an extreme form of the idea that an individual should assume personal responsibility for his or her health. People with most behavior-related diseases are treated as sympathetically and compassionately as those with other kinds of illness. People with HIV-AIDS are more apt to be treated as moral deviants for whom others have little sympathy and compassion. In a 1991 nationwide *New York Times*/CBS poll, only 39 percent said they had a lot or some sympathy for "people who get AIDS from homosexual activity," and only 30 percent said this for "people who get AIDS from sharing needles while using illegal drugs" (Kagay, 1991:B-8). This view has implications for the medical treatment and prevention of HIV-AIDS.

Deviance as a Deterrent to Treatment

Since medical treatment is based on the scientific conception of disease, such treatment would presumably not be affected by nonscientific views of disease. This is the ideal, but medical practice is never immune to nonscientific beliefs in society. Otherwise medical treatments for the same conditions in England, France, Germany, and the United States would not vary so much (Payer, 1988). A particularly good example of the role of nonscientific social beliefs in medical treatment is the ensemble of respiratory diseases, known as black lung disease, frequently contracted by coal miners. From about 1920 to World War II, physicians typically considered this to be an "ordinary condition" for miners and believed that miners' complaints were due to "well-known" attributes of miners, such as alcoholism, "fear of the mines," "hurtful forms of recreation," or "malingering" (Smith, 1981). Physicians' views were thus shaped by wider social beliefs about coal miners (e.g., that miners commonly malinger). Considering the social stigma associated with HIV-AIDS, it would be surprising if physicians were not influenced by the pariah status of most persons who have this disease. Evidence indicates that they are.

A 1990 study by Barbara Gerbert et al. (1991) of a nationwide sample of primary care physicians found that only 68 percent felt they had a responsibility to treat people with AIDS, only 42 percent would welcome people with HIV as patients, 50 percent would not treat AIDS patients if they had a choice, and 32 percent did not even want to treat people who just had a high risk of contracting AIDS. Since the major high-risk groups are homosexuals and drug addicts, it is not surprising that responses were related to physician attitudes toward homosexuals and drug addicts, which reflected attitudes in the wider society (e.g., "homosexuality is a threat to many of our basic institutions"). Although a very high proportion of the physicians were certainly knowledgeable about the cause of AIDS in 1990, the moral status of people with AIDS still impeded many doctors from accepting them as patients. Other studies have also revealed prejudicial attitudes of physicians toward persons with AIDS (Douglas et al., 1985; Kelly et al., 1987; Hayward and Shapiro, 1991).

Such data are only for physician attitudes. There is little systematic evidence showing that physicians actually discriminate against persons with HIV-AIDS by denying them treatment or providing inferior care. However, Weitz's study is strongly suggestive in this regard. She (1991:82) found that when receiving care from someone other than their regular physician, HIV-AIDS patients feared "either rejection or receiving poor-quality care."

A major tenet of medical sociology concerns the distinction between disease and illness. Disease refers to a specific biological state and is defined in terms of the medical model, which usually means according to the medical science conception of disease. Illness refers to the way these biological states (real or merely perceived) are understood and experienced by ill persons and other members of society and are thus defined in terms of a sociomedical model, which includes societal reactions to disease (Mishler, 1981a, 1981b; Conrad, 1987). Sociologists contend that too little attention is given to illness in the treatment process, and it may be ignored altogether. Since patients must cope not only with physical impairment but frequently also with the negative attitudes, avoidance, and hostile actions of others, efforts to help patients cope with these reactions should be part of the treatment process. But the foregoing reveals that for HIV-AIDS, there is another dimension to the problem. Patients may need to cope with the negative reactions of professionals who do the treating.

The problem is not limited to physicians but extends also to other providers of health care. A 1988 study of emergency medical service professionals in Michigan revealed that 25 percent felt they should be able to refuse services to a patient who was a known or suspected carrier of HIV (Smyser et al., 1990), and some hospital nurses have been reported to ignore patients with AIDS (Hancock and Carim, 1986:90). The significance of HIV-AIDS being viewed as deviance for the person with HIV-AIDS is particularly sharp in a case cited by Weitz (1991:64). A gay attempted suicide after learning he had HIV-AIDS, after which he was placed in a maximum security ward at a state mental hospital. He told Weitz:

> I was treated worse than a caged leopard. I was put in solitary confinement. I wasn't allowed to use the same bathroom, as anybody else. I wasn't allowed to eat with the regular patients. All of my food came in disposable Styrofoam containers and they'd write in the container, "Calvin _____, isolation, AIDS." And the staff were very abusive, [telling me,] "Stay away from me. I don't want you near me. ... " The first night ... two of them threw their keys down and quit. They weren't about to work with a faggot with AIDS.

Beliefs that people with HIV-AIDS are moral deviants may hinder treatment in a more subtle way than by outright denial of treatment. In a review of several unpublished studies of educational efforts, Conrad (1986:55) concluded that negative attitudes toward persons with AIDS "creates resistance and barriers to taking in accurate knowledge about AIDS," even among health care providers. The view that victims of HIV-AIDS are moral deviants may be difficult to change by facts. When they are contrary to unfounded beliefs, people, including health care providers, frequently choose to ignore the facts.

Deviance as a Deterrent
to Prevention

Few, if any, experts question that rates of HIV transmission could be significantly reduced by educating gays to practice safe sex and, if necessary, distributing condoms to gays and providing IDUs with access to clean needles, either through a doctor's prescription, legalization of over-the-counter sales, or exchange programs. Such programs have been publicly and officially recommended since 1985, and all along they have been strongly resisted on moral grounds (Bayer, 1989:207–231). Many people believe, quite simply, that the programs would support and encourage deviant behavior (gay sex and drug use). Even biomedical research has been opposed for this reason (Hancock and Carim, 1986:30–39). For example, *Commentary* editor Norman Podhoretz was quoted in the *New York Times* on March 16, 1986 (Dershowitz, 1986:A-27), as saying that when government officials spend money for research to find a vaccine (or cure) for HIV-AIDS, they are giving "social sanction to what can only be described as brutish degradation." Opposition to government funding of research to seek a vaccine began to erode in the mid-1980s,[9] but programs promoting safe sex and sterile drug injection are still vigorously opposed.

To many people, HIV-AIDS is the result of deviant behavior and a problem of morality more than a viral disease and a problem of medicine. Gays and IDUs who have HIV-AIDS are seen as moral deviants, not just people who are sick. Even if they avoid contracting HIV by being careful and responsible (engaging in safe sex and using clean needles), they are still immoral. The problem is to stop their immorality (to correct for their immunodeficiency in values). Prevention programs that protect them from getting a virus do not change the immorality of their behavior. Even if they are careful and responsible, male homosexuals and IDUs are still bad people.

Moral opposition to prevention programs is particularly clear in programs for IDUs. Even though programs in needle exchange and legalization of over-the-counter sales have been shown to reduce HIV infections among drug users in cities around the world (Des Jarlais and Friedman, 1994:86–88), few such programs have been implemented in the United States. Des Jarlais and Friedman (1994) observed that this is due to a lack of political will. But political will is weak precisely because moral opposition is so strong: Public officials fear that in sponsoring prevention programs, they would promote deviant (immoral) behavior or that they would be accused of doing so. (In fact, however, there is no evidence to support the contention that such programs do increase drug use [Des Jarlais and Friedman, 1994: 87].)

Moral attitudes also impede sex education for gays. Such efforts are opposed because safe or careful gay sex (e.g., using condoms) is just as immoral as risky gay sex. The only morally correct behavior is to abstain from such sex. Despite the fact that moral preachment may have limited effect on sexual practices with respect to contracting STDs (Brandt, 1987), moral warnings continue to be issued with respect to HIV. The ineffectiveness of such efforts in preventing HIV-AIDS should be obvious to anyone who stops and thinks about the issue. Gays know how most people feel about them. To remind them of their immorality (as viewed by so many people) does not tell them anything they do not already know. (The same is true for moral preachment to drug injectors. They already know that in the eyes of society their use of drugs is wrong. That is why they conceal what they do.)

Moral attitudes may impede safe-sex efforts for gays in another way. Sex education in general may be opposed because it is interpreted as promoting homosexuality. For example, in September 1990 the school chancellor of New York City, Joseph Fernandez, recommended to the Board of Education that public schools make condoms available to students on request in an effort to reduce the spread of HIV-AIDS (*New York Times,* September 30, 1990:E-7). Opposition to the plan emerged. A crowd demonstrated at City Hall carrying placards, one of which stated, "STOP FERNANDEZ FROM TEACHING OUR KIDS GAY SEX" (*Time,* January 21, 1991:66).

To charge or imply, as many have, that opposition to HIV-AIDS prevention programs, especially for gays, comes from bigoted and mean-spirited leaders of "the extreme political and religious Right" oversimplifies greatly. In all societies people condemn what they define as morally deviant behavior. Sociologically, it would be surprising indeed if many people did not oppose HIV-AIDS preventive programs, which assist individuals to engage safely in what many in society define as morally repugnant behavior. Simply to charge moral opponents with bigotry, homophobia, and mean-spirited behavior fails to recognize that their opposition stems from the fact that their moral norms of behavior are being violated.[10] And far from being extremists, moral opponents are in the mainstream of much American religious tradition and indeed general cultural tradition. Many are fair-minded people who are no more mean-spirited and bigoted than Pope John Paul.[11] And even though many of the leaders are vocal in their moral opposition, many of the followers are not. In the same sense that politicians and political analysts speak of a silent majority, we may certainly speak of a silent majority, fair-minded or not, that is opposed to programs that promote safe gay sex and hygienic drug use.

Therefore, when programs of sex education are introduced, they are apt to be structured in accordance with the expectations of moral opponents (silent and vocal). Gays are apt to be excluded. For example, in 1987 Congress amended a health appropriations bill to preclude the use of funds by the CDC for sex educational programs in which the approach could be regarded as promoting male homosexual activities (Institute of Medicine, 1988). Thus, safe-sex programs must be directed to heterosexuals, who are not a high-risk group. Understandably, then, funding for prevention programs that target men who have sex with other men has been very limited. In 1993 *AIDS Alert* (8, 1993:62) reported that according to the Washington-based AIDS Action Council, some CDC prevention programs were not even attempting to reach gays: Some states provided no funding at all for male homosexuals, and in other states the funding was meager. For example, Connecticut devoted only 2 percent of its budget on prevention to gays. And for

California, where gays account for 80 percent of AIDS cases, gays receive less than 10 percent of AIDS prevention funds (Gross, 1993:8; Odets, 1994: 4).

Television news programs about HIV-AIDS commonly ignore the fact that anal sex between males and drug use (especially the former) are the primary means of contracting HIV. Warnings are more often than not directed to heterosexuals, particularly to women and adolescents. Members of these groups do face risks, of course, but we have the spectacle of television news commentators searching for groups that are at high risk when the high-risk groups are obvious to anyone who cares to look. But they seem not to want to discuss social deviants and their high-risk behavior. For example, on the evening of February 2, 1992, on "Peter Jennings Reporting," ABC presented a ninety-minute program, "Growing-up in the Age of AIDS." A viewer who did not know better would have been led to believe that HIV-AIDS was widespread among young heterosexuals, who, unless they abstained or used condoms, were at high risk of contracting HIV. That the risk was especially high among gays who engaged in anal sex with multiple partners and IDUs who exchanged needles with other users (and persons who had heterosexual intercourse with members of these two groups) was hardly mentioned. Several nationally and internationally known medical scientists and epidemiologists as well as the U.S. surgeon general appeared on the program. Although none stated that AIDS was increasing rapidly through heterosexual intercourse, none countered the general thrust of the program either. Of course, the decision about what appeared and was said on the show rested with network officials and Peter Jennings, and the participants' statements were responses to specific questions put to them by Jennings. But regardless of who was responsible, the program simply distorted the problem of HIV-AIDS in the United States. The point here is not that HIV-AIDS cannot be contracted through heterosexual intercourse—it can—but rather that discussion of the far more risky forms of deviant behavior was avoided. (To the program's credit, the idea that HIV could be contracted through casual contact was downplayed.)

Even agencies responsible for prevention may use the media to present HIV-AIDS as though mainstream white middle-class young people are most at risk. The Public Health Service condom commercials that appeared in early 1994, after the Clinton administration had announced it was going to attack HIV-AIDS head-on by providing, among other things, "frank and accurate information on AIDS" (*AIDS Alert*, 8, 1994:62), is an example. The commercials were more entertaining than earlier ones (some commentators said they were "cute"), but the message and audience to which it was directed were the same: Most potential victims are young white middle-class heterosexuals, and penile-vaginal intercourse is a major mode of transmitting HIV in the United States. The commercials did not mention anal sex or male homosexuals or drug injectors (or the fact that minorities and marginal social groups are especially at risk). Paradoxically, by calling attention to the problem of HIV-AIDS but avoiding discussion of what millions of people consider morally deviant aspects of the disease, the commercials deflected attention away from where the problem is. They were the topic of CNN's "Crossfire," January 6, 1994, in a ludicrous debate, moderated by Michael Kinsley and John Sununu, between the Clinton administration's AIDS "czar," or coordinator of AIDS programs, Kristine Gebbie, and Gary Bauer of the Family Research Council. The debate revolved around what percentage of condoms failed (Gebbie argued very few) and whether the commercials encouraged people to have sex (Bauer argued they did). Little was said about HIV-AIDS, male homosexuality and anal sex were not even addressed, and the increasing concentration of HIV-AIDS among African Americans was not mentioned. The way the commercials avoided, and Bauer, Gebbie, Kinsley, and Sununu worked to avoid, addressing deviant aspects of HIV-AIDS was amusing sociologically, but for enlightenment about how to prevent HIV-AIDS, the effect of the commercials and the debate must have been close to zero. Meanwhile, the spread of HIV in the gay and IDU populations continues (80 percent of the cases of AIDS reported in 1993 came from these two groups) (CDC, 1994a:8), and its disproportionate concentration among African Americans and probably lower-socioeconomic groups grows right along.

Moral opposition to safe-sex education is not limited to sex between males. Programs that would prevent the heterosexual transmission of HIV are also opposed. Many people consider premarital and extramarital sex as deviant and immoral, and moral admonishment to abstain from such sex is the only form of sex "education" they will approve. The strength of this attitude for some people may be seen from the fact that it prevails in some of the very places where we might expect HIV-AIDS to be viewed largely, if not entirely, as a medical problem: in hospitals. Personnel in Catholic hospitals in New York City know that safe sex will reduce the transmission of HIV but are prohibited from advising patients who are *already* infected with HIV-AIDS about safe-sex practices to prevent them from infecting others (Navarro, 1993a). Since Catholic institutions are major nonprofit providers of medical care, including care for patients with HIV-AIDS, persons who set hospital policy are certainly not uncaring people; the contrary is the case. (This belies the argument that opposition to HIV-AIDS prevention programs comes only from vocal homophobic extremists.) But they are morally committed to abolishing certain behavior they define as deviant, not just caring for sick people, and the former is at least as important to them as the latter. Since many of these people view prevention programs as encouraging deviant behavior, to them prevention of HIV-AIDS is worse than the disease itself.[12]

Conclusion

An archaic conception of disease in which disease is viewed as a visitation by spirits is ancient and probably dates to the beginning of human existence. Yet this conception emerged as a major explanation of HIV-AIDS in the 1980s when a medical science conception of disease was well established in the minds of people throughout the population. Most people with HIV-AIDS were (and are) viewed as normative deviants and bad. This view not only questioned one of the most important sociological ideas (those associated with Parsons) about the deviant properties of sickness; it also impeded (and continues to impede) the treatment and prevention of the disease. But simply to label such problems as the work of extremists and bigots oversimplifies how deeply and widespread an archaic conception of HIV-AIDS is entrenched in the minds of much of the population. The institutionalization of the medical science conception of disease does not mean that an archaic conception will disappear for all diseases. Just as any number of unknown biological microbes lurk in the environment and appear when the conditions are right, archaic conceptions of disease are latent in society and emerge to define a particular disease when certain social conditions exist. HIV-AIDS was such a disease.

NOTES

1. There is no one-to-one correspondence between type or severity of illness and exemption. Exemption for the same condition may vary depending on the social and cultural context (Parsons, 1979:123–125). Children with broken arms are not normally exempt from attending school, but workers may be exempt from work, depending on the social characteristics of the work (Yelin et al., 1980). In addition, some social units are more lenient than others in exempting individuals because of illness. For example, military units are stricter than prisons. When a soldier is hospitalized, it may inconvenience his or her comrades and bring the unit under threat, but when a prisoner is hospitalized, it has no adverse consequences for other prisoners, guards, and the overall functioning of the prison (Waitzkin and Waterman, 1974:46–54).

2. Parsons's focus was clearly on acute conditions that can be successfully treated. Consequently, some writers have questioned whether Parsons's formulation applies to chronic and incurable conditions (Cogswell and Weir, 1964; Stewart and Sullivan, 1982). Parsons (1975) answered by noting that even for diseases that cannot be cured, individuals are still expected to seek medical care and that with proper treatment, as with diabetes, individuals can frequently return to normal role functioning.

3. Like other agents of social control, physicians are not always successful. For example, in a study of workers who had been disabled, Sybil Better et al. (1979) found that after severity of disability had been controlled for, workers who received Social Security disability insurance and/or supplemental security income were less apt to

have been rehabilitated (to have returned to work) than workers without those benefits. The economic incentives of the sick role apparently overrode social expectations of the sick role.

4. For a discussion that recognizes the cultural bias in Parsons's formulation, see Freidson (1970).

5. HIV-AIDS is not exactly a unique disease in this respect. Other diseases are also stigmatized, and some are considered morally deviant. For example, people who are mental patients are often stigmatized (Scheff, 1984), which may deter them from seeking treatment and adopting the sick role (Denzin and Spitzer, 1966; Petroni, 1972), and many consider alcoholics as irresponsible persons rather than as people with a disease. However, the stigma attached to such conditions and moralizing about them do not begin to approach those of HIV-AIDS. (Even though many view alcoholism in moral, rather than medical, terms, few view it as a form of divine punishment.)

6. The permanency of the impairment would be made visible by a policy recommended by the editor of the *National Review,* William Buckley Jr. (1986), among others. People who are infected with HIV would have AIDS tattooed on their buttocks or the upper portion of their forearms, depending on how they contracted HIV. Buckley's argument—that this would not be a form of stigma but a public health measure since the tattoo would be seen only by potential gay sexual partners or IDUs who might share needles—is faulty. A man's buttocks are seen in places other than in a sexual context (e.g., in athletic dressing rooms), and a tattoo on an arm is visible for all to see unless covered by clothing.

7. For example, Mary Fisher, a prominent Republican who was apparently infected by her former husband, a drug user, spoke at the Republican National Convention in 1992. Columnist Robert Novak, in commenting during CNN's August 22 "Capital Gang" on Fisher's appearance, said, "She didn't have any business on the podium" as a representive of people with AIDS since most people who get AIDS are prostitutes, drug addicts, and homosexuals.

8. Those who have unhealthy (deviant) habits should, in the words of the secretary of health, education, and welfare in the Carter administration, Joseph Califano (1986:201), "pay more to the insurance company or Blue Cross/Blue Shield." Furthermore, "if a family member smoked, the annual payment would be higher. The payment would also be increased for obesity, for not bringing down high cholesterol levels within a reasonable time, for excessive drinking of alcoholic beverages, and for failure to get the appropriate physical exams and tests."

9. This erosion was due in large part to the activism of what some have called the "AIDS lobby" (Fumento, 1990:326–331), which is composed of leaders of the gay community, medical scientists, concerned public officials, and some persons who fear that HIV will spread to the heterosexual population.

10. Even Harvard sociologist David Reisman appears not to have got this point. He was quoted in the *Wall Street Journal* (Ansberry, 1987:A-5) as saying that negative reactions to gay victims are forms of "mean-spiritedness" and "bigotry" and not in keeping with the compassion and tolerance cultivated by advances in civil rights during the 1960s, in which "we're supposed to be good, egalitarian citizens." The point is not that such treatment of gay victims is justified but rather that tolerance is

rare and mean-spirited and bigoted reactions are common when people violate the moral norms of society. An increase in civil rights and egalitarianism need not change people's view that certain types of behavior are deviant.

11. Verghese (1994:49, 39) captured the Janus-faced quality of many people in his description of the people of Johnson City, Tennessee, where he treated AIDS patients. In Johnson City Jerry Falwell's pronouncement that gays would "one day be utterly annihilated and there would be celebration in heaven" was taken as "a self-evident truth." But the typical person in Johnson City was also "someone who would give you the shirt off his back."

12. HIV-AIDS is not the only disease in history that has evoked moral opposition to prevention. McNeill (1976:236) wrote, "The doctrine that disease came from God could easily be interpreted to mean that it was impious to intervene with God's purpose by trying to take conscious precaution against disease." Opposition to HIV-AIDS may be less explicitly linked to this doctrine than many diseases in the past, but the doctrine is far from dead. In 1982 evangelist Billy Graham, in talking about STDs, stated, "We have conquered VD with penicillin. But then along comes Herpes Simplex. Nature itself lashes back when we go against God" (Brandt, 1987:180). Using this archaic moral logic, we could say, "Then along comes HIV-AIDS."

Sociology and the Eradication and Control of HIV-AIDS

There are two general ways to combat an infectious disease: eradication and control (Dubos, 1965:369–384). Eradication relies on drugs (e.g., vaccines, antibiotics), or "magic bullets," that prevent the infection or cure the disease after the infection has occurred. The goal of eradication is to eliminate the microbe altogether. Programs of control aim to limit the spread of the disease. Control stresses the need to change environmental conditions and the behavior of populations with the aim of making it harder for the agent to survive and be transmitted from host to host. Of course, eradication programs may incorporate control measures, and control programs may rely on magic bullets by making them available throughout the population, especially to persons at greatest risks, such as infants and children. Nevertheless, the aims of the two approaches differ, with one emphasizing complete elimination of the disease and the other, a limit to its spread.

Because magic bullets frequently have dramatic, visible, and immediate effects, they have special appeal for medical professionals and the lay public alike. And social status and money, fame and fortune, are powerful motivators for scientists to discover these drugs. Therefore, over the years much effort and money have gone into discovering more and more drugs that, it is hoped, will eradicate various infectious diseases.

Everyone agrees that eradication is a desired state since once the infectious agent has been eradicated, we need not worry about the microbe and constantly monitor the environment to be certain the microbe is under control. Unfortunately, eradication is much simpler in theory than in practice. Unless environmental changes are also made and/or the host population behavior changes, with rare exceptions magic bullets alone do not eliminate the agent. For example, tetracycline and the intravenous or oral consumption of lots of liquid containing salt can cure cholera, and a vaccine (requiring boosters) also exists, but to eradicate the disease, all major sources of filth and contaminated water would have to be eliminated. This would require widespread control over environmental conditions (especially the chlorination of

227

water supplies) and population behavior. Since as a practical matter all adverse conditions and behaviors would never be completely eliminated, as evidenced by the appearance of cholera in several regions of the world in recent years, the cholera bacillus will probably never be eradicated. However, adverse conditions and behaviors are controlled to a considerable extent and cholera is kept under reasonable control even in places where medication and vaccine for treating and preventing the disease are not available. Control, with its focus on changing the environment and host behavior, is more relevant to sociology than is eradication. Nevertheless, a few problems of eradication programs are worthy of mention, particularly as they relate to HIV-AIDS.

Problems of Eradication and HIV-AIDS

Eradication requires that every single agent be killed worldwide, once and for all (Cockburn, 1961:1050–1051). The speed of intercontinental travel makes it virtually impossible to limit an infectious microbe to a certain region. Consequently, if an effective vaccine for HIV were developed, its distribution worldwide would be essential before HIV could be eradicated. But many developing countries do not have the social and economic resources for effective distribution programs, and it is not certain that richer countries would provide them with the resources.

Moreover, the result of an effective vaccine for HIV could be catastrophic. In the struggle for survival, HIV may currently enjoy a competitive advantage over other microbes, whose proliferation is suppressed by HIV. But if drugs eradicated or drastically suppressed HIV, other microbes might find the environment more nourishing and thus proliferate rapidly. The death of HIV might mean opportunities for other microbes. Some might be just as deadly as HIV or might be relatively benign agents that become extremely virulent in an HIV-free environment. (The worst fear is that such agents might be airborne.) An effective drug for HIV might lead to mutant forms of HIV against which the drug would be ineffective (Garrett, 1992:835–836). (For a general discussion of how drugs against a microbe may have such adverse consequences, see Dubos, 1965:370–382; Grmek, 1989:168–171.)

Because of the possible iatrogenic effects of drugs and other problems in eradication, Dubos (1965:381–382, 379), among others, argued that control programs are superior to eradication programs. This, after all, is the way many infectious diseases of the past, before the age of vaccines and antibiotics, were made manageable. Changing the environment to reduce conditions under which a microbe thrives and changing the behavior of host populations to reduce transmission are better strategies, Dubos argued, than relying on magic bullets to eradicate the pest, which is most likely an elusive goal anyway.

Theoretically, drugs could be used to fight HIV-AIDS in three ways. Antiviral drugs, such as AZT, could suppress or kill HIV after infection had occurred. Immune-corrective drugs could be used to boost immune systems and increase host resistance to opportunistic infections. The ultimate weapon, a vaccine, would make people immune to HIV. Although virologists, immunologists, and other biomedical scientists do not agree on the best approach, once AIDS was identified as an infectious disease with HIV as its cause, many became characteristically optimistic: As with so many other infectious diseases, effective drugs to combat HIV would be developed; efforts in one or more of the three areas would be successful (Radetsky, 1991: 343–351).

Despite this optimism, and even ignoring the socioeconomic problems and possible iatrogenic effects, the fact is, there is no assurance that any of these efforts will succeed. The history of antiviral drugs does not inspire optimism that eradication will come from this route. Some antiviral drugs do inhibit a viral agent for some strains of certain diseases, and they may destroy the virus in some individuals. In general, however, there is no antiviral drug that cures a viral disease. Antibiotics are generally ineffective against viral diseases, and the antiviral equivalent of penicillin, which cures a variety of bacterial infections, simply does not exist. As for immune-boosting drugs, they may help resist certain infections, but they do not kill the microbe, so carriers might still pass HIV on to other hosts. Few viruses have been eradicated with vaccines (smallpox is the well-known exception). We must wonder, therefore, to what extent the optimism that HIV-AIDS will eventually be brought to its knees with magic bullets is really warranted.

As was noted in Chapter 7, some scientists believe the scientific consensus that HIV is a necessary and sufficient cause of AIDS is premature. Root-Bernstein (1993), in particular, believed that the biological etiology of AIDS is multifactorial and that this has major implications for research to develop drugs to treat and/or prevent HIV-AIDS. Moreover, Harvard microbiologist Bernard Fields (1994:96) wrote that after a decade of research, fundamental gaps in knowledge about HIV still exist and that approaches to developing drugs "have not shown great promise." He maintained that research strategy has been on the wrong track and that a new direction is needed. And others believe that even if an effective vaccine or cure were developed, its effectiveness might be short-lived. The nature of HIV is such that a vaccine or cure for HIV-AIDS might become ineffective shortly after being put to clinical use (Ewald, 1994:179–180). Thus, there are good reasons to wonder if HIV will ever be eradicated and even more reasons to question whether drugs that cure or prevent the infection will be developed anytime soon.

Control Programs and HIV-AIDS

Meanwhile, millions of people worldwide are infected, and many more will be infected in the years ahead. For the foreseeable future, the only feasible approach to HIV-AIDS is to reduce the conditions that facilitate its spread. This would require that more resources be devoted to education about how HIV is spread in certain sexual and drug use practices, to condom and clean needle distribution, and to HIV testing (so infected persons and the persons who may have infected them can be identified and counseled to take care not to infect others). In the United States much has already been accomplished, of course. In particular, safe-sex practices by gays and hygienic needle use by drug injectors have increased, and public health education (even if primarily through the mass media) has contributed to this. Yet experts agree that the accomplishments are much less than they could be.

Deficiencies are not due to insufficient knowledge since the ways to reduce the risk of contracting HIV are well known. And they are not due to too few resources: The economic cost of adequate prevention programs would be a pittance of all health care expenditures and only a fraction of what we are spending to develop drugs against HIV-AIDS. Deficiencies are due instead to the resistance of certain people to changing their high-risk habits and to the social attitudes and behavior of people who oppose preventive measures on moral grounds.

It goes without saying that explicitly directing education efforts to high-risk groups is essential (Kolata, 1993b). However, as we have seen, the moral opposition to informational programs about HIV-AIDS may cause the information to get distorted so that persons who are not at high risk (white middle-class heterosexuals) end up being the targets. Moral opponents—the silent moderates no less than the vocal extremists—will not readily accept the idea that gays and IDUs should be taught safe sex and drug use practices, much less making condoms and clean needles easily available to them. Consequently, prevention efforts tend to focus on heterosexuals rather than members of groups that are at greatest risk.

Societal reactions to HIV-AIDS lead to curious results and strange bedfellows. The position taken by some of those who are scientifically most informed about HIV-AIDS and its spread in the population probably encourages a result that the moral opponents of gays and IDUs demand, namely, that high-risk groups not be the focus of prevention. For example, physicians David Rogers and June Osborn (1993:494) of the National Commission on AIDS object to the emphasis on high-risk groups and prefer instead that prevention "focus more broadly on the universality of risk among all people." They believe that only if HIV-AIDS is recognized as a universal threat will the public give prevention the political support it needs. To contend that HIV-AIDS is limited largely to groups about which society cares very little conveys the idea that it "will disappear into the socially invisible substrata of American society without [society] having to lift a finger" (Rogers and Osborn, 1993:494; Kolata, 1993a).

Rationalists like Rogers and Osborn oppose the moralists as vehemently as anyone, but paradoxically they end up in the same camp. There is a difference, of course. The rationalists want prevention efforts to emphasize that white middle-class heterosexuals are at risk, whereas the moralists object to a policy in which high-risk groups (gays and IDUs) are the focus, so that white middle-class heterosexuals actually become the primary targets of prevention efforts. But it is the moralists who do so much damage because they impede efforts at prevention for persons from high-risk groups. The rationalists support prevention programs in general but oppose specific programs in which high-risk groups are the primary focus. Since it is the moralists who are so strongly opposed to targeting high-risk groups for prevention in the first place, the rationalists' opposition is a reaction to the moralists' reaction.[1] Before prevention efforts will realize maximum effectiveness, the attitudes of moralists must be changed.

Obviously, this is easier said than done. To challenge the position of moral opponents (e.g., to accuse them of homophobia and racism) will certainly not make them receptive to certain measures to control the spread of HIV any more than challenging the morals of gays and IDUs will make them receptive to certain changes in their behavior. Even to argue that moral attitudes are in conflict with medical science will fall on many deaf ears. No matter how forceful the logic, arguments will not likely move many moral opponents closer to the view that HIV-AIDS is a medical problem with natural causes rather than a moral problem with irresponsible human (or even supernatural) causes. Furthermore, for public health educators to engage in moral education entails political risks, which may actually undermine support for programs designed to contain the spread of HIV.

An alternative is to make the benefits that such programs have for society overall the centerpiece of prevention efforts. If the number of HIV-AIDS cases were reduced, medical and economic resources would be saved and the danger, however remote, of HIV-AIDS becoming widespread beyond the gay, IDU, low-socioeconomic, and racial minority populations would decline. Some moral opponents might therefore realize that society would be better off if gays, IDUs, and heterosexual "sinners" did not transmit HIV than if they did, even if this amounted to a policy of educating them to do safely what the moralists oppose. This would be no easy task, of course, but it is a morally neutral strategy and certainly an appropriate one for public health officials to adopt.

In any case, the point is that before prevention programs can be truly effective, they must change not only the high-risk behavior of high-risk groups but also the societal reaction of the moral enemies of high-risk groups. Only then will preventive measures be supported and information about the risks of contracting HIV flow more directly to persons who are at greatest risk.

Nevertheless, even though information that polygamous behavior, anal sex, sex with members of high-risk groups, and needle sharing increase the chances of infection is sufficient to increase prevention for many people, the "information model" is inadequate for many others (Patton, 1990a; Odets, 1994). Scientific information is mediated by social meanings and cultural symbols and hence interpreted by persons according to their social and cultural backgrounds. Thus, for example, to public health educators bathhouses and polygamous sex mean high-risk behavior and the danger of HIV transmission, but to many gays they mean other things as well or instead. The professional educator may view the exchange of semen in anal intercourse is very high-risk behavior, but to many gays the exchange of semen promotes intimacy and social bonding with other gays (Odets, 1994:13). (Corresponding differences may hold for shooting galleries and drug injectors.) Professional behaviorist educators who use scientific information about HIV-AIDS to try and modify the behavior of gays, IDUs, and marginal persons (the poor, uneducated, and jobless) from racial-ethnic minorities may be ineffective simply because they fail to understand a fundamental point: The symbolic meaning of certain customs and institutions may have a greater impact on the behavior of such persons than does the fear of knowing that behaving in accordance with these customs and institutions increases the risk of contracting HIV (Patton, 1990a:41, 71, 100; Odets, 1994). The effectiveness of formal safe-sex education has yet to be proven, but one problem is that sex educators may assume that the rationalization process is more entrenched in society than it is; their effectiveness may be impaired because they do not understand the attitudes of members of high-risk groups and the social meanings that certain acts, customs, and institutions have for them. In fact, research on prevention programs for gays in the Netherlands indicates that unless health educators understand attitudes that gays have about certain sexual practices and their social meaning, changes in high-risk sexual behavior may not be sustained (de Wit et al., 1993). Odets (1994) argues that the failure of professional safe-sex educators to understand the social meaning that certain sexual acts have for gays explains much of the relapse in preventive behavior among gays.

Patton (1990a:43, 41) contends that in the early 1980s, when most prevention programs were organized and implemented by gays, the problem was not as serious. Then programs educating gays to change their sexual practices "trained [gay] bartenders as educators" and sent "leatherclad hunks [to raid] bars to pass out condoms and AIDS literature." Such persons understood the attitudes of other gays. They could therefore discuss prevention measures in terms of the social meaning and symbolic significance certain sexual acts had for their listeners, without admonishing them to be responsible or implicitly raising moral questions about gay sex. The grassroots nature of early prevention programs may explain why the decline in high-risk behavior in the early 1980s was so substantial, particularly among gays. Therefore, some prevention programs sponsored and staffed by gays as well as drug injectors may deserve public funding and support; and the effectiveness of other programs might be raised if such persons were incorporated into those programs.

Of course, the moral opponents would not take kindly to public-health funds being used this way. The problem may be highlighted by way of an example. The exchange of semen in oral sex may have significant emotional and social value for many gays (Odets, 1994:13) and carries low risk for contracting HIV (though potential risk does exist) (Levy, 1993:91). In an effort to reduce high-risk anal sex, preventive programs for gays could build on social rewards that appear to be motivating factors in gay sex by emphasizing the joy and relative safety of oral sex. Nevertheless, in a preventive education campaign for gays that also emphasized the joy of gay sex, professional educators of the private San Francisco AIDS Foundation considered but then rejected using "Enjoy Oral Sex" as a "tag line" (Odets, 1994:10–11). One can imagine the outrage of the public, and certainly the moral opponents of gays, if publically funded programs even considered endorsing oral gay sex. This underscores the importance of the societal reaction to controlling the spread of HIV. But unless control efforts develop strategies with oppositional moral attitudes and behavior as well as high-risk behavior in mind, the containment of the HIV-AIDS epidemic will move at a tragically slower pace than knowledge and resources warrant.

African Americans and Control of Heterosexual AIDS

Efforts to prevent the heterosexual transmission of HIV among African Americans are complicated by other problems. As was noted in Chapter 4, heterosexual and especially secondary transmission of HIV-AIDS from IDUs will be slowed as heterosexuals become increasingly careful in choosing their sexual partners. However, African Americans who live in economically depressed communities and neighborhoods may find it difficult to be very choosy. Opportunities for females, in particular, to be selective in choosing sexual partners are very limited. And the greater social acceptance of polygamous behavior by African Americans, which may derive from a combination of the drug subculture, the socioeconomics of the culture of the underclass and welfare dependence, and possibly cultural tradition, further complicates the problem.

Results of a study of women, most of them African American, who were attending a prenatal clinic in Belle Glade, Florida, which is almost 100 percent African American, suggest just how serious the problem may be. The average number of sexual partners was twenty-seven for women who were HIV positive but only five for women who were HIV negative (Ellerbrock et al., 1992:1706). Although the identity of the male partners was not reported in the study, it is not improbable that a high proportion of the partners of HIV-infected women were IDUs; the finding that the HIV-positive women were more apt to have exchanged sex for drugs suggests this is the case. And given the large number of partners they had had, these women were obviously not very discriminating in the men with whom they had sex, which suggests sexual norms of polygamous behavior.

These structural features of predominantly low socioeconomic African-American communities and neighborhoods along with the high prevalence of non-HIV STDs may make it very hard indeed to slow the heterosexual transmission of HIV in the African-American population. The secondary transmission from IDUs may be especially difficult to slow. Thus the racial difference in heterosexual HIV-AIDS will continue and probably increase.

Control of HIV-AIDS in Africa

As serious as the foregoing problems are, they pale in comparison to the problems of control in Africa. The economies of most African countries are in shambles, and inflation is rampant; the national wealth of many countries has been plundered by corrupt officials and military dictators; and foreign debts are so high that virtually all exports must go to pay down debt. Fifteen of the twenty poorest countries in the world are in Africa (and poorer today than in the 1970s [O'Connor, 1991:3]). That African governments on average spend only about $3.50 per capita on health care each year (by way of comparison, Scandinavian countries spend about $1,000) (Barnett and Blaikie, 1992:167) illustrates the magnitude of the problem. There are simply few economic resources for public health programs.[2]

Problems of social organization abound. The numerous clans and tribes create divisions that are difficult, if not impossible, to bridge. Different groups frequently speak different languages. Individuals tend to identify more with clan and tribe than nation-state, thus draining support from the programs that central governments may try to establish (Cockcroft, 1990: 99–103). Problems are especially acute in the cities, where HIV-AIDS is so prevalent. There, social division combines with allegiance to traditional customs to produce anomie on a wide scale, making coherent government programs, including public health programs to control the spread of HIV-AIDS, almost impossible to mount and sustain.[3]

In addition, political turmoil is widespread, as the media make clear almost any day. More than a few countries and regions border on anarchy, several are gripped by fierce civil wars and savage clan-tribal conflicts, and many are ruled by bandits, thugs, and warlords, who strengthen their rule by controlling the distribution of food and economic resources among distrusting clans and tribes, which the rulers play off against each other, thus strengthening clan-tribal conflict.[4]

But health care programs would face a daunting task in controlling HIV-AIDS even if economic resources were available, social divisions bridged, and political stability achieved. In the final analysis, whether the HIV-AIDS epidemic in Africa slows down will depend on millions of people changing their behavior. And since behavior is anchored in cultural norms, social institutions, and the structure of social rewards, changes will be hard for health care professionals to bring about. It will be most difficult to reduce risky sexual practices in cultures where sex is viewed as recreational and enjoyable; contributes so much to sex identity; produces children and hence increases individual social status as well as the strength of family, clan, and tribe; and allows women to escape the domination of men. Actions that hold the most promise for slowing the spread of HIV are simply beyond the purview of medical programs, narrowly defined.

For example, the social empowerment of women through statutory change is central to the control of HIV-AIDS in Africa. Land reform that gives women greater access to and control of land might do more than any other single factor to change polygamous behavior and hence the transmission of HIV. Social programs that elevate the education and occupational skills of women would also help. These are not matters with which the health care profession is usually concerned; they are far removed from the administering of magic bullets. But African programs must be adapted to the traditional social practices and culture of Africa. Whether we wish to call such programs health care or not, these are the ways communal health *effects* are most apt to be registered.

Of course, land and other reforms that would empower women would be opposed by clan and tribal elders and men in general. Also, most educational efforts aimed at changing behavior directly would be opposed. For example, advocating the use of condoms may be socially explosive, and governments must address the issue very delicately, if at all (Barnett and Blaikie, 1992: 161). Such a policy is apt to be viewed as contrary to the valued outcomes of individuals. And since use of condoms reduces population growth, government advocacy of them may be interpreted as an effort to weaken the power of certain clans and tribes. Condom use may also be viewed as a racial conspiracy against all Africans (Barnett and Blaikie, 1992:160). This is most apparent in South Africa, where some groups view the use of condoms in terms of reduction in fertility, which would emasculate the indigenous culture and allow the white culture to become dominant (Green, 1994:77).[5]

This does not mean that all efforts at public health education would be resisted. To be most effective, however, education must be adapted to social and cultural features of African society. To start, health care professionals must accept the fact that magico-religious and other nonscience-based explanations of disease and HIV-AIDS are powerful social forces. Africans' faith in explanations of disease that are embedded in African culture is just as strong as Westerners' faith in explanations derived from medical science. To instill HIV-preventive behaviors, health care workers must sometimes develop explanations of HIV-AIDS that merge magico-religious myths with science, or what Barnett and Blaikie (1992:43) called "syncretic explanations." A good example of this can be seen in a health problem, unrelated to HIV-AIDS, in northern Nigeria. Missionaries were alarmed about the level of infant mortality resulting from mothers giving their infants contaminated water to drink:

> They explained to "converts" at the mission that the deaths were due to animals in the water, and that these animals would be killed if they only boiled it before giving it to the children. Talk of invisible animals produced only a tolerant skepticism: the babies went on dying. Finally a visiting anthropologist suggested a remedy. There were, he said, evil spirits in the water; boil the water and you could see them going away, bubbling out to escape the heat. This time the message worked. (Okri, 1991:134–135)

Many Africans will accept scientific explanations of disease and corresponding preventive measures if they can be squared with traditional magico-religious beliefs.

With specific reference to HIV-AIDS, the view that HIV is transmitted through sexual intercourse must be synthesized with a variety of myths about sex and disease. Barnett and Blaikie (1992:156) suggested such a course with respect to the sexual cleansing ritual, in which symbolic actions would replace physical intercourse. Sally Scott and Mary Mercer (1994) suggested merging scientific explanation of HIV with the Zimbabwean belief that HIV-AIDS is due to *runyoka* (transmitted only through sex that is culturally taboo). Unfortunately, however, these authors did not indicate what the syncretic explanations or specific preventive measures would be. Similarly, Thurow (1986) reported that in their fight against HIV-AIDS, physicians in South Africa enlisted the help of local healers, some of whom believed AIDS was caused by wizards. He did not say how the notion of wizards was integrated with the medical science explanation.

Of course, simply making people aware of the scientific explanation of how HIV is transmitted will have some positive effect. Some African anthropologists have suggested that the fear of getting AIDS may have already caused a decline in casual sex (Bennett, 1987:532; Caldwell et al., 1989:

226), and some success in getting prostitutes to use condoms has been reported (Mann et al., 1992:18, 401). In general, however, little increase in preventive behavior (or attitudes) seems to have occurred, particularly among men (Barnett and Blaikie, 1992:44–46, 49–50, 83; Green, 1994:1, 108–110). Certainly, in contrast to a highly rationalized society like the United States, where the dissemination of scientific information alone increases preventive behavior, for the masses of Africans much more is needed. Just because Africans fear HIV-AIDS does not mean they will be guided in their behavior by a scientific explanation if it is inconsistent with explanations based on ancestral magico-religious beliefs.

This is not to suggest that philosophically the scientific and rational values of the West are superior to cultural values derived from African beliefs in spirits and other invisible entities. (The inherent superiority of science and rational values continues to be debated as a philosophical issue in the West. Indeed, at least one author wondered whether it is even desirable for Africans to give up beliefs in invisible agents as causes of disease [Okri, 1991: 135].) However, from the standpoint of preventing the spread of HIV, people are obviously on safer grounds adapting their behavior to the way science says HIV behaves than to the way they think witches, spirits, and wizards behave. Crucial to limiting the transmission of HIV in Africa is getting people to adapt their behavior to the way HIV behaves *as well as* to the way they think mystical agents (e.g., spirits associated with widowhood, *runyoka,* wizards), which bear on sex and HIV-AIDS in a variety of ways, also behave.

In any society it is far more difficult to eradicate than to control and limit an infectious disease, but in Africa social and cultural forces present unusually strong obstacles to programs designed to limit the transmission of HIV. We need not subscribe to the hyperbole sometimes heard, that "AIDS is depopulating an entire continent," to realize that these forces will determine the extent to which HIV-AIDS in Africa will be controlled for years to come. To counter them, medical professionals must work very hard to invent any number of explanations in which myth and science are combined.

Unlike scientific medicine, in which there is usually one dominant explanation for a disease (particularly for an infectious disease), many syncretic explanations would be needed for HIV-AIDS because explanations for a disease vary from group to group. In developing these explanations, medical professionals must solicit the views of local healers and incorporate these healers in prevention programs (Green, 1994). It is they who are most knowledgeable about tribal explanations of disease. Also, since they command the faith of people and can convey the message about prevention in terms that people understand, local healers are frequently the best persons to implement prevention programs. For example, Western-trained professionals might convince healers that using condoms may prevent HIV-AIDS.

Then when diviner-medium healers see patients with STDs, they could divine that spirits want the patients to use condoms. This advice would probably elicit much greater compliance than the recommendations of Western-trained doctors or nurses, particularly since Africans believe indigenous healers are superior to Western-trained doctors in treating STDs (Green, 1994). Local healers would also be more effective in advising people to stick to single partners or, in the case of polygamous marriage, to confine sexual relations to marital partners (Green, 1994:112). For some groups, such advice might be made in terms of *runyoka*. This would have no scientific basis, of course, but it could still be effective. It is the health effect produced that makes an action effective, not the rationale (scientific or otherwise) on which the action is based.[6]

A Final Note

The globalization of AIDS is now well known. Many infectious disease experts view this as they have viewed other infectious diseases, particularly those that are air- or waterborne. In 1987 Dr. Jonathan M. Mann, then director of the World Health Organization's AIDS programs, was reported to have stated, "There is a global epidemic of AIDS that leaves no country untouched. We can't stop AIDS anywhere until we stop it everywhere" (Corey, 1987:13). This implies that the prevalence of AIDS depends on HIV alone and suggests that AIDS will continue its spread unless stopped by vaccines or other drugs. No population is safe until HIV has been stopped, that is, eradicated everywhere.

A central theme of this book leads to another view, namely, that HIV-AIDS can be controlled with preventative measures even if it is not eradicated. The transmission of HIV reflects the behavior of populations. Such behavior, in turn, is embedded in the social and cultural forces that characterize those populations and the wider societies of which they are a part. Therefore, the prevalence of AIDS depends on the behavior of populations and hence the social and cultural characteristics that cause such behavior. By the same token, the transmission of HIV can be slowed by changes in population behavior and social attitudes and cultural beliefs with respect to the way HIV is transmitted. But because societies differ in the ease with which such changes can be effected, HIV-AIDS may be slowed in some populations, while its increase continues unabated, and even increases rapidly, in others. The idea of the global village is valid with respect to many infectious diseases. And it is certainly relevant to HIV-AIDS, as the global spread of the disease reveals. Nevertheless, social and cultural barriers impede the transmission of HIV in ways that they do not impede the transmission of many other infectious microbes. It is no doubt true that eradication of HIV-AIDS anywhere depends on its eradication everywhere. But to slow HIV-AIDS anywhere does not depend on its being slowed everywhere.[7]

NOTES

1. Another paradoxical social alignment occurs with respect to mandatory testing for HIV. Whether testing would reduce the spread of HIV is subject to debate, but testing is vigorously opposed on grounds that have nothing to do with its effectiveness in reducing HIV-AIDS and by persons who otherwise hold radically different views about HIV-AIDS and high-risk groups. On the one hand, some Christian groups that are morally opposed to homosexuality oppose mandatory testing because if pregnant women knew they were infected with HIV, this would increase abortion, which these groups also oppose on moral grounds. On the other hand, others oppose testing because of civil rights concerns and the fear that individuals identified as HIV positive would be subjected to social stigma, which, of course, the moral interpretation of HIV-AIDS creates in the first place. (These views were expressed on ABC's "60 Minutes" on September 18, 1994.) As in other instances, this paradox reveals that simply to charge that preventive measures are impeded by mean-spirited bigots and moral zealots grossly oversimplifies the social complexities involved.

2. This reflects the priorities of governments and not just limited economic resources. For example, governments give airlines higher priority than expenditures for health care: "The first priority for most governments at independence, even before expenditures on education and health, was a spanking new airport and an international carrier bearing a new flag." All the airlines lose money (Lamb, 1987:230–231).

3. In discussing Central African Republic, Shoumatoff (1988:102) wrote that it is more "an anarchic collection of [about 80] tribes" than a country. In describing the anomie ("African Madness") in sub-Saharan urban areas (where "the old ways of Africa [are] no good anymore"), he (1988:170, xiv) stated, "When large cities begin to appear ... a societal madness begins to occur," and "detribalized young men [are] lost souls wandering in the vast space between the traditional and modern worlds." They "can be heard howling in the streets of downtown Nairobi in the middle of the night," and "stark naked *alienes* can be seen rummaging in the ditches of Bangui." Shoumatoff's work is an excellent journalistic description of Africans living in an anomic void between the tribal and urban worlds, with specific reference to HIV-AIDS (Shoumatoff, 1988:131–202).

4. For insightful journalistic accounts of the interrelation of economic scarcity, social divisiveness, and political anarchy in Liberia, Zaire, and Natal (South Africa), see Berkeley (1992, 1993, 1994).

5. On CNN's "Moneyline" (June 7, 1993), two black South African social workers said that programs promoting condoms to prevent HIV-AIDS were really intended to control the black population, one stating they were intended to reduce the number of black voters.

6. Incorporating indigenous explanations and healers this way resembles to some extent the strategy of incorporating members of high-risk groups in prevention programs in the United States. There is a vast difference, however. Members of high-risk groups in the United States would be incorporated in order to integrate the social meanings and attitudes of these groups in education to avoid high-risk behavior; such meanings and attitudes have nothing to do with myth (e.g., gay sex may in fact give a greater sense of identity; semen exchange, a greater sense of belonging). In themselves, they are not inconsistent with science. In the case of Africa, however, magico-religious explanations are inconsistent with science. Preventive efforts must therefore not just recognize the social meaning that certain acts and beliefs have for people but also be based on explanations that somehow make science and myth consistent with each other.

7. Statements and works by Dr. Mann since 1987 (Mann, 1988; Mann et al., 1992) indicate that he subscribes to this position today.

Appendix
Bisexual Transmission and the Efficiency of Heterosexual Transmission of HIV

Some believe that male bisexuals are a major source of secondary transmission. However, the possible number of bisexuals is usually never addressed in such discussions, though the assumption of a relatively large number seems to be based on statistics reported by Kinsey and associates from their study in the 1930s and 1940s in what became known as the Kinsey Report. One of Kinsey's arguments is that heterosexuality and homosexuality exist on a continuum. Some men are exclusively heterosexual, some are exclusively homosexual, and some fall in between and hence are bisexual.

Kinsey et al. (1948) reported that 10 percent of males said they had been predominantly homosexual for at least three years and that 4 percent were exclusively homosexual. (Kinsey et al. also reported that 37 percent had had some same-gender sex.) If these figures are approximately correct, up to 6 percent of the male population could be bisexual. This would be a substantial potential reservoir of secondary transmission of HIV and would lend credence to the assertion that HIV-AIDS is a serious threat to many heterosexuals. But it is hard to know how to interpret the statistics in the Kinsey Report. They are not based on a representative sample of the population but on volunteers who came disproportionately from hospitals, universities, and prisons.

Statistics from surveys based on representative national samples in recent years are not uniform, but they do indicate the 10 percent figure is an exaggeration. Based on surveys from 1978 to 1991, the percentage of American males who have had any homosexual experience in the recent past (up to ten years) may be no higher than 2–4 percent and those who are exclusively homosexual may be as low as 1 percent (Fay et al., 1989; Billy et al., 1993; Rogers, 1993). (Similar conclusions are indicated by the results of surveys in Great Britain and France in the early 1990s [Johnson et al., 1992; ACSF Investigators, 1992].) A 1993 survey found that 5.7 percent of men and women described themselves "as homosexual" (Elliott, 1994), but in a more comprehensive survey conducted in 1992, only 2.8 percent of men and 1.4 percent of women eighteen to fifty-nine years old identified themselves as homosexual or bisexual (Laumann et al., 1994:291). Findings for bisexuals are especially significant. Billy et al. (1993:59) found that only 0.6 percent of married men and 1.1 percent of formerly married men—men who definitely were having or had had sexual experience with women—reported having had *any* same-gender sexual contact in the previous ten years; in the survey by Laumann et al. (1994:311) only 0.8 percent of men identified themselves as bisexual and only 0.7 percent said they had had sex with a man and a woman in the previous twelve months. Therefore, contrary to Osborn's (1993:S230) claim that there is a "large group of bisexual men" in the United States, bisexuals are a small minority within a small minority. Opportunities for secondary transmissions of HIV from homosexual (bisexual) men are far less than some have assumed. Through 1992 only 1,389 female cases had reported sexual contact with a bisexual male; this accounted for only 3.1 percent of all female cases (0.30 percent of all cases). The absolute numbers are very small. Although they increased from 109 in 1989 to 174 in 1992, as a percentage of all female cases there was virtually no change, being about 3.0 percent from 1989 through 1992 (CDC, 1991d:9, 1992:9, 1993a: 9, 1994a:8).

In addition, it is not clear how transmission from bisexuals actually occurs when it does occur. Bisexuals may prefer anal intercourse even with females, so a high proportion of bisexual transmission may occur this way. Evidence for heterosexuals suggests that anal intercourse may be a major mode of heterosexual transmission. A study of lower-socioeconomic heterosexuals from New York City who were infected with HIV showed that 27 percent of women and 35 percent of men had engaged in anal sex during the previous twelve months (Kim et al., 1993), and studies of couples in which the male had HIV showed that the risk of male-to-female transmission increased significantly if the couples engaged in anal intercourse (European Study Group, 1989; Seidlin, et al. 1993; Root-Bernstein, 1993:33). At the same time, anal intercourse appears not to be very frequent among heterosexuals. Studies of sexually active women in Canada, Denmark, and the United States suggest that 20–40 percent experiment with anal sex at least once in their lives (for a review, see Root-Bernstein 1993:315–339), but data for Americans indicate that this form of sex does not occur on a regular basis and in fact is most uncommon (Laumann et al., 1994:107–109, 158).

Several lines of evidence indicate that HIV is difficult to transmit in penile-vaginal intercourse. According to one estimate (Booth, 1988), the risk of transmission is 1 in 100 million sexual episodes with a person who tests negative for HIV (a negative result could be erroneous) and has no history of high-risk behavior and 1 in 5 billion if the couple uses a condom. If the HIV status of the partner is unknown and he or she does not belong to a high-risk category, the risks are still only 1 in 5 million contacts or 1 in 50 million if a condom is used (see also Hearst and Hully, 1988). Studies of couples in which a partner was known to be infected (e.g., as a result of hemophilia) showed that, on average, sex led to infection in just 1 out of 500 episodes (Root-Bernstein, 1993:32). And if anal heterosexual intercourse were avoided, the risk of male-to-female transmission (from IDUs, bisexuals, or members of other high-risk group) would be even lower. If such intercourse were to decline substantially, secondary or tertiary transmission would also probably decline.

Nevertheless, the risks of penile-vaginal transmission appear to vary widely between individuals. One individual may not get infected even after thousands of sexual episodes with an infected person, whereas for another individual a single encounter may suffice. This does not mean that "sex remains as chancy as roulette" (Johnston and Hopkins, 1990:69). It only means that in having sex with an HIV-infected partner, a person may, in some very rare instances, contract infection after only a few episodes of penile-vaginal sex.

However, the presence of an STD increases the efficiency of HIV transmission in penile-vaginal intercourse greatly, as the experience in Africa indicates. A European study of male AIDS patients and their sexual partners found that the female partner had a significantly higher chance of being HIV infected if she had a history of STD (European Study Group, 1989). Although the CDC does not report a history of STD as a risk category, for all cases reported through June 30, 1993, 36 percent of heterosexuals for whom no risk was identified reported a history of venereal disease (CDC, 1993b: 17). It is possible, also, that some had had sex with a partner infected with an STD. It is not unreasonable to assume, therefore, that for a significant proportion of heterosexuals classified as having sex with an HIV-infected person ("risk not specified"), a sexually transmitted disease may have been a significant factor in HIV transmission.

One reason there has been no heterosexual HIV-AIDS epidemic in the United States may simply be that HIV is hard to transmit in penile-vaginal sex in the absence of another STD and that STDs are not very prevalent in the overall heterosexual population in the United States (Rolfs and Nakashima, 1990). Nevertheless, some contend that heterosexual transmission of HIV is not this difficult and that heterosexual HIV-AIDS will escalate in the 1990s (Johnston and Hopkins, 1990; Anderson and May, 1992). For example, Johnston and Hopkins (1990:69) argued that figures "suggest that the chances of one person's being infected over a five-year relationship with one infected individual are as high as two-thirds or more." This is simply at odds with the analysis of biomedical scientists and statisticians (Booth, 1988; Hearst and Hully, 1988; Root-Bernstein, 1993:312–326).

References

Aboulker, J., and A. Swart. 1993. "Preliminary Analysis of the Concorde Trials." *Lancet,* 341:889–890.

Ackerknecht, E. 1971. *Medicine and Ethnology: Selected Essays.* Edited by H. Walser and H. Koelbing. Baltimore: Johns Hopkins University Press.

_____. 1982. *A Short History of Medicine.* Rev. ed. Baltimore: Johns Hopkins University Press.

ACSF Investigators. 1992. "AIDS and Sexual Behaviour in France." *Nature,* 360: 407–409.

Adam, B. 1992. "Sex and Caring Among Men: Impacts of AIDS in Gay People." Pp. 175–183 in K. Plummer (ed.), *Modern Homosexualities: Fragments of Lesbian and Gay Experience.* London: Routledge.

Adams, S. 1947. "That Was Up-state New York: My Grandfather and the Plague." *New Yorker* (October 18):82–88.

Adib, S., J. Joseph, D. Ostrow et al. 1991. "Relapse in Sexual Behavior Among Homosexual Men: A 2-Year Follow-up from the Chicago MAC/CCC." *AIDS,* 5: 757–760.

Aguilar, S., and A. Hardy. 1993. "AIDS Knowledge and Attitudes for 1991: Data from the National Health Interview Survey." *Advance Data from Vital and Health Statistics.* No. 225. Hyattsville, Md.: National Center for Health Statistics.

Ahmed, R. 1991. "Women in Egypt and the Sudan." Pp. 107–134 in L. Adler (ed.), *Women in Cross-Cultural Perspective.* New York: Praeger.

Akers, R. 1987. *Deviant Behavior: A Social Behavior Approach.* 3d ed. Belmont, Calif.: Wadsworth.

Albert, E. 1986. "Illness and Deviance: The Response of the Press to AIDS." Pp. 163–178 in D. Feldman and T. Johnson (eds.), *The Social Dimensions of AIDS: Method and Theory.* New York: Praeger.

Alcorn, K. 1988. "Illness, Metaphor and AIDS." Pp. 65–82 in P. Aggleton and H. Homans (eds.), *Social Aspects of AIDS.* London: Falmer Press.

Allen, S., C. Lindan, and A. Serufilira. 1991. "Human Immunodeficiency Virus Infection in Urban Rwanda." *Journal of the American Medical Association,* 266: 1657–1663.

Altman, D. 1982. *The Homosexualization of America.* New York: St. Martin's Press.

_____. 1986. *AIDS in the Mind of America.* Garden City, N.Y.: Anchor/ Doubleday.

Altman, L. 1990. "2 AIDS Infections Deepen Florida Mystery." *New York Times* (September 22):8.

_____. 1993. "U.S. Survey Finds 550,000 Are Infected with H.I.V. Outside Risk Groups." *New York Times* (December 14):B-7.

_____. 1994. "AIDS Mystery That Won't Go Away: Did a Dentist Infect 6 Patients?" *New York Times* (July 5):B-6.

Amundsen, D. 1977. "Medical Deontology and Pestilential Disease in the Late Middle Ages." *Journal of the History of Medicine,* 32:403–421.

Anderson, R. 1993. "AIDS: Trends, Predictions, Controversy." *Nature,* 363:393–394.

Anderson, R., and R. May. 1992. "Understanding the AIDS Pandemic." *Scientific American,* 266:58–67.

Anderson, R., R. May, M. Boily et al. 1991. "The Spread of HIV-1 in Africa: Sexual Contact Patterns and the Predicted Demographic Impact of AIDS." *Nature,* 352:581–589.

Ansberry, C. 1987. "AIDS, Stirring Panic and Prejudice, Test Nation's Character." *Wall Street Journal* (November 13):A-1, 5.

Antonio, G. 1986. *The AIDS Cover-up: The Real and Alarming Facts About AIDS.* San Francisco: Ignatius.

Antonovsky, A. 1972. "Social Class, Life Expectancy, and Overall Mortality." Pp. 5–30 in E. Jaco (ed.), *Patients, Physicians and Illness: A Sourcebook in Behavioral Science and Health.* 2d ed. New York: Free Press.

Applebome, P. 1990. "After Dentist's AIDS Death, Florida City Is Sad But Uneasy." *New York Times* (September 8):1, 9.

Ardener, E. 1961. "Social and Demographic Problems of the Southern Cameroon's Plantation Area." Pp. 83–97 in A. Southall (ed.), *Social Change in Modern Africa.* New York: Oxford University Press.

Arluke, A., L. Kennedy, and R. Kessler. 1979. "Re-examining the Sick Role Concept: An Empirical Assessment." *Journal of Health and Social Behavior,* 20:30–36.

Arya, O., and F. Bennett. 1976. "Role of the Medical Auxiliary in the Control of Sexually Transmitted Disease in a Developing Country." *British Journal of Venereal Disease,* 52:116–121.

Ascher, M., H. Sheppard, W. Winkelstein et al. 1993. "Does Drug Use Cause AIDS?" *Nature,* 362:103–104.

Bailey, J., and R. Pillard. 1991. "A Genetic Study of Male Sexual Orientation." *Archives of General Psychiatry,* 48:1089–1096.

Bailey, N. 1957. *The Mathematical Theory of Epidemics.* New York: Hafner.

Baker, A. 1986. "The Portrayal of AIDS in the Media: An Analysis of Articles in *New York Times.*" Pp. 179–194 in D. Feldman and T. Johnson (eds.), *The Social Dimensions of AIDS: Method and Theory.* New York: Praeger.

Barnett, T., and P. Blaikie. 1992. *AIDS in Africa: Its Present and Future Impact.* New York: Guildorm Press.

Barrett, D. 1992. "Supreme Court Refuses to Hear Appeal of Benefit Cost for Workers of AIDS." *Wall Street Journal* (November 10):A-4.

Barringer, F. 1991. "The Sting of AIDS, the Scorn of Strangers." *New York Times* (September 9):l, 10.

Bartlett, J. 1993. "Zidovudine Now or Later?" *New England Journal of Medicine,* 329:351–352.

Bateson, M., and R. Goldsby. 1988. *Thinking AIDS.* New York: Addison-Wesley.

Bayer, R. 1985. "AIDS and the Gay Community: Between the Specter and the Promise of Medicine." *Social Research*, 52:581–606.

_____. 1989. *Private Acts, Social Consequences: AIDS and the Politics of Public Health*. New York: Free Press.

Beauchamp, D. 1990. "Morality and the Health of the Body Politic." Pp. 604–619 in N. McKenzie (ed.), *The Crisis in Health Care: Ethical Issues*. New York: Penguin.

Becker, G. 1984. "The Social Regulation of Sexuality: A Cross-cultural Perspective." *Current Perspectives in Social Theory*, 5:45–69.

Becker, M., and J. Joseph. 1988. "AIDS and Behavioral Change to Reduce Risk: A Review." *American Journal of Public Health*, 78:394–410.

Begley, S. 1994. "The End of Antibiotics." *Newsweek* (March 28):47–51.

Bell, A., and M. Weinberg. 1978. *Homosexualities: A Study of Diversity Among Men and Women*. New York: Simon and Schuster.

Bennett, F. 1987. "AIDS as a Social Phenomenon." *Social Science and Medicine*, 25: 329–339.

Berger, P., and T. Luckmann. 1966. *The Social Construction of Reality*. Garden City, N.Y.: Doubleday.

Berke, R. 1991. "AIDS Battle Reverting to Us Against Them." *New York Times* (October 6):IV-1, 14.

Berkeley, B. 1992. "Liberia: Between Repression and Slaughter." *Atlantic Monthly*, 270 (December):52–64.

_____. 1993. "Zaire: An African Horror Story." *Atlantic Monthly*, 272 (August): 20–28.

_____. 1994. "The Warlords of Natal." *Atlantic Monthly*, 273 (March):85–100.

Berkman, L. 1985. "The Relationship of Social Networks and Social Support to Morbidity and Mortality." Pp. 241–262 in S. Cohen and L. Syman (eds.), *Social Support and Health*. Orlando, Fla.: Academic Press.

Better, S., P. Fine, D. Simison et al. 1979. "Disability Benefits as Disincentive to Rehabilitation." Milbank Memorial Fund Quarterly/*Health and Society*, 57:412–427.

Billy, J., K. Tanfer, W. Grady et al. 1993. "The Sexual Behavior of Men in the United States." *Family Planning Perspectives*, 25:52–60.

Black, D. 1986. *The Plague Years*. New York: Simon and Schuster.

Black, F. 1975. "Infectious Diseases in Primitive Societies." *Science*, 187:515–518.

Bledsoe, C. 1990. "Transformation in Sub-Saharan African Marriage and Fertility." *Annals of the American Academy of Political and Social Science*, 510:115–125.

Blumstein, P., and P. Schwartz. 1983. *American Couples: Money, Work, and Sex*. New York: William Morrow.

Boccaccio, G. 1971. "Plague in Florence: A Literary Description." Pp. 7–12 in W. Bowsky (ed.), *The Black Death: A Turning Point in History?* New York: Holt, Rinehart and Winston, 1971.

Booth, W. 1988. "Heterosexual AIDS: Setting the Odds." *Science*, 240:597.

Bowen, O. 1988. "Widespread Heterosexual Epidemic Not Foreseen by Secretary of HHS." *Aids Policy and Law* (January 270:1.

Brandt, A. 1987. *No Magic Bullet: A Social History of Venereal Disease in the United States Since 1880*. Exp. ed. New York: Oxford University Press.

_____. 1988a. "AIDS and Metaphor: Toward the Social Meaning of Epidemic Disease." *Social Research,* 44:412–432.

_____. 1988b. "AIDS in Historical Perspective: Four Lessons from the History of Sexually Transmitted Diseases." *American Journal of Public Health* 78:367–371.

_____. 1988c. "AIDS: From Social History to Social Policy." Pp. 147–171 in E. Fee and D. Fox (eds.), *AIDS: The Burdens of History.* Berkeley and Los Angeles: University of California Press.

Braudel, F. 1981. *Civilization and Capitalism, 15th–18th Century.* Vol. 1: *The Structure of Everyday Life: The Limits of the Possible.* London: Collins.

Bregman, D., and A. Langmuir. 1990. "Projecting the Incidence of AIDS." *Journal of the American Medical Association,* 263:1522–1525.

Breo, D. 1993. "The Dental AIDS Cases—Murder or an Unsolvable Mystery." *Journal of the American Medical Association,* 270:2732–2734.

Briggs, A. 1961. "Cholera and Society in the Nineteenth Century." *Past and Present,* 19:76–96.

Brookmeyer, R. 1991. "Reconstruction and Future Trends of the AIDS Epidemic in the United States." *Science,* 253:37–42.

Brunham, R., and A. Ronald. 1991. "Epidemiology of Sexually Transmitted Diseases in Developing Countries." Pp. 61–80 in J. Wasserheit, S. Aral, K. Holmes et al. (eds.), *Research Issues in Human Behavior and Sexually Transmitted Diseases in the AIDS Era.* Washington, D.C.: American Society for Microbiology.

Buchanan, P. 1983. "AIDS Disease: It's Nature Fighting Back." *New York Post* (May 24):31.

_____. 1991. "A Gay St. Paul? So Says This Bishop." *Tennessean* (February 6):A9.

Buckley, W. 1986. "Identify All the Carriers." *New York Times* (March 18):A-27.

Bucyendore, A., P. Van de Perre, E. Karita et al. 1993. "Estimating the Seroincidence of HIV-1 in the General Adult Population in Kigali, Rwanda." *AIDS,* 7:275–277.

Bullough, V., and B. Bullough. 1987. *Women and Prostitution: A Social History.* Buffalo, N.Y.: Prometheus Books.

Burgess, E. 1949. "The Sociologic Theory of Psychosexual Behavior." Pp. 222–241 in P. Hoch and J. Zubin (eds.), *Psychological Development in Health and Disease.* New York: Grove and Stratton.

Burnet, M., and D. White. 1972. *Natural History of Infectious Diseases.* 4th ed. Cambridge: Cambridge University Press.

Byne, W. 1994. "The Biological Evidence Challenged." *Scientific American,* 270:50–55.

Caldwell, J., P. Caldwell, and P. Quiggin. 1989. "The Social Context of AIDS in Sub-Saharan Africa." *Population and Development Review,* 15:185–234.

Califano, J. Jr. 1986. *America's Health Care Revolution: Who Lives? Who Dies? Who Cares?* New York: Random House.

Carlson, R. 1975. *The End of Medicine.* New York: John Wiley and Sons.

Cartwright, F. 1972. *Disease and History.* New York: Thomas Y. Crowell.

Cary, L. 1992. "Why It's Not Just Paranoia." *Newsweek* (April 6):23.

Cassidy, C. 1980. "Nutrition and Health in Agriculturalists and Hunter-Gatherers." Pp. 117–145 in N. Jerome, R. Kandel, and G. Pelton (eds.), *Nutritional Anthro-*

pology: Contemporary Approaches to Diet and Culture. Pleasantville, N.Y.: Regrave.

Catania, J., T. Coates, S. Kegeles et al., 1992. "Condom-Use in Multi-ethnic Neighborhoods in San Francisco." *American Journal of Public Health,* 82:284–287.

Catania, J., T. Coates, R. Stall et al., 1992. "Prevalence of AIDS-Related Risk Factors and Condom Use in the United States." *Science,* 258:1101–1106.

Centers for Disease Control (CDC). 1985. *Morbidity and Mortality Weekly Report,* 34 (October 11):613–614. Atlanta: U.S. Public Health Service.

_____. 1990a. *Morbidity and Mortality Weekly Report,* 39 (February 9):81–86. Atlanta: U.S. Public Health Service.

_____. 1990b. *Morbidity and Mortality Weekly Report,* 39 (February 23):110–119. Atlanta: U.S. Public Health Service.

_____. 1990c. *Morbidity and Mortality Weekly Report,* 39 (April 27):273–276. Atlanta: U.S. Public Health Service.

_____. 1991a. *HIV/AIDS Surveillance Report: Year-End Edition* (January). Atlanta: U.S. Public Health Service.

_____. 1991b. *Morbidity and Mortality Weekly Report,* 40 (June 7):357–369. Atlanta: U.S. Public Health Service.

_____. 1991c. *Morbidity and Mortality Weekly Report,* 40 (November 22):792–794. Atlanta: U.S. Public Health Service.

_____. 1991d. *Morbidity and Mortality Weekly Report,* 40 (December 13):855–860. Atlanta: U.S. Public Health Service.

_____. 1992. *HIV/AIDS Surveillance Report: Year-End Edition* (January). Atlanta: U.S. Public Health Service.

_____.1993a. *HIV/AIDS Surveillance Report: Year-End Edition* (February). Atlanta: U.S. Public Health Service.

_____. 1993b. *HIV/AIDS Surveillance Report: Second Quarter Edition* (July). Atlanta: U.S. Public Health Service.

_____. 1993c. *HIV/AIDS Surveillance Report: Third Quarter Edition* (October). Atlanta: U.S. Public Health Service.

_____. 1993d. "Update: Mortality Attributable to HIV Infection Among Persons Aged 25–44 Years—United States, 1991 and 1992." *Morbidity and Mortality Weekly Report,* 45 (November 19): 869–872.

_____. 1993e. "HIV Transmission Between Two Adolescent Brothers with Hemophilia." *Morbidity and Mortality Weekly Report,* 42 (December 17):948–951. Atlanta: U.S. Public Health Service.

_____. 1994a. *HIV/AIDS Surveillance Report: Year-End Edition.* Atlanta: U.S. Public Health Service.

_____. 1994b. *HIV/AIDS Surveillance Report: Mid-Year Edition.* Atlanta: U.S. Public Health Service.

Chandra, R. 1983. "Nutrition Immunity and Infection: Present Knowledge and Future Directions." *Lancet*:688–691.

Chase, M. 1988. "Corporations Urge Peers to Adopt Humane Policies for AIDS Victims." *Wall Street Journal* (January):31.

Check, W. 1987. "Beyond the Political Model of Reporting: Nonspecific Symptoms in Media Communication About AIDS." *Reviews of Infectious Diseases,* 9:987–1000.

Chirimuuta, R., and R. Chirimuuta. 1987. *AIDS, Africa, and Racism*. Derbyshire, England: Richard Chirimuuta.

Clark, M., M. Coswell, D. Witherspoon et al. 1985. "AIDS." *Newsweek* (August 12):20–27.

Clumeck, N., P. Van de Perre, M. Carael et al. 1985. "Heterosexual Promiscuity Among African Patients with AIDS." *New England Journal of Medicine*, 313:182.

Cockburn, T. 1961. "Eradication of Infectious Disease." *Science*, 133:1050–1058.

———. 1977. "Infectious Disease in Ancient Populations." Pp. 83–95 in D. Landy (ed.), *Culture, Disease, and Healing: Studies in Medical Anthropology*. New York: Macmillan.

Cockcroft, L. 1990. *Africa's Way: A Journey from the Past*. London: I. B. Tauris.

Cockerham, W. 1986. *Medical Sociology*. 3d ed. Englewood Cliffs, N.J.: Prentice-Hall.

Cogswell, B., and D. Weir. 1964. "A Role in Process: The Development of Medical Professions' Role in Long-Term Care of Chronically Diseased Patients." *Journal of Health and Social Behavior*, 5:95–103.

Colebunders, R., H. Taelman, and P. Piot. 1984. "AIDS: An Old Disease from Africa?" *British Medical Journal*, 289:765.

Collins, R., and M. Makowsky. 1989. *The Discovery of Society*. 4th ed. New York: Random House.

Conrad, L. 1992. "Epidemic Disease in Formal and Popular Thought in Early Islamic Society." Pp. 77–99 in T. Ranger and P. Slack (eds.), *Epidemics and Ideas: Essays on the Historical Perception of Pestilence*. Cambridge: Cambridge University Press.

Conrad, P. 1986. "The Social Meaning of AIDS." *Social Policy*, 16:51–56.

———. 1987. "The Experience of Illness: Recent and New Directions." *Research in the Sociology of Health Care*, 6:1–31.

Conrad, P., and J. Schneider. 1980. *Deviance and Medicalization: From Badness to Sickness*. St. Louis: C. V. Mosby.

Cook, K. (ed.). 1987. *Social Exchange Theory*. Newbury Park, Calif.: Sage.

Cooper, D., J. Gatell, S. Kroon et al. 1993. "Zidovudine in Persons with Asymptomatic HIV Infection and CD4+ Cell Counts Greater Than 400 per Cubic Millimeter." *New England Journal of Medicine*, 329:298–303.

Cooper, M., and G. Ferguson. 1990. "The Return of the Paranoid Style in American Politics." *U.S. News and World Report* (March 12):30–31.

Corey, J. 1987. "And Now, a Worldwide War Against AIDS." *U.S. News and World Report* (April 6):13.

Corey, J., B. Quick, and R. Riley. 1987. "AIDS: A Time of Testing." *U.S. News and World Report* (April 20):56–58.

Cornell, J. 1982. *The Great International Disaster Book*. 3d ed. New York: Charles Scribner's Sons.

Courtwright, D. 1980. "Public Health and Public Wealth: Social Costs as a Basis for Restrictive Policies. Milbank Memorial Fund Quarterly/*Health and Society*, 58: 268–282.

Coxon, T. 1988. "The Numbers Game—Gay Lifestyles, Epidemiology of AIDS and Social Science." Pp. 126–138 in P. Aggleton and H. Homans (eds.), *Social Aspects of AIDS*. London: Falmer Press.

Crawford, R. 1977. "You Are Dangerous to Your Health: The Ideology and Politics of Victim Blaming." *International Journal of Health Services,* 8:663–681.

Crosby, A. 1989. *America's Forgotten Pandemic: The Influenza of 1918.* New York: Cambridge University Press.

Culliton, B. 1992. "The Mysterious Virus Called 'Isn't.'" *Nature,* 358:619.

Curran, J., H. Jaffe, A. Hardy et al. 1988. "Epidemiology of HIV Infection and AIDS in the United States." *Science,* 239:610–616.

Curran, J., W. Morgan, A. Hardy et al., 1985. "The Epidemiology of AIDS: Current Status and Future Prospects." *Science,* 229:1352–1357.

Cutrufelli, M. 1983. *Women of Africa: Roots of Oppression.* Translated by N. Romano. London: Zed Press.

Dallabetta, G., P. Miotti, J. Chiphangwi et al. 1993. "High Socioeconomic Status Is a Risk Factor for Human Immunodeficiency Virus Type I (HIV-1) Infection But Not for Sexually Transmitted Disease in Women in Malawi: Implications for HIV-1 Control." *Journal of Infectious Diseases,* 167:36–42.

Dank, B. 1971. "Coming Out in the Gay World." *Psychiatry,* 34:180–197.

Darrow, W. 1991. "AIDS: Socioepidemiologic Response to an Epidemic." Pp. 82–99 in R. Ulack and W. Skinner (eds.), *AIDS and the Social Sciences: Common Threads.* Lexington: University of Kentucky Press.

Darrow, W., E. Gorman, and B. Glick. 1986. "The Social Origins of AIDS: Social Change, Sexual Behavior, and Disease Trends." Pp. 95–107 in D. Feldman and T. Johnson (eds), *The Social Dimensions of AIDS: Method and Theory.* New York: Praeger .

Davenport, D. 1977. "Sex in Cross-cultural Perspective." Pp. 115–163 in F. Beach (ed.), *Human Sexuality in Four Perspectives.* Baltimore: Johns Hopkins University Press.

Davidson. B. 1955. *The African Awakening.* London: Jonathan Cape.

———. 1985. "AIDS Germs Warfare, Need Media Probe, Gregory Says." *San Antonio Express-News* (October 9):A-10.

Davison, J. 1988a. "Land and Women's Agricultural Production: The Contest." Pp. 1–32 in J. Davison (ed.), *Agriculture, Women and the Land: The African Experience.* Boulder: Westview Press.

———. 1988b. "Who Owns What? Land Registration and Tensions in Gender Relations of Production in Kenya." Pp. 157–201 in J. Davison (ed.), *Agriculture, Women and the Land: The African Experience.* Boulder: Westview Press.

———. (ed.). 1988. *Agriculture, Women and the Land: The African Experience.* Boulder: Westview Press.

Dawson, N., M. Cynamon, and J. Fitti. 1987. "AIDS Knowledge and Attitudes: Provisional Data from the National Health Interview Survey—United States." *Advance Data from Vital and Health Statistics.* No. 146. Hyattsville, Md.: National Center for Health Statistics.

Day, L. 1991. *AIDS: What the Government Isn't Telling You.* Palm Desert, Calif.: Rockform Press.

D'Costa, L., F. Plummer, I. Bowmer et al., 1985. "Prostitutes Are a Major Reservoir of Sexually Transmitted Diseases in Nairobi, Kenya." *Sexually Transmitted Diseases,* 12:64–67.

De Cock, K. 1984. "AIDS: An Old Disease from Africa?" *British Medical Journal,* 298:306–308.

De Venette, J. 1971. "The Chronicle of a French Cleric." Pp. 15–18 in W. Bowsky (ed.), *The Black Death: A Turning Point in History?* New York: Holt, Rinehart and Winston.

De Wit, J., G. Friensvenm, G. Kok et al. 1993. "Why Do Homosexual Men Relapse into Unsafe Sex? Predictors of Resumption of Unprotected Anogenital Intercourse with Casual Partners." *AIDS,* 7:1113–1118.

DeBuono, B., S. Zinner, M. Daamen et al. 1990. "Sexual Behavior of College Women in 1975, 1986, and 1989." *New England Journal of Medicine,* 322:821–825.

Del Grasso, A. 1971. "Plague in Siena: An Italian Chronicle." Pp. 13–14 in W. Bowsky (ed.), *The Black Death: A Turning Point in History?* New York: Holt, Rinehart and Winston.

DeLancey, M. 1978. "Health and Disease on the Plantations of Cameroon, 1884–1939." Pp. 153–179 in G. Hartwig and K. Patterson (eds.), *Disease in African History: An Introductory Survey and Case Studies.* Durham, N.C.: Duke University Press.

Delaporte, F. 1986. *Disease and Civilization: The Cholera in Paris, 1832.* Cambridge, Mass.: MIT Press.

D'Emilio, J. 1992. "Gay Politics, Gay Community: San Francisco's Experience." Pp. 85–113 in W. Dynes and S. Donaldson (eds.), *History of Homosexuality in Europe and America.* New York: Garland.

Denzin, N., and S. Spitzer. 1966. "Paths to the Mental Hospital and Staff Predictions of Patient Role Behavior." *Journal of Health and Social Behavior,* 7:265–271.

Dershowitz, A. 1986. "Emphasize Scientific Information." *New York Times* (Late edition) (March 18):A-27.

Des Jarlais, D., S. Friedman, and D. Strug. 1986. "AIDS and Needle Sharing Within the Intravenous Drug Use Subculture." Pp. 111–125 in D. Feldman and T. Johnson (eds.), *The Social Dimensions of AIDS: Method and Theory.* New York: Praeger.

Des Jarlais, D., S. Friedman, D. Novick et al. 1989. "HIV-1 Infection Among Intravenous Drug Users in Manhattan, New York City, from 1977 Through 1987." *Journal of the American Medical Association,* 261:1008–1012.

Des Jarlais, D., and S. Friedman. 1994. "AIDS and the Use of Injected Drugs." *Scientific American,* 270:82–88.

Dirasse, L. 1991. *The Commoditization of Female Sexuality: Prostitution and Socio-Economic Relations in Addis Ababa, Ethiopia.* New York: AMS Press.

Dolcini, M., J. Catania, T. Coates et al. 1993. "Demographic Characteristics of Heterosexuals with Multiple Partners: The National AIDS Behavioral Surveys." *Family Planning Perspectives,* 25:208–214.

Dols, M. 1977. *The Black Death in the Middle East.* Princeton: Princeton University Press.

Douglas, C., C. Kalman, and T. Kalman. 1985. "Homophobia Among Physicians and Nurses: An Empirical Study. *Hospital and Community Psychiatry,* 36:1309–1311.

Douglas, G. 1976. *Health, Sickness and Society.* St. Lucia, Queen Island: University of Queensland.

Dover, K. 1978. *Greek Homosexuality.* Cambridge, Mass.: Harvard University Press.

Dowling, H. 1977. *Fighting Infection: Conquests of the Twentieth Century.* Cambridge, Mass.: Harvard University Press.

Du Bois, V. 1967. *Prostitution in the Ivory Coast: A Social Problem and Its Treatment.* Vol. 10, no. 2 of West African Series. New York: American Universities Field Staff.

Dubos, R. 1959. *Mirage of Health: Utopia, Progress, and Biological Change.* New York: Harper and Row.

_____. 1965. *Man Adapting.* New Haven: Yale University Press.

_____. 1968. *Man, Medicine, and Environment.* London: Pall Mall Press.

Dubos, R., and J. Dubos. 1987. *The White Plague: Tuberculosis, Man, and Society.* New Brunswick: Rutgers University Press.

Duesberg, P. 1988. "HIV Is Not the Cause of AIDS." *Science,* 241:514, 517.

_____. 1990. "AIDS: Noninfectious Deficiencies Acquired by Drug Consumption and Other Risk Factors." *Research in Immunology,* 141:5–11.

_____. 1992. "The Role of Drugs in the Origin of AIDS." *Biomedical Pharmacotherapy,* 46:3–15.

Duh, S. 1991. *Blacks and AIDS.* Newbury Park, Calif.: Sage.

Dumond, D. 1977. "The Limitation of Human Population: A Natural History." Pp. 299–310 in D. Landy (ed.), *Culture, Disease, and Healing: Studies in Medical Anthropology.* New York: Macmillan.

Durey, M. 1979. *The Return of the Plague: British Society and Cholera, 1831–32.* Dublin: Gill and Macmillan.

Durkheim, E. 1949. *Suicide.* Translated by J. C. Spaulding and G. Simppson. Glencoe: Free Press.

Dynes, W., and S. Donaldson. 1992. "Introduction." Pp. vii–xix in W. Dynes and S. Donaldson (eds.), *History of Homosexuality in Europe and America.* New York: Garland.

Eckholm, E. 1990a. "What Makes the 2 Sexes So Vulnerable to Epidemic." *New York Times* (September 16): A1–11.

_____. 1990b. "Confronting the Cruel Reality of Africa's AIDS Epidemic." *New York Times* (September 20):A-1, 10.

_____. 1990c. "Cut Down as They Grow Up: AIDS Stalks Gay Teenagers." *New York Times* (December 13):A-1, 14.

Eckholm, E., and J. Tierney. 1990. "AIDS in Africa: A Killer Rages On." *New York Times* (September 16):I-1, 10.

Ellerbrock, T., S. Lieb, P. Harrington et al. 1992. "Heterosexually Transmitted Human Immunodeficiency Virus Infection Among Pregnant Women in a Rural Florida Community." *New England Journal of Medicine* 327:1704–1709.

Elliott, S. 1994. "A Sharper View of Gay Consumers." *New York Times* (June 9): C-1, 17.

Epstein, P. 1991. "Condoms in School: The Right Lesson." *New York Times* (January 19):19.

Essex, M., and P. Kanki. 1988. "The Origins of the AIDS Virus." *Scientific American,* 259:64–71.

European Study Group. 1989. "Risk Factors for Male to Female Transmission of HIV." *British Medical Journal,* 298:411–415.

Evans, R. 1987. *Politics of a Plague: Society and Politics in the Cholera Years, 1830–1910.* London: Oxford University Press.

———. 1992. "Epidemics and Revolutions: Cholera in Nineteenth-Century Europe." Pp. 149–173 in T. Ranger and P. Slack (eds.), *Epidemics and Ideas: Essays on the Historical Perception of Pestilence.* Cambridge: Cambridge University Press.

Eversley, D. 1965. "Population, Economy and Society." Pp. 23–69 in D. Glass and D. Eversley (eds.), *Population in History: Essays in Historical Demography.* Chicago: Aldine.

Ewald, P. 1994. *Evolution of Infectious Disease.* New York: Oxford University Press.

Fauci, A. 1983. "The Acquired Immune Deficiency Syndrome." *Journal of the American Medical Association,* 249:2375-2376.

Fay, R., C. Turner, A. Klassen et al. 1989. "Prevalence and Patterns of Same Gender Sexual Contact Among Men." *Science,* 243:338–348.

Fettner, A., and W. Check. 1984. *The Truth About AIDS: Evaluation of an Epidemic.* New York: Holt, Rinehart and Winston.

Fields, B. 1994. "AIDS: Time to Turn to Basic Science." *Nature,* 369:95–96.

Fineberg, H. 1986. "A Way to Tackle AIDS Education." *New York Times* (Late edition) (July 13):IV-29.

———. 1988. "Education to Prevent AIDS: Prospects and Obstacles." *Science,* 239:592–595.

Fisher, J. 1994. *The Plague Makers: How We Are Creating Catastrophic Epidemics—and What We Must Do to Avert Them.* New York: Simon and Schuster.

Fletcher, J. 1984. "Homosexuality: Kick and Kickback." *Southern Medical Journal* (February):149–150.

Flinn, W. 1965. "Introduction." Pp. 1–73 in E. Chadwick, "Report on the Sanitary Condition of Labouring Population of Great Britain [1842]." Edinburgh: Edinburgh University Press.

Fortes, M. 1978. "Family, Marriage and Fertility in West Africa." Pp. 17–54 in C. Oppong, G. Ababa, M. Bekombo et al., *Marriage, Fertility, and Parenthood in West Africa.* Canberra: National University Press.

Fox, D. 1986. "AIDS and the American Health Polity: The History and Prospects of a Crisis of Authority." Milbank Memorial Fund Quarterly/*Health and Society,* 64:7–33.

Freeman, H., and S. Levine (eds.). 1989. *Handbook of Medical Sociology.* 4th ed. Englewood Cliffs, N.J.: Prentice-Hall.

Freidson, E. 1970. *Profession of Medicine: A Study in the Sociology of Applied Knowledge.* New York: Harper and Row.

Frieden, T., T. Sterling, A. Pablos-Mendez et al. 1993. "The Emergence of Drug-Resistant Tuberculosis in New York City." *New England Journal of Medicine.* 328:521–526.

Friedland, G., and R. Klein. 1987. "Transmission of the Human Immunodeficiency Virus." *New England Journal of Medicine,* 317:1125–1135.

Friedland, G., B. Saltzman, M. Rogers et al. 1986. "Lack of Transmission of HTLV-III/LAV Infection to Household Contacts of Patients with AIDS or AIDS-Related Complex with Oral Candidiasis." *New England Journal of Medicine,* 314:344–349.

Friedman, S., D. Des Jarlais, and C. Sterk. 1990. "AIDS and the Social Relations of Intravenous Drug Users." Milbank Memorial Fund Quarterly/*Health and Society,* 68:85–109.

Fujikawa, L., A. Palestine, R. Nussenblatt et al. 1985. "Isolation of Human T-Lymphotropic Virus Type III from the Tears of a Patient with the Acquired Immunodeficiency Syndrome." *Lancet*:529–530.

Fukasawa, M., T. Miura, A. Hasegawa et al. 1988. "Sequence of Simian Immunodeficiency Virus from African Green Monkey, a New Member of the HIV/SIV Group." *Nature,* 233:457–461.

Fullilove, R., M. Thompson, B. Bowser et al. 1990. "Risk of Sexually Transmitted Disease Among Black Adolescent Crack Users in Oakland and San Francisco, Calif." *Journal of the American Medical Association,* 263:851–855.

Fumento, M. 1990. *The Myth of Heterosexual AIDS.* New York: Basic Books.

Furnas, J. 1969. *The Americans: A Social History of the United States, 1587–1914.* New York: G. P. Putnam's.

Gail, M., and R. Brookmeyer. 1990. "Projecting the Incidence of AIDS." *Journal of the American Medical Association,* 263:1538–1539.

Gallo, R. 1987. "The First Human Retrovirus." *Scientific American,* 257:88–98.

———. 1988. "The AIDS Virus." *Scientific American,* 258:47–56.

Gallo, R., and L. Montagnier. 1988. "The AIDS Epidemic." Pp. 1–12 in J. Piel (ed.), *The Science of AIDS: Readings from Scientific American.* New York: W. H. Freeman.

Garrett, L. 1992. "The Next Epidemic." Pp. 825–839 in J. Mann, D. Tarantola, and T. Netter (eds.), *AIDS in the World.* Cambridge, Mass.: Harvard University Press.

Garrison, F. 1929. *An Introduction to the History of Medicine.* Philadelphia: W. B. Saunders.

Garry, R., M. Witte, A. Gottlieb et al. 1988. "Documentation of an AIDS Virus Infection in the United States in 1968." *Journal of the American Medical Association,* 260:2085–2087.

Gerbert, B., B. Maguire, T. Bleecker et al. 1991. "Primary Care Physicians and AIDS: Attitudinal Structural Barriers to Care." *Journal of the American Medical Association,* 266:2837–2842.

Getchell, J., D. Hicks, A. Svinivasan et al. 1987. "Human Immunodeficiency Virus Isolated from a Serum Sample Collected in 1976 in Central Africa." *Journal of Infectious Diseases,* 156:833–836.

Gibbs, P. 1989. *Social Control: Sociology's Central Notion.* Urbana: University of Illinois Press.

Gilks, C. 1991. "AIDS, Monkeys and Malaria." *Nature,* 354:262.

Glasscote, R., J. Sussex, J. Jaffe et al. 1974. *The Treatment of Drug Abuse: Programs, Problems, Prospects.* Washington, D.C.: American Psychiatric Association.

Gluckman, J. 1993. "AIDS Virus History." *Science,* 259:1809.

Goldsmith, M. 1985. "Many Groups Offer AIDS Information, Support." *Journal of the American Medical Association,* 254:2522–2523.

Goodwin, J. 1989. *More Man Than You'll Ever Be: Gay Folklore and Acculturation in Middle Class America.* Bloomington: Indiana University Press.

Gorman, C. 1993. "Are Some People Immune to AIDS?" *Time* (March 22):49–51.

Gould, S. 1987. "The Exponential Spread of AIDS Underscores the Tragedy of Our Delay in Fighting One of Nature's Plagues." *New York Times Sunday Magazine* (April 19):33.

Greenberg, D. 1988. *The Construction of Modern Homosexuality.* Chicago: University of Chicago Press.

Gregersen, E. 1983. *Sexual Practices: The Story of Human Sexuality.* New York: Franklin Watts.

Grinstead, O., B. Faigeles, D. Binson et al. 1993. "I. Sexual Risk for Human Immunodeficiency Virus Infection Among Women in High-Risk Cities." *Family Planning Perspectives,* 25:252–256, 277.

Grmek, M. 1989. *History of AIDS: Emergence and Origin of a Modern Pandemic.* Translated by R. C. Maulitz and J. Duffin. Princeton: Princeton University Press.

Gross, J. 1993. "Second Wave of AIDS Feared by Officials in San Francisco." *New York Times* (Late edition) (December 11):1, 8.

Gugler, J., and W. Flanagan. 1978. *Urbanization and Social Change in West Africa.* Cambridge: Cambridge University Press.

Guyer, J. 1984. "Women in the Rural Economy: Contemporary Variations." Pp. 19–32 in M. Hay and S. Stichter (eds.), *African Women South of the Sahara.* London: Longman.

Haggard, H. 1929. *Devils, Drugs, and Doctors: The Story of the Science of Healing from Medicine-Man to Doctor.* New York: Blue Ribbon Books.

Hahn, R., L. Magder, S. Aral et al. 1989. "Race and the Prevalence of Syphilis Seroactivity in the U.S. Population." *American Journal of Public Health,* 79:467–470.

Hallowell, A. 1941. "The Social Function of Anxiety in a Primitive Society." *American Sociological Review,* 7:869–881.

Hamer, D., S. Victoria, H. Nan et al. 1993. "A Linkage Between DNA Markers on the X Chromosome and Male Sexual Orientation." *Science,* 261:321–327.

Hancock, G., and E. Carim. 1986. *AIDS: The Deadly Epidemic.* London: Victor Gollancz.

Hanna, W., and J. Hanna. 1981. *Urban Dynamics in Black Africa: An Interdisciplinary Approach.* 2d rev. ed. New York: Aldine.

Hanson, B., G. Beschner, J. Walters et al. 1985. *Life with Heroin: Voices from the Inner City.* Lexington, Mass.: Lexington Books.

Hardy, A. 1990. "National Health Interview Survey Data on Adult Knowledge of AIDS in the United States." *Public Health Reports,* 105:629–634.

Harris, J. 1990. "The AIDS Epidemic: Recent Trends and Future Prospects." Pp. 22–27 in V. Fransen (ed.), *Proceedings: AIDS Prevention and Services Workshop.* Princeton: Robert Wood Johnson Foundation.

Harry, J., and W. DeVall. 1978. *The Social Organization of Gay Males*. New York: Praeger.

Hartwig, G. 1978. "Social Consequences of Epidemic Diseases: The Nineteenth Century in Eastern Africa." Pp. 25–45 in G. Hartwig and K. Patterson (eds.), *Disease in African Society: An Introductory Survey and Case Studies*. Durham, N.C.: Duke University Press.

Hay, J. 1989. "Is Too Much Being Spent on AIDS? *Wall Street Journal* (October 3): A17.

Hayward, P., and M. Shapiro. 1991. "A National Study of AIDS and Residency Training: Experiences, Concerns, and Consequences." *Annals of Internal Medicine*, 114:23–32.

Hearst, N., and S. Hulley. 1988. "Preventing the Heterosexual Spread of AIDS: Are We Giving Our Patients the Best Advice?" *Journal of the American Medical Association*, 259:2428–2432.

Heath, A. 1976. *Rational Choice and Social Exchange*. Cambridge: Cambridge University Press.

Henig, R. 1983. "AIDS: A New Disease's Deadly Odyssey." *New York Times Sunday Magazine* (February 6):28–35.

_____. 1992. "Flu Pandemic." *New York Times Sunday Magazine* (November 29): 28–31, 55, 64–65.

Henn, J. 1984. "Women in the Rural Economy: Past, Present, and Future." Pp. 1–18 in M. Hay and S. Stichter (eds.), *African Women South of the Sahara*. London: Longman.

Hevesi, D. 1988. "AIDS Carriers Win a Court Ruling." *New York Times* (July 9):8.

Hilts, P. 1991. "Experts Oppose AIDS Tests for Doctors." *New York Times* (September 20):A-ll.

_____. 1992. "Doctor Accused Anew in AIDS Studies." *New York Times* (June 25): A-18.

_____. 1993. "Misconduct Charges Dropped Against AIDS Scientist." *New York Times* (November 13):1, 9.

Ho, D., A. Neumann, A. Perelson, et al. 1994. "Rapid Turnover of Plasma Virions and CD4 Lymphocytes in HIV-1 Infection." *Nature*, 373:123–126.

Hochswender, W. 1990. "High Fashion at Low Prices in an AIDS Benefit." *New York Times* (November 30):B-7.

Hollander, C. 1993. "Publicity About Magic Johnson May Have Led Some to Reduce Their Risky Behavior, Require HIV Testing." *Family Planning Perspectives*, 25:192–193.

Holleran, A. 1978. *Dancer from the Dance*. New York: New American Library.

_____. 1988. *Ground Zero*. New York: William Morrow.

Homans, G. 1961. *Social Behavior: Its Elementary Forms*. 2d ed. New York: Harcourt Brace Jovanovich.

House, J., K. Landis, and D. Umberson. 1988. "Social Relationships and Health." *Science*, 241:540–545.

Hrdy, D. 1987. "Cultural Practices Contributing to the Transmission of Human Immunodeficiency Virus in Africa." *Reviews of Infectious Diseases*, 9:1109–1119.

Huber, J., and B. Schneider. 1992. *The Social Context of AIDS.* Newbury Park, Calif.: Sage.

Humphreys, L. 1970. *Tearoom Trade: Impersonal Sex in Public Places.* Chicago: Aldine.

Hunt, C. 1989. "Migrant Labor and Sexually Transmitted Disease: AIDS in Africa." *Journal of Health and Social Behavior,* 30:353–373.

Iliffe, J. 1987. *The African Poor: A History.* Cambridge: Cambridge University Press.

Illich, I. 1976. *Medical Nemesis: The Expropriation of Health.* New York: Random House.

Inciardi, J. 1992. *The War on Drugs II: The Continuing Epic of Heroin, Cocaine, Crack, Crimes, AIDS, and Public Policy.* Mountain View, Calif.: Mayfield.

Ingrassia, M. 1994. "Virgin Cool." *Newsweek* (October 17):58–62, 64, 69.

Institute of Medicine. 1986. *Confronting AIDS.* Washington, D.C.: National Academy Press.

———. 1988. *Confronting AIDS: Update.* Washington, D.C.: National Academy Press.

Ippolito, M. 1993. "Tuskegee Study Cited in AIDS Plot Fear." *Tennessean* (February 6):B-1, 2.

Jacobson, J. 1993. "Closing the Gender Gap in Development." Pp. 61–79 in L. Brown (ed.), *State of the World—1993.* New York: W. W. Norton.

Jaffe, H., C. Keewhan, P. Thomas et al. 1983. "National Case-Control Study of Kaposi's Sarcoma and *Pneumocystis carinii* Pneumonia in Homosexual Men: Part 1, Epidemiologic Results." *Annals of Internal Medicine,* 99:145–151.

Johnson, A., J. Wadsworth, K. Wellings et al. 1992. "Sexual Lifestyles and HIV Risk." *Nature,* 360:410–412.

Johnston, W., and K. Hopkins. 1990. *The Catastrophe Ahead: AIDS and the Case for a New Public Policy.* New York: Praeger.

Jonsen, A., and J. Stryker (eds.). 1993. *The Social Impact of AIDS in the United States.* Washington, D.C.: National Academy Press.

Joseph, C. 1988. "Current and Future Trends in AIDS in New York City." *Advances in Alcohol and Substance Abuse,* 7:159–174.

Kagay, M. 1991. "Fear of AIDS Has Altered Behavior, Poll Shows." *New York Times* (June 18):B-5, 8.

Katner, H., and G. Pankey. 1987. "Evidence for a Euro-American Origin of HIV." *Journal of the National Medical Association,* 79:1069–1072.

Kegeles, S., N. Adler, and C. Irwin. 1988. "Sexually Active Adolescents and Condoms: Changes over One Year in Knowledge, Attitudes and Use." *American Journal of Public Health,* 78:460–461.

Kelly, J., J. St. Lawrence, S. Smith Jr. et al., 1987. "Stigmatization of AIDS Patients by Physicians." *American Journal of Public Health,* 77:789–791.

Kestler, H., L. Yen, Y. Naidu et al. 1988. "Comparison of Simian Immunodeficiency Virus Isolates." *Nature,* 331:619–622.

Khare, R. 1977. "Ritual Purity and Pollution in Relation to Domestic Sanitation." Pp. 242–250 in D. Landy (ed.), *Culture, Disease, and Healing: Studies in Medical Anthropology.* New York: Macmillan.

Kim, M., M. Marmor, N. Dubin et al. 1993. "HIV Risk-Related Sexual Behaviors Among Heterosexuals in New York City: Associations with Race, Sex, and Intravenous Drug Use." *AIDS,* 7:409–474.

Kinsella, J. 1989. *Covering the Plague: AIDS and the American Media.* New Brunswick: Rutgers University Press.

Kinsey, A., W. Pomeroy, and C. Martin. 1948. *Sexual Behavior in the Human Male.* Philadelphia: W. B. Saunders.

Kirk, M., and H. Madsen. 1989. *After the Ball: How America Will Conquer Its Fear and Hatred of Gays in the 90's.* New York: Doubleday.

Kleiman, M. 1987. "Prostitution Isn't Victimless with AIDS Here." *Wall Street Journal* (June 1):22.

Kleinberg, S. 1980. *Alienated Affections: Being Gay in America.* New York: St. Martin's Press.

Klepinger, D., J. Billy, K. Tanfer et al. 1993. "Perceptions of AIDS Risk and Severity and Their Association with Risk-Related Behavior Among Men." *Family Planning Perspectives,* 25:74–82.

Knowles, J. 1976. "The Struggle to Stay Healthy." *Time* (August 9):60–62.

_____. 1977. "The Responsibility of the Individual." Pp. 75–80 in J. Knowles (ed.), *Doing Better and Feeling Worse: Health in the United States.* New York: W. W. Norton.

Koblin, B., J. Morrison, P. Taylor et al. 1992. "Mortality Trends in a Cohort of Homosexual Men in New York City, 1978–1988." *American Journal of Epidemiology,* 136:646–656.

Kolata, G. 1991. "For Heterosexuals, Diagnosis of AIDS Is Often Unmercifully Late." *New York Times* (November 9):I-34.

_____. 1993a. "Report Saying AIDS Impact Is Small Is Causing Dismay." *New York Times* (February 7):I-19.

_____. 1993b. "Targeting Urged in Attacks on AIDS." *New York Times* (March 7): A-1.

Kost, K., and J. Forrest. 1992. "American Women's Sexual Behavior and Exposure to Risk of Sexually Transmitted Diseases." *Family Planning Perspectives,* 24:244–254.

Kramer, L. 1977. *Faggots.* New York: St. Martin's Press.

_____. 1989. *Reports from the Holocaust.* New York: St. Martin's Press.

Kramer, M. 1987. "Facing Life in the AIDies." *U.S. News and World Report* (June 15):13.

Kraut, A. 1994. *Silent Travelers: Germs, Genes and the "Immigrant Menace."* New York: Basic Books.

Kreiss, J., D. Koech, F. Plummer et al., 1986. "AIDS Virus Infection in Nairobi Prostitutes: Spread of the Epidemic to East Africa." *New England Journal of Medicine,* 314:414–418.

Krieger, L. 1992. "City Hall Comes to Accept Gay Sex Clubs." *San Francisco Examiner* (July 22):A-1, 15.

Kurland, M. 1988. *Coping with AIDS: Facts and Fears.* New York: Rosen.

La Fontaine, J. 1974. "The Free Women of Kinshasa: Prostitution in a City in Zaire." Pp. 89–113 in J. Davis (ed.), *Choice and Change: Essays in Honour of Lucy Mair.* New York: Humanities Press.

Lamb, D. 1987. *The Africans*. New York: Vintage Books.

Lamb, G., and L. Liebling. 1989. "The Role of Education in AIDS Prevention." Pp. 315–322 in P. O'Malley (ed.), *The AIDS Epidemic: Private Rights and the Public Interest*. Boston: Beacon Press.

Lambert, B. 1984. "Numbers 'Don't Add Up': AIDS Forecasts Are Grim—and Disparate." *New York Times* (October 25):IV-24.

————. 1988. "AIDS in Prostitutes Not as Prevalent as Believed, Studies Find." *New York Times* (September 20):B-1, 6.

————. 1990. "Prisons Criticized on AIDS Program." *New York Times* (August 19): A-12.

Landesman, S., H. Ginzberg, and S. Weiss. 1985. "The AIDS Epidemic." *New England Journal of Medicine*, 312:521–525.

Lange, W., F. Snyder, D. Lozowsky et al. 1988. "Geographic Distribution of Human Immunodeficiency Virus Markers in Parenteral Drug Abusers." *American Journal of Public Health*, 78:443–446.

Langer, W. 1958. "The Next Assignment." *American Historical Review*, 63:283–304.

————. 1973. "The Black Death." Pp. 106–111 in K. Davis (ed.), *Cities: Their Origin, Growth, and Human Impact: Readings from Scientific American*. San Francisco: W. H. Freeman.

Langone, J. 1988. *AIDS: The Facts*. Boston: Little, Brown.

Larson, A. 1989. "Social Context of Human Immunodeficiency Virus Transmission in Africa: Historical and Cultural Bases of East and Central African Sexual Relations." *Reviews of Infectious Diseases*, 11:716–731.

Lasagna, L. 1975. *The VD Epidemic: How It Started, Where It's Going, and What to Do About It*. Philadelphia: Temple University Press.

Laumann, E., J. Gagnon, R. Michael et al. 1994. *The Social Organization of Sexuality: Sexual Practices in the United States*. Chicago: University of Chicago Press.

Lauritsen, J. 1994. "Explaining Race and Gender Differences in Adolescent Sexual Behavior." *Social Forces*, 72:859–883.

Lee, F. 1994. "On a Harlem Block, Hope Is Swallowed by Decay." *New York Times* (September 8):A-1, 14–15.

Leishman, K. 1987. "Heterosexuals and AIDS: The Second Stage of the Epidemic." *Atlantic Monthly* (February):39–58.

Lerner, R. 1982. "The Black Death and Western European Eschatological Mentalities." Pp. 77–97 in D. Williman (ed.), *The Black Death: The Impact of the Fourteenth-Century Plague*. Binghamton, N.Y.: Center for Medieval and Early Renaissance Studies.

Lester, D. 1988. "Prejudice Toward AIDS Patients Versus Other Terminally Ill Patients." *American Journal of Public Health*, 78:854.

LeVay, S. 1991. "A Difference in Hypothalamic Structure Between Heterosexual and Homosexual Men." *Science*, 253:1034–1037.

LeVay, S., and D. Hamer, 1994. "Evidence for a Biological Influence in Male Homosexuality." *Scientific American*, 270:44–49.

Levine, S., and M. Kozloff. 1978. "The Sick Role: Assessment and Overview." *Annual Review of Sociology*, 4:317–343.

Levy, J. 1993. "The Transmission of HIV and Factors Influencing Progression to AIDS." *American Journal of Medicine*, 95:86–100.

Lewin, T. 1992. "Sex Partners Increase Among Teen-Age Girls." *New York Times* (December 10):A-14.

Leznoff, M., and W. Westley. 1956. "The Homosexual Community." *Social Problems*, 3:257–263.

Lieban, R. 1977. "The Field of Medical Anthropology." Pp. 13–31 in D. Landy (ed.), *Culture, Disease, and Healing: Studies in Medical Anthropology*. New York: Macmillan.

Lifson, A. 1988. "Do Alternate Modes of Transmission of Human Immunodeficiency Virus Exist? A Review." *Journal of the American Medical Association*, 239:1353–1356.

Linden, L. 1993. "Megacities." *Time* (January 11):28–38.

Lipset, M., and B. Wattenberg (eds.). 1988. "Opinion Roundup." *Public Opinion*, 11:36–39.

Little, K. 1965. *West African Urbanization: A Study of Voluntary Associations and Social Change*. Cambridge: Cambridge University Press.

_____. 1971. *Some Aspects of African Urbanization South of the Sahara*. Reading, Mass.: Addison-Wesley.

_____. 1973. *African Women in Towns: An Aspect of Africa's Social Revolution*. Cambridge: Cambridge University Press.

_____. 1974. *Urbanization, Migration, and the African Family*. Reading, Mass.: Addison-Wesley.

Lofland, J. 1981. "Collective Behavior: Its Elementary Forms." Pp. 411–466 in M. Rosenberg and R. Turner (eds.), *Social Psychology: Sociological Perspectives*. New York: Basic Books.

Longrigg, J. 1992. "Epidemics, Ideas and Classical Athenian Society." Pp. 21–44 in T. Ranger and P. Slack (eds.), *Epidemics and Ideas: Essays on the Historical Perception of Pestilence*. Cambridge: Cambridge University Press.

Lundberg, G. 1985. "The Age of AIDS: A Great Time for Defensive Living." *Journal of the American Medical Association*, 253:3440–3441.

Lyons, A., and R. Petrucelli. 1987. *Medicine: An Illustrated History*. New York: Harry N. Abrams.

Mack, A. (ed.). 1991. *In Time of Plague: The History and Social Consequences of Lethal Epidemic Disease*. New York: New York University Press.

Maddox, J. 1994. "Study Confirms AZT's Lack of Prophylactic Effect." *Nature*, 368:577.

Mair, L. 1974. *African Societies*. London: Cambridge University Press.

Malamba, S., H. Wagner, G. Maude et al. 1994. "Risk Factors for HIV-1 Infection in Adults in a Rural Ugandan Community: A Case-Controlled Study." *AIDS*, 8:253–257.

Malinowski, B. 1954. *Magic, Science, and Religion and Other Essays*. New York: Anchor Books.

Mann, J. 1988. "AIDS Epidemiology, Impact, Prevention, and Control: The World Organization Perspective." *AIDS and Social Policy Journal*, 3:10–13.

Mann, J., D. Tarantola, and T. Netter (eds.). 1992. *AIDS in the World*. Cambridge, Mass.: Harvard University Press.

Margolick, D. 1992. "Legal System Is Assailed on AIDS Crisis." *New York Times* (January 19):I-10.

Marks, G., and W. Beatty. 1976. *Epidemics*. New York: Charles Scribner's Sons.

Marotta, T. 1981. *The Politics of Homosexuality*. Boston: Houghton Mifflin.

Masters, W., V. Johnson, and R. Kolodny. 1988. *Crisis: Heterosexual Behavior in the Age of AIDS*. New York: Grove Press.

Matarazzo, J. 1984. "Behavioral Health: A 1990 Challenge for the Health Sciences Professions." Pp. 3–10 in J. Matarazzo, S. Weiss, J. Herd et al. (eds.), *Behavioral Health: A Handbook of Health Enhancement and Disease Prevention*. New York: John Wiley and Sons.

Mbiti, J. 1969. *African Religions and Philosophy*. Garden City, N.Y.: Doubleday.

McAuliffe, K., J. Carey, S. Wells et al. 1987. "AIDS: At the Dawn of Fear." *U.S. News and World Report* (January 12):60–69.

McCord, C., and H. Freeman. 1990. "Excess Mortality in Harlem." *New England Journal of Medicine*, 322:173–177.

McGrew, R. 1960. "The First Cholera Epidemic and Social History." *Bulletin of the History of Medicine*, 34:61–73.

_____. 1962. "The First Russian Cholera Epidemic: Themes and Opportunities." *Bulletin of the History of Medicine*, 36:220–244.

_____. 1965. *Russia and the Cholera, 1823–1832*. Madison: University of Wisconsin Press.

McKeown, T. 1979. *The Role of Medicine: Dream, Mirage, or Nemesis?* Princeton: Princeton University Press.

McKeown, T., and R. Brown. 1965. "Medical Evidence Related to English Population Changes in the Eighteenth Century." Pp. 285–307 in D. Glass and D. Eversley (eds.), *Population in History: Essays in Historical Demography*. Chicago: Aldine.

McKinlay, J., and S. McKinlay. 1977. "The Questionable Contribution of Medical Measures to the Decline of Mortality in the United States in the Twentieth Century." Milbank Memorial Fund Quarterly/*Health and Society*, 55:405–428.

McKusick, L., W. Horstman, and T. Coates. 1985. "AIDS and Sexual Behavior Reported by Gay Men in San Francisco." *American Journal of Public Health*, 75: 493–496.

McLaughlin, L. 1989. "AIDS: An Overview." Pp. 15–35 in P. O'Malley (ed.), *The AIDS Epidemic: Private Rights and the Public Interest*. Boston: Beacon Press.

McNeill, W. 1976. *Plagues and People*. New York: Oxford University Press.

_____. 1983. "The Plague of Plagues." *New York Review of Books* (July 21):28–29.

Meheus, A., A. De Clercq, and R. Prat. 1974. "Prevalence of Gonorrhoea in Prostitutes in a Central African Town." *British Journal of Venereal Disease*, 50:50–52.

Melnick, S., R. Jeffery, G. Burke et al. 1993. "Changes in Sexual Behavior by Young Urban Heterosexual Adults in Response to the AIDS Epidemic." *Public Health Reports*, 108:582–588.

Merton, R. 1938. "Social Theory and Social Structure." *American Sociological Review*, 3:672–682.

———. 1957. *Social Theory and Social Structure.* Rev. and enlr. ed. Glencoe, Ill.: Free Press.

———. 1970. *Science, Technology and Society in Seventeenth-Century England.* New York: Howard Pertig/Harper and Row.

Mishler, E. 1981a. "The Social Construction of Illness." Pp. 141–168 in E. Mishler, R. Amarasingham, S. Hauser et al. (eds.), *Social Contexts of Health, Illness, and Patient Care.* Cambridge: Cambridge University Press.

———. 1981b. "Viewpoint: Critical Perspectives on the Biomedical Model." Pp. 1–23 in L. Mishler, R. Amarasingham, S. Hauser et al. (eds.), *Social Contexts of Health, Illness, and Patient Care.* Cambridge: Cambridge University Press.

Molnos, A. 1968. *Attitudes Towards Family Planning in East Africa.* London: C. Hurst.

Montgomery, S., and J. Joseph. 1989. "Behavioral Change in Homosexual Men at Risk for AIDS: Intervention and Policy Implications." Pp. 323–333 in P. O'Malley (ed.), *The AIDS Epidemic: Private Rights and the Public Interest.* Boston: Beacon Press.

Moore, A., and R. Le Baron. 1986. "The Case for a Haitian Origin of the AIDS Epidemic." Pp. 77–94 in D. Feldman and T. Johnson (eds.), *The Social Dimensions of AIDS: Method and Theory.* New York: Praeger.

Moore, J., E. Cone, and S. Alexander. 1985. "HTLV-III Seropositivity in 1971–1972 Parenteral Drug Abusers—a Case of False Positives or Evidence of Viral Exposure?" *New England Journal of Medicine,* 314:1387–1388.

Moran, J., S. Aral, W. Jenkins et al. 1989. "The Impact of Sexually Transmitted Diseases on Minority Populations." *Public Health Reports,* 104:560–565.

Morgan, M., J. Curran, and R. Berkelman. 1990. "The Future Course of AIDS in the United States." *Journal of the American Medical Association,* 203:1539–1540.

Morgan, S., A. McDaniel, A. Miller et al. 1993. "Racial Differences in Household and Family Structure at the Turn of the Century. *American Journal of Sociology,* 98:799–828.

Morganthau, T., with M. Hager, B. Cohn et al. 1986. "Future Shock." *Newsweek* (November 24):30–34, 36, 39.

Morganthau, T., with M. Mabry, F. Washington et al. 1992. "Losing Ground: New Fears and Suspicions as Black America's Outlook Grows Bleaker." *Newsweek* (April 6):20–22.

Morris, R. 1976. *Cholera 1832: The Social Response to an Epidemic.* New York: Holmes and Meier.

Mosher, W., and W. Pratt. 1993. "AIDS-Related Behavior Among Women 15–44 Years of Age: United States, 1988 and 1990." *Advance Data from Vital and Health Statistics.* No. 239. Hyattsville, Md.: National Center for Health Statistics.

Moss, A., K. Vranizan, R. Gorter et al. 1994. "HIV Seroconversion in Intravenous Drug Users in San Francisco, 1985–1990." *AIDS,* 8:223–232.

Muchmore, W., and W. Hanson. 1991. *Coming Out Right: A Handbook for the Gay Male.* Rev. ed. Boston: Alyson.

Mulder, C. 1988a. "A Case of Mistaken Non-Identity." *Nature,* 333:562–563.

———. 1988b. "Human AIDS Virus Not from Monkeys." *Nature,* 333:396.

Mulder, D., A. Nunn, H. Wagner et al. 1994. "HIV-1 Incidence and HIV-1 Associated Mortality in a Rural Ugandan Population Cohort." *AIDS,* 8:87–92.

Murdock, G. 1934. *Our Primitive Contemporaries.* New York: Macmillan Company.

_____. 1952. "Anthropology and Its Contribution to Public Health." *American Journal of Public Health,* 42:7–11.

_____. 1980. *Theories of Illness: A World Survey.* Pittsburgh: University of Pittsburgh Press.

Murdock, G., S. Wilson, and V. Frederick. 1978. "World Distribution of Theories of Illness." *Ethnology,* 17:449–470.

Musto, D. 1986. "Quarantine and the Problem of AIDS." Milbank Memorial Fund Quarterly/*Health and Society,* 64, Supplement 1:97–117.

Myers, W. 1987. "AIDS: A Presidential Issue." *Wall Street Journal* (December 30): 12.

National Center for Health Statistics (NCHS). 1989. *Health, United States, 1988.* Washington, D.C.: GPO.

_____. 1991. *Health, United States, 1990.* Washington, D.C.: GPO.

_____. 1994. *Health, United States, 1993.* Washington, D.C.: GPO.

Navarro, M. 1990. "AIDS Children's Foster Care: Hope Conquers Fears." *New York Times* (December 7):A-17.

_____. 1992. "Trials and Triumphs Emerge for H.I.V.-Infected Workers." *New York Times* (November 23):A-1, B-12.

_____. 1993a. "Ethics of Giving AIDS Advice Troubles Catholic Hospitals." *New York Times* (January 3):I-3, 15.

_____. 1993b. "Healthy, Gay, Guilt-Stricken: AIDS' Toll on the Virus-Free." *New York Times* (January 11):A-1, 11.

_____. 1993c. "Despite AIDS's Continuing Spread, Sex Clubs Are Proliferating Again." *New York Times* (March 3):A-15.

Nelkin, D., and S. Hilgartner. 1986. "Disputed Dimensions of Risk: A Public School Controversy over AIDS." Milbank Memorial Fund Quarterly/*Health and Society,* 64:118–142.

Newall, V. 1973. "The Jew as a Witch Figure." Pp. 95–124 in V. Newall (ed.), *The Witch Figure.* London: Routledge and Kegan Paul.

Noble, B. 1992. "AIDS Awareness Goes to Office." *New York Times* (December 6): IV-25.

_____. 1993. "Clashing over AIDS Coverage." *New York Times* (October 10): IV-23.

Nunn, A., J. Dengeya-Kayondo, S. Malamba et al. 1993. "Risk Factors for HIV-1 Infection in Adults in a Rural Ugandan Community: A Population Study." *AIDS,* 8: 81–86.

Obbo, C. 1980. *African Women: Their Struggle for Economic Independence.* London: Zed Press.

O'Connor, A. 1983. *The African City.* New York: Holmes and Meier.

_____. 1991. *Poverty in Africa: A Geographical Approach.* London: Belhaven Press.

Odets, W. 1994. "AIDS Education and Harm Reduction for Gay Men: Psychological Approaches for the 21st Century." *AIDS and Social Policy Journal,* 9:3–15.

Okafor, N, 1991. "Some Traditional Aspects of Nigerian Women." Pp. 135–142 in L. Adler (ed.), *Women in Cross-cultural Perspective*. New York: Praeger.

Okri, B. 1991. *The Famished Road*. New York: Oxford University Press.

Oleske, J., A. Minnefor, R. Cooper et al. 1983. "Immune Deficiency Syndrome in Children." *Journal of the American Medical Association*, 249:2345–2349.

Oliver, R. 1991. *The African Experience*. New York: Harper Collins.

Osborn, J. 1993. "AIDS Prevention: Issues and Strategies." *AIDS*, 2(Supplement): S229–S233.

Osoba, A. 1981. "Sexually Transmitted Diseases in Tropical Africa: A Review of the Present Situation." *British Journal of Venereal Disease*, 57:89–94.

Ostrow, D., T. Sandholzer, and Y. Felman (eds.). 1983. *Sexually Transmitted Disease in Homosexual Men*. New York: Plenum Medical Book.

Padgug, R. 1989. "Gay Villain, Gay Hero: Homosexuality and the Social Construction of AIDS." Pp. 293–313 in K. Peiss and C. Simmons (eds.), *Passion and Power: Sexuality in History*. Philadelphia: Temple University Press.

Padian, N., and J. Pickering. 1986. "Female-to-Male Transmission of AIDS: A Reexamination of the African Sex Ratio of Cases." *Journal of the American Medical Association*, 256:590.

Padian, N., S. Shiboski, and N. Jewell. 1990. "The Effect of Number of Exposures on Risk of Heterosexual HIV Transmission." *Journal of Infectious Diseases*, 161: 883–887.

_____. 1991. "Female-to-Male Transmission of Human Immunodeficiency Virus." *Journal of the American Medical Association*, 266:1664–1667.

Page, W. 1987. "Water and Health." Pp. 105–138 in M. Greenberg (ed.), *Public Health and the Environment: The United States Experience*. New York: Guilford Press.

Pankhurst, D., and S. Jacobs. 1988. "Land Tenure, Gender Relations, and Agricultural Production: The Case of Zimbabwe's Peasantry." Pp. 202–227 in J. Davison (ed.), *Agriculture, Women, and the Land: The African Experience*. Boulder: Westview Press.

Pape, W., B. Liautaud, F. Thomas et al. 1983. "Characteristics of the Acquired Immunodeficiency Syndrome (AIDS) in Haiti." *New England Journal of Medicine*, 309:945–950.

Parran, T. 1937. *Shadow on the Land: Syphilis*. New York: Reynal and Hitchcock.

Parsons, T. 1951a. "Illness and the Role of the Physician: A Sociological Perspective." *American Journal of Orthopsychiatry*, 21:452–460.

_____. 1951b. *The Social System*. Glencoe, Ill.: Free Press.

_____. 1975. "The Sick Role and the Role of the Physician Reconsidered." Milbank Memorial Fund Quarterly/*Health and Society*, 53:257–278.

_____. 1979. "Definitions of Health and Illness in Light of American Values and Social Structure." Pp. 120–144 in E. Jaco (ed.), *Patients, Physicians and Illness*. 3d ed. New York: Free Press.

Parsons, T., and R. Fox. 1952. "Illness, Therapy, and the Modern Urban American Family." *Journal of Social Issues*, 8:31–44.

Parsons, T., and E. Shils. 1951. *Toward a General Theory of Action*. Glencoe, Ill.: Free Press.

Patterson, K., and G. Hartwig. 1978. "The Disease Factors: An Introductory Overview." Pp. 3-24 in G. Hartwig and K. Patterson (eds.), *Disease in African History: An Introductory Survey and Case Studies.* Durham, N.C.: Duke University Press.

Patton, C. 1990a. *Inventing AIDS.* London: Routledge, Chapman Hall.

———. 1990b. "What Science Knows: Formations of AIDS Knowledge." Pp. 1–18 in P. Aggleton, P. Davies, and G. Hart (eds.), *AIDS: Individual, Cultural, and Policy Dimensions.* London: Falmer Press.

Paul, B. 1977. "The Role of Beliefs and Customs in Sanitation Programs." Pp. 233–236 in D. Landy (ed.), *Culture, Disease, and Healing: Studies in Medical Anthropology.* New York: Macmillan.

Payer, L. 1988. *Medicine and Culture: Varieties of Treatment in the United States, England, West Germany, and France.* New York: Henry Holt.

Penny, D. 1988. "Origins of the AIDS Virus." *Nature,* 333:494–495.

Perlez, J. 1990. "AIDS Virus and Its Stigma Plaguing Women in Zambia." *New York Times* (April 28):5.

Petroni, F. 1972. "Correlates of the Psychiatric Sick Role." *Journal of Health and Social Behavior,* 13:47–54.

Piot, P., F. Plummer, M. Rey et al. 1987. "Retrospective Seroepidemiology of AIDS Virus Infection in Nairobi Populations." *Journal of Infectious Diseases,* 155:1108–1112.

Piot, P., F. Plummer, F. Mhalu et al., 1988. "AIDS: An International Perspective. *Science,* 239:573–579.

Piot, P., B. Kapita, E. Ngugi et al. 1992. *AIDS in Africa: A Manual for Physicians.* Geneva: World Health Organization.

Plourde, P., F. Plummer, J. Pepin et al. 1992. "Human Immunodeficiency Virus Type 1 Infection in Women Attending a Sexually Transmitted Disease Clinic in Kenya." *Journal of Infectious Diseases,* 166:86–92.

Plummer, F., J. Simonsen, D. Cameron et al. 1991. "Cofactors in Male-Female Sexual Transmission of Human Immunodeficiency Virus Type 1." *Journal of Infectious Disease,* 163:233–239.

Plummer, K. 1975. *Sexual Stigma: An Interactionist Approach.* Boston: Routledge and Kegan Paul.

———. 1988. "Organizing AIDS." Pp. 20–51 in P. Aggleton and H. Homans (eds.), *Social Aspects of AIDS.* London: Falmer Press.

Preson, R. 1994. *The Hot Zone.* New York: Random House.

Preston, S. 1976. *Mortality Patterns in National Populations.* New York: Academic Press.

Preston, S., S. Lim, and S. Morgan. 1992. "African-American Marriage in 1910: Beneath the Surface of Census Data." *Demography,* 29:1–15.

Quindlen, A. 1993. "The Other Side." *New York Times* (December 9):A-23.

Radcliffe-Brown, A. 1950. "Introduction." Pp. 1–85 in A. R. Radcliffe-Brown and D. Forde (eds.), *African Systems of Kinship and Marriage.* London: Oxford University Press.

Radetsky, P. 1991. *The Invisible Invaders: The Story of the Emerging Age of the Viruses.* Boston: Little, Brown.

Ranger, T. 1992. "Plagues of Beasts and Men: Prophetic Responses to Epidemic in Eastern and Southern Africa." Pp. 241–268 in T. Ranger and P. Slack (eds.), *Epidemics and Ideas: Essays on the Historical Perception of Pestilence*. Cambridge: Cambridge University Press.

Ranger, T., and P. Slack (eds.). 1992. *Epidemics and Ideas: Essays on the Historical Perception of Pestilence*. Cambridge: Cambridge University Press.

Richards, L., and E. Carroll. 1970. "Illicit Drug Use and Addiction in the United States." *Public Health Reports*, 85:1035–1042.

Ricklefs, R. 1987. "AIDS Cases Prompt a Host of Lawsuits." *Wall Street Journal* (October 7):32.

Riesenberg, D., and M. Fishbein. 1986. "AIDS-Prompted Behavior Changes Reported." *Journal of the American Medical Association*, 255:171–172.

Risse, G. 1988. "Epidemics and History: Ecological Perspectives and Social Responses." Pp. 33–64 in E. Fee and D. Fox (eds.), 1988. *AIDS: The Burdens of History*. Berkeley and Los Angeles: University of California Press.

Ritzer, G. 1988. *Sociological Theory*. 2d ed. New York: Alfred A. Knopf.

Robertson, C. 1984. "Women in the Urban Economy." Pp. 33–49 in M. Hay and S. Stichter (eds.), *African Women South of the Sahara*. London: Longman.

Rogers, D., and J. Osborn. 1993. "AIDS Policy: Two Divisive Issues." *Journal of the American Medical Association*, 270:494–495.

Rogers, P. 1993. "How Many Gays Are There?" *Newsweek* (February 15):46.

Rolfs, R., and A. Nakashima. 1990. "Epidemiology of Primary and Secondary Syphilis in the United States, 1981 Through 1989." *Journal of the American Medical Association*, 264:1432–1437.

Rompalo, A., and H. Handsfield. 1989. "Overview of Sexually Transmitted Diseases in Homosexual Men." Pp. 3–11 in P. Ma and D. Armstrong (eds.), *AIDS and Infections of Homosexual Men*. 2d ed. Boston: Butterworths.

Root-Bernstein, R. 1993. *Rethinking AIDS: The Tragic Cost of Premature Consensus*. New York: Free Press.

Rosenberg, C. 1959. "The Cholera Epidemic of 1832 in New York City." *Bulletin of the History of Medicine*, 33:37–49.

————. 1962. *The Cholera Years: The United States in 1832, 1849, and 1866*. Chicago: University of Chicago Press.

Rosenkrantz, B. 1987. "Introductory Essay: Rene Dubos and Tuberculosis, Master Teacher." Pp. xiii–xxxiv in R. Dubos and J. Dubos, *The White Plague: Tuberculosis, Man, and Society*. New Brunswick: Rutgers University Press.

Rosenthal, E. 1990. "The Spread of AIDS: A Mystery Unravels." *New York Times* (August 28):B-5, 6.

Roth, T. 1985. "Many Firms Fire AIDS Victims, Citing Health Risk to Co-Workers." *Wall Street Journal* (August 12):19.

Rothenberg, R. 1988. *The New Lexicon Illustrated Medical Encyclopedia and Guide to Family Health*. New York: Lexicon.

Rubinstein, A., M. Sicklick, A. Gupta et al. 1983. "Acquired Immunodeficiency with T_4/T_8 Ratios in Infants Born to Promiscuous and Drug-Addicted Mothers." *Journal of the American Medical Association*, 249:2350–2356.

Rueda, E., and M. Schwartz. 1987. *Gays, AIDS and You*. Old Greenwich, Conn.: Devian Adair.

Ruggles, S. 1994. "The Origins of African-American Family Structure." *American Sociological Review,* 59:136–151.

Rushing, W. 1972. *Class, Culture, and Alienation: A Study of Farmers and Farm Workers.* Lexington, Mass.: Lexington Books.

Sabatier, R. 1989. *AIDS in the Third World.* London: Panos Institute/New Society Publishers.

Sack, K. 1990. "Court Rejects HIV-Test Ban in a Health-Insurance Case." *New York Times* (December 12):A-17.

Sande, M. 1986. "The Transmission of AIDS: The Case Against Casual Contagion." *New England Journal of Medicine,* 314:380–382.

Sandholzer, T. 1983. "Factors Affecting the Incidence and Management of Sexually Transmitted Diseases in Homosexual Men." Pp. 3–12 in D. Ostrow, T. Sandholzer, and Y. Felman (eds.), *Sexually Transmitted Disease in Homosexual Men: Diagnosis, Treatment, and Research.* New York: Plenum Medical Book.

Scheff, T. 1984. *Being Mentally Ill.* Rev. ed. Chicago: Aldine.

Schmalz, J. 1993a. "Poll Finds an Even Split on Homosexuality Cause." *New York Times* (March 5):A-11.

_____. 1993b. "Whatever Happened to AIDS?" *New York Times Magazine* (November 28):56–61, 81, 85–86.

Schneider, B. 1992. "AIDS and Class, Gender, and Race Relations." Pp. 19–43 in J. Huber and B. Schneider (eds.), *The Social Context of AIDS.* Newbury Park, Calif.: Sage.

Schneider, D. 1953. "Social Dynamics of Physical Disability in Army Basic Training." Pp. 386–397 in C. Kluckhohn, H. Murray, and D. Schneider (eds.), *Personality in Nature, Society, and Culture.* 2d ed., rev. New York: Alfred A. Knopf.

Schoepf, B. 1992. "Women at Risk: Case Studies from Zaire." Pp. 259–286 in G. Herdt and S. Lindenbaum (eds.), *Time of AIDS: Social Analysis, Theory, and Method.* Newbury Park, Calif.: Sage.

Schuster, I. 1979. *New Women of Lusaka.* Palo Alto, Calif.: Mayfield.

Schwartz, E., V. Kofie, M. Rivo et al. 1990. "Black/White Comparisons of Deaths Preventable by Medical Intervention: United States and the District of Columbia, 1980–1986." *International Journal of Epidemiology,* 19:591–598.

Scott, S., and M. Mercer. 1994. "Understanding Cultural Obstacles to HIV-AIDS Prevention in Africa." *AIDS Education and Prevention,* 6:81–89.

Seidlin, M., M. Vogler, E. Lee et al. 1993. "Heterosexual Transmission of HIV in a Cohort of Couples in New York City." *AIDS,* 7:1247–1254.

Seligmann, J., and N. Greenberg. 1985. "Only a Month to Live and No Place to Die." *Newsweek* (August 12):26.

Seligmann, J., and M. Reese. 1985. "A Family Gives Refuge to a Son Who Has AIDS." *Newsweek* (August 12):24.

Senelick, L. 1992. "Mollies or Men of Mode? Sodomy and the Eighteenth Century London Stage." Pp. 287–322 in W. Dynes and S. Donaldson (eds.), *History of Homosexuality in Europe and America.* New York: Garland.

Serwadda, D., N. Sewankambo, J. Carswell et al. 1985. "Slim Disease: A New Disease in Uganda and Its Association with HTLV-III Infection." *Lancet:*849–852.

Shannon, G. 1991. "AIDS: A Search for Origins." Pp. 8–29 in R. Ulack and W. Skinner (eds.), *AIDS and the Social Sciences: Common Threads.* Lexington: University of Kentucky Press.

Sharp, P., and W. Li. 1988. "Understanding the Origins of AIDS Viruses." *Nature,* 336:315.

Shaw, M., and P. Costanzo. 1982. *Theories of Social Psychology.* 2d ed. New York: McGraw-Hill.

Shillington. K. 1989. *History of Africa.* New York: St. Martin's Press.

Shilts, R. 1987. *And the Band Played On: Politics, People, and the AIDS Epidemic.* New York: St. Martin's Press.

Shoumatoff, A. 1988. *African Madness.* New York: Alfred A. Knopf.

Simonsen, J. et al. 1988. "Human Immunodeficiency Virus Infection Among Men with Sexually Transmitted Diseases: Experience from a Center in Africa." *New England Journal of Medicine,* 319:274–278.

Singer, E., T. Rogers, and M. Corcoran. 1987. "The Polls—a Report." *Public Opinion Quarterly,* 50:580–595.

Siraisi, N. 1982. "Introduction." Pp. 9–19 in D. Williman (ed.), *The Black Death: The Impact of the Fourteenth-Century Plague.* Binghamton, N.Y.: Center for Medieval and Early Renaissance Studies.

Sittitrai, W., T. Brown, and J. Sterns. 1990. "Opportunities for Overcoming the Continuing Restraints in Behavior Change and HIV Risk Reduction." *AIDS,* 4(Supplement 1):S269–276.

Sivard, R. 1985. *Women—a World Survey.* Washington, D.C.: World Priorities.

Slack, P. 1992. "Introduction." Pp. 1–20 in T. Ranger and P. Slack (eds.), *Epidemics and Ideas: Essays on the Historical Perception of Pestilence.* Cambridge: Cambridge University Press.

Smith, B. 1981. "Black Lung: The Social Production of Disease." *International Journal of Health Services,* 11:343–359.

Smothers, R. 1993. "In Florida, Girl Discovers Chill of Life with AIDS." *New York Times* (January 9):7.

Smyser, M., J. Bryce, and J. Joseph. 1990. "AIDS-Related Knowledge, Attitudes, and Precautionary Behaviors Among Emergency Medical Professionals." *Public Health Reports,* 105:496–503.

Sonenschein, D. 1968. "The Ethnography of Male Homosexual Relations." *Journal of Sex Research,* 4:69–83.

Sontag, S. 1978. *Illness as Metaphor.* New York: Farrar, Straus and Giroux.

———. 1988. "AIDS as Metaphor." *New York Review of Books* (October 27):89–99.

Southall, A. 1961. "Introductory Summary." Pp. 1–66 in A. Southall (ed.), *Social Change in Modern Africa.* London: Oxford University Press.

Specter, M. 1992. "Neglected for Years, TB Is Back with Strains That Are Deadlier." *New York Times* (October 11):I-1, 20.

Stall, R., D. Coates, and C. Hoff. 1988. "Behavioral Risk Reduction of HIV Infection Among Gay and Bisexual Men." *American Psychologist,* 43:878–885.

Stevens, C., P. Taylor, E. Zang et al. 1986. "Human T-Cell Lymphotropic Virus Type III Infection in a Cohort of Homosexual Men in New York City." *Journal of the American Medical Association,* 255:2167–2172.

Stewart, D., and T. Sullivan. 1982. "Illness Behavior and the Sick Role in Chronic Disease: The Case of Multiple Sclerosis." *Social Science and Medicine,* 16:1397–1404.

Stipp, H., and D. Kerr. 1989. "Determinants of Public Opinion About AIDS." *Public Opinion Quarterly,* 53:98–106.

Strobel, M. 1984. "Women in Religion and Secular Ideology." Pp. 87–101 in M. Hay and S. Stichter (eds.), *African Women South of the Sahara.* New York: Longman.

Sudarkasa, N. 1981. "Interpreting the African Heritage in Afro-American Family Organization." Pp. 37–53 in H. McAdoo (ed.), *Black Families.* Beverly Hills, Calif.: Sage.

_____. 1987. " 'The Status of Women' in Indigenous African Societies." Pp. 25–44 in R. Terborg-Penn, S. Harley, and A. Rushing (eds.), *Women in Africa and the African Diaspora.* Washington, D.C.: Howard University Press.

Syme, A., and L. Berkman. 1976. "Social Class, Susceptibility, and Sickness." *American Journal of Epidemiology,* 104:1–8.

Tessina, A. 1989. *Gay Relationships.* Los Angeles: Jeremy P. Tarcher.

Thompson, D. 1990. "A Losing Battle with AIDS." *Time* (July 2):42–43.

Thurow, R. 1986. "Physicians Enlisting 100 Witch Doctors in War on AIDS." *Wall Street Journal* (December 16):38.

Tierney, J. 1990a. "AIDS Tears Lives of African Family." *New York Times* (September 17):A-1, 6.

_____. 1990b. "Newark's Spiral of Drugs and AIDS." *New York Times* (December 16):I-1, 23.

Trachenberg, A. 1994. *Living in the Shadow of Death: Tuberculosis and the Social Experience of Illness in American Society.* New York: Basic Books.

Trager, O. 1988. *AIDS: Plague or Panic?* New York: Facts on File.

Treichler, P. 1987. "AIDS, Homophobia, and Biomedical Discourse: An Epidemic of Signification." *Cultural Studies,* 1:263–305.

Tuchman, B. 1978. *A Distant Mirror: The Calamitous 14th Century.* New York: Random House.

Turque, B., with C. Friday, J. Gordon et al. 1992. "Gays Under Fire." *Newsweek* (September 14):35–40.

Ulijaszek, S. 1990. "Nutritional Status and Susceptibility to Infectious Disease." Pp. 137–154 in G. Harrison and J. Waterlow (eds.), *Diet and Disease in Traditional and Developing Societies.* Cambridge: Cambridge University Press.

Ungar, S. 1989. *Africa: The People and Politics of an Emerging Continent.* Rev. ed. New York: Simon and Schuster.

Urdang, S. 1989. *And Still They Dance: Women, War, and the Struggle for Change in Mozambique.* New York: Monthly Review Press.

U.S. Bureau of the Census. 1975. *Historical Statistics of the United States, Colonial Times Bicentennial Edition, Part I.* Washington, D.C.: GPO.

_____. 1988. *Statistical Abstract of the United States, 1988.* Washington, D.C.: GPO.

_____. 1991. *World Population Profile: 1991.* Washington, D.C.: GPO.

_____. 1992. *1990 Census of Population: General Population Characteristics—United States.* Washington, D.C.: GPO.

U.S. Public Health Service. 1986a. *Acquired Immune Deficiency Syndrome.* Washington, D.C.: GPO.

_____. 1986b. "Coolfont Report: A PHS Plan for Prevention and Controls of AIDS and the AIDS Virus." *Public Health Reports,* 101:341–348.

_____. 1988. "Understanding AIDS." Washington, D.C.: GPO.

Vanderveen, E. 1991. "Federal Funding in AIDS Activity." Pp. 149–157 in R. Ulack and W. Skinner (eds.), *AIDS and the Social Sciences: Common Threads.* Lexington: University of Kentucky Press.

Verghese, A. 1994. *My Own Country: A Doctor's Story of a Town and Its People in the Age of AIDS.* New York: Simon and Schuster.

Verghese, A., S. Berk, and F. Sarubbi. 1989. "*Urbs in Rure:* Human Immunodeficiency in Rural Tennessee." *Journal of Infectious Diseases,* 160:1051–1055.

Waddle, R. 1992. "Bible and Homosexuality: Mixed Message." *Tennessean* (May 7):D-1, 2.

Wade, N. 1988. "Why the Curse of AIDS Is Defying Africa's Precedent." *New York Times* (February 21):IV-6.

Wagner, H., A. Kamali, A. Nunn et al. 1993. "General and HIV-1–Associated Morbidity in a Rural Ugandan Community." *AIDS,* 7:1461–1467.

Waitzkin, H., and B. Waterman. 1974. *The Exploitation of Illness in Capitalist Society.* Indianapolis: Bobbs-Merrill.

Walker, R. 1991. *AIDS—Today, Tomorrow: An Introduction to the HIV Epidemic in America.* London: Humanities Press International.

Wallace, J. 1989. "Case Presentation of AIDs in the United States." Pp. 285–295 in P. Ma and D. Armstrong (eds.), *AIDS and Infections of Homosexual Men.* 2d ed. Boston: Butterworth.

Wallis, C. 1985. "AIDS: A Growing Threat." *Time* (August 12):40–47.

Watney, S. 1988. "The Spectacle of AIDS." Pp. 71–88 in D. Crimp (ed.), *AIDS: Cultural Analysis/Cultural Activism.* Cambridge, Mass.: MIT Press.

Weber, M. 1964. *The Theory of Social and Economic Organization.* New York: Free Press.

Webster, L., and T. Rolfs. 1993. "Surveillance for Primary and Secondary Syphilis—United States, 1991." *Morbidity and Mortality Report: Surveillance Summaries,* 42:13–19.

Weeks, J. 1988. "Male Homosexuality: Cultural Perspectives." Pp. 1–14 in M. Adler (ed.), *Diseases in the Male Homosexual.* London: Springer-Verlag.

_____. 1990. *Coming Out: Homosexual Politics in Britain from the Nineteenth Century to the Present.* Rev. ed. London: Quartet Books.

Wei, X., S. Ghost, M. Taylor, et al. 1994. "Viral Dynamics in Human Immunodeficiency Virus Type 1 Infection." *Nature,* 373:117–122.

Weinberg, M., and C. Williams. 1974. *Male Homosexuals: Their Problems and Adaptations.* New York: Oxford University Press.

_____. 1975. "Gay Baths and the Social Organization of Impersonal Sex." *Social Problems,* 23:124–136.

_____. 1988. "Black Sexuality." *Journal of Sex Research,* 25:197–218.

Weintraub, B. 1991. "Hollywood Called Hypocritical by Actor Who Died of AIDS." *New York Times* (September 12):B-1.

Weitz, R. 1991. *Life with AIDS.* New Brunswick: Rutgers University Press.

Wellings, K. 1988. "Perceptions of Risk—Media Treatment of AIDS." Pp. 83–105 in P. Aggleton and H. Homans (eds.), *Social Aspects of AIDS.* London: Falmer House.

Wenzel, S. 1982. "Pestilence and Middle English Literature: Friar John Grimestone's Poems of Death." Pp. 131–159 in D. Williman (ed.), *The Black Death: The Impact of the Fourteenth-Century Plague.* Binghamton, N.Y.: Center for Medieval and Early Renaissance Studies.

Wertz, D., J. Sorenson, L. Liebling et al. 1987. "Knowledge and Attitudes of AIDS Health Care Providers Before and After Education Programs." *Public Health Reports,* 102:248–254.

West, P. 1972. *Land Policy in Buganda.* Cambridge: Cambridge University Press.

Westby, D. 1991. *The Growth of Sociological Theory: Human Nature, Knowledge, and Social Change.* Englewood Cliffs, N.J.: Prentice-Hall.

White, E. 1980. *States of Desire: Travels in Gay America.* New York: E. P. Dutton.

White, L. 1983. "A Colonial State and an African Petty Bourgeoisie: Prostitution, Property, and Class Struggle in Nairobi, 1936–1940." Pp. 167–194 in F. Cooper (ed.), *Struggle for the City: Migrant Labor, Capital, and the State in Urban Africa.* Beverly Hills, Calif.: Sage.

_____. 1984. "Women in the Changing African Family." Pp. 53–68 in M. Hay and S. Stichter (eds.), *African Women South of the Sahara.* London: Longman.

Williams, A. 1992. *AIDS: An African Perspective.* Boca Raton, Fla.: CRC Press.

Williams, D. 1990. "Socioeconomic Differentials in Health: A Review and Redirection." *Social Psychology Quarterly,* 53:81–99.

Williams, M. 1990. "Polygamy and the Declining Male to Female Ratio in Black Communities: A Social Inquiry." Pp. 171–193 in H. Cheatman and J. Stewart (eds.), *Black Families: Interdisciplinary Perspectives.* New Brunswick, N.J.: Transaction.

Wilson, W. 1978. *The Declining Significance of Race: Blacks and Changing American Institutions.* Chicago: University of Chicago Press.

Winkelstein, J., M. Samuel, N. Padian et al. 1987. "Selected Sexual Practices of San Francisco Heterosexual Men and Risk of Infection by the Human Immunodeficiency Virus." *Journal of the American Medical Association,* 257:1471–1472.

Winkelstein, J., J. Wiley, N. Padian et al. 1988. "The San Francisco Men's Study: Continued Decline in HIV Seroconversion Among Homosexual/Bisexual Men." *American Journal of Public Health,* 78:1472–1474.

Winslow, R. 1968. *Crime in a Free Society: Selections from the President's Commission on Law Enforcement and Administration of Justice.* Belmont, Calif.: Dickenson.

Wipper, A. 1984. "Women's Voluntary Associations." Pp. 659–686 in M. Hay and S. Strichter (eds.), *African Women South of the Sahara.* London: Longman.

Wirth, L. 1938. "Urbanism as a Way of Life." *American Journal of Sociology,* 44:1–24.

Witte, M., C. Witte, L. Minnich et al. 1984. "AIDS in 1968." *Journal of the American Medical Association,* 251:1657.

Wojnarowicz, D. 1991. *Close to the Knives: A Memoir of Disintegration.* New York: Vintage Books.

Wolff, C. 1991. "New Rules on AIDS Produce First Resignation of Doctor." *New York Times* (July 26):10.

Wolinsky, F. 1988. *The Sociology of Health: Principles, Practitioners and Issues.* Belmont, Calif.: Wadsworth.

Woolhandler, S., D. Himmelstein, R. Silber et al. 1985. "Medical Care and Mortality: Racial Differences in Preventable Deaths." *International Journal of Health Services,* 15:1–22.

World Health Organization (WHO). 1992. *World Health Statistics Annual, 1991.* Geneva: World Health Organization.

Wormser, G., and C. Joline. 1988. "Would You Eat Cookies Prepared by an AIDS Patient?" *Postgraduate Medicine,* 86:174–175, 178–191.

Yelin, D., M. Nevitt, and W. Epstein. 1980. "Toward an Epidemiology of Work Disability." Milbank Memorial Fund Quarterly/*Health and Society,* 58:386–415.

Ziegler, P. 1969. *The Black Death.* London: Collins.

Zilbergeld, B., and M. Evans. 1990. "The Inadequacy of Masters and Johnson." *Psychology Today,* 14:29–30.

Zinsser, H. 1938. *Rats, Lice, and History.* Boston: Little, Brown.

Zola, I. 1978. "Medicine as an Institution of Social Control." Pp. 80–100 in J. Ehrenreich (ed.), *The Cultural Crisis of Modern Medicine.* New York: Monthly Review Press.

Zuckerman, L. 1988. "Open Season on Gays." *Time* (March 7):24.

Zurcher, L., and D. Snow. 1981. "Collective Behavior: Social Movements." Pp. 447–482 in M. Rosenberg and R. Turner (eds.), *Social Psychology: Sociological Perspectives.* New York: Basic Books.

About the Book and Author

This comprehensive introduction to the problem of AIDS lays out the medical facts and social epidemiology of the disease and illuminates the complex social problems this disease poses for the United States and other nations. Each chapter introduces a key sociological approach that clarifies how social scientists understand and explain important social aspects of the AIDS epidemic. The author's use of historical comparisons of other deadly epidemics sets in relief the social problems presented by AIDS today.

William A. Rushing is professor of sociology at Vanderbilt University and former chair of the Section on Medical Sociology of the American Sociological Association.

Index

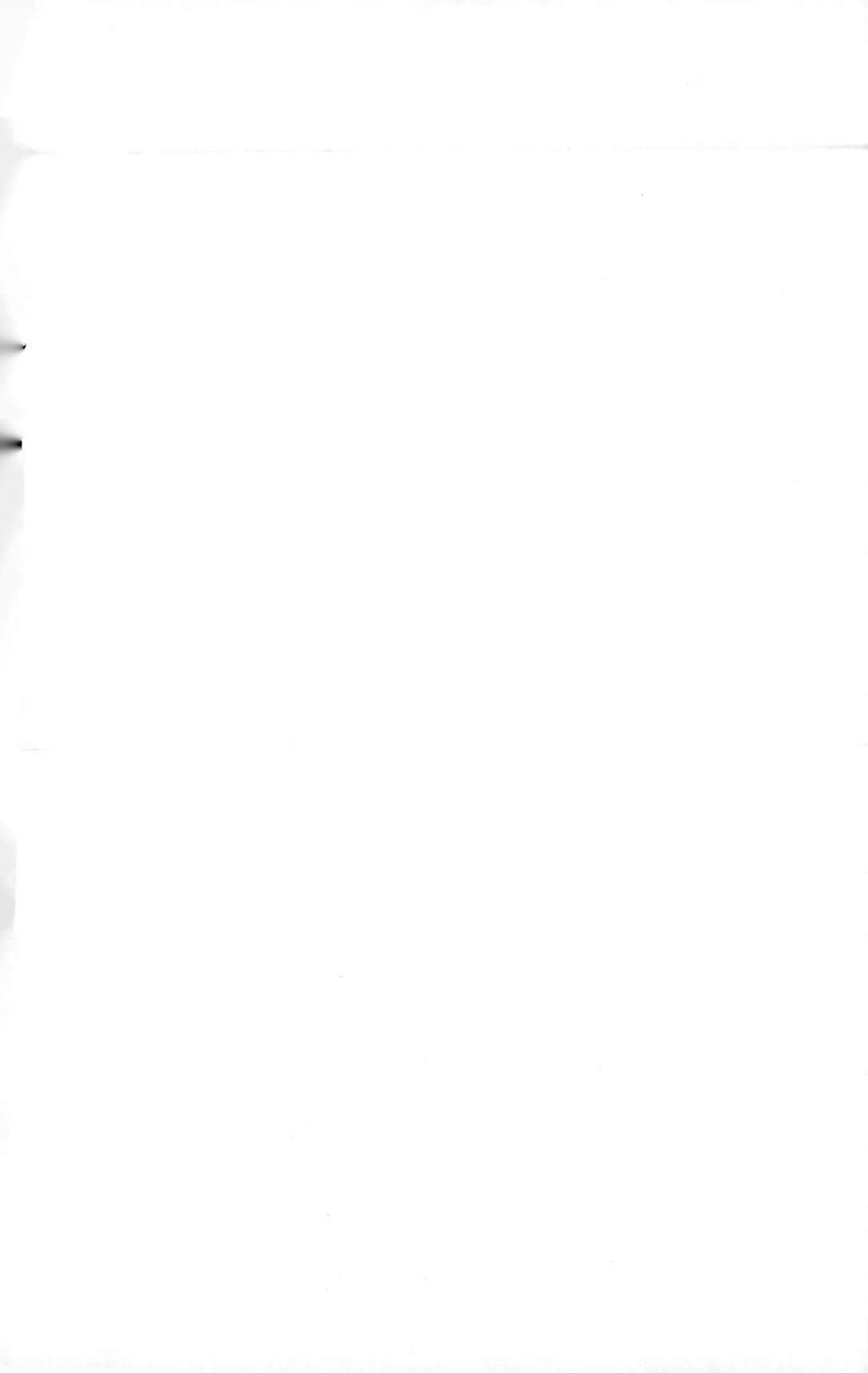